Fundamentals of Sectional Anatomy: An Imaging Approach

Fundamentals of Sectional Anatomy: An Imaging Approach

Denise L. Lazo, MA, RT (R) (M)
Assistant Professor and Clinical Coordinator
Community College of Rhode Island
Lincoln, Rhode Island

THOMSON
™
DELMAR LEARNING

Australia   Canada   Mexico   Singapore   Spain   United Kingdom   United States

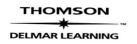

Fundamentals of Sectional Anatomy: An Imaging Approach
by Denise L. Lazo, MA, RT (R), (M)

Vice President, Health Care Business Unit:
William Brottmiller

Editorial Director:
Cathy L. Esperti

Acquisitions Editor:
Maureen Rosener

Developmental Editor:
Darcy M. Scelsi

Editorial Assistant:
Elizabeth Howe

Marketing Director:
Jennifer McAvey

Marketing Coordinator:
Christopher Manion

Project Editor:
Jennifer Luck

Production Coordinator:
Bridget Lulay

Art and Design Coordinators:
Alexandros Vasilakos
Bridget Lulay

For permission to use material from this text or product, contact us by
Tel   (800) 730-2214
Fax (800) 730-2215
www.thomsonrights.com

Library of Congress Cataloging-in-Publication Data
Lazo, Denise L.
   Fundamentals of sectional anatomy : an imaging approach / Denise L. Lazo.
       p. cm
   Includes index.
   ISBN 0-7668-6172-4
   1. Human anatomy—Atlases. 2. Tomography—Atlases.
   3. Magnetic resonance imaging—Atlases. I. Title.

QM25.L39 2005
611'.0022'2—dc22

2004049848

NOTICE TO THE READER

Publisher does not warrant or guarantee any of the products described herein or perform any independent analysis in connection with any of the product information contained herein. Publisher does not assume, and expressly disclaims, any obligation to obtain and include information other than that provided to it by the manufacturer.

The reader is expressly warned to consider and adopt all safety precautions that might be indicated by the activities described herein and to avoid all potential hazards. By following the instructions contained herein, the reader willingly assumes all risks in connection with such instructions.

The publisher makes no representations or warranties of any kind, including but not limited to, the warranties of fitness for particular purpose or merchantability, nor are any such representations implied with respect to the material set forth herein, and the publisher takes no responsibility with respect to such material. The publisher shall not be liable for any special, consequential, or exemplary damages resulting, in whole or part, from the reader's use of, or reliance upon, this material.

This book is dedicated to my husband, Michael,
To my beautiful and talented daughters,
Natasha and Christiana,
Who are undoubtedly my life's greatest work,
And to those people in my life who have inspired me to be the best I can be,
Including, but not limited to,
My mother, Gloria Paquette,
Whose greatest legacy is her extraordinary work ethic.

Contents

Figure Credits

Pages xx–xxiv:

All MR images provided by Roger Williams Medical Center, Diagnostic Imaging Department, Providence, Rhode Island

All CT images provided by Our Lady of Fatima Hospital, Division of St. Joseph's Health Services, North Providence, Rhode Island

Chapter 1:

All MR and CT images provided by Roger Williams Medical Center, Diagnostic Imaging Department, Providence, Rhode Island

Chapter 2:

All MR and CT images provided by Roger Williams Medical Center, Diagnostic Imaging Department, Providence, Rhode Island

Chapter 3:

All MR and CT images provided by Roger Williams Medical Center, Diagnostic Imaging Department, Providence, Rhode Island

Chapter 4:

All MR and CT images provided by Our Lady of Fatima Hospital, Division of St. Joseph's Health Services, North Providence, Rhode Island

Chapter 5:

All MR images provided by Roger Williams Medical Center, Diagnostic Imaging Department, Providence, Rhode Island

All CT images provided by Our Lady of Fatima Hospital, Division of St. Joseph's Health Services, North Providence, Rhode Island

Chapter 6:

All MR images provided by Roger Williams Medical Center, Diagnostic Imaging Department, Providence, Rhode Island

All CT images provided by Our Lady of Fatima Hospital, Division of St. Joseph's Health Services, North Providence, Rhode Island

Chapter 7:

All MR and CT images provided by Roger Williams Medical Center, Diagnostic Imaging Department, Providence, Rhode Island

Chapter 8:

All MR images provided by Roger Williams Medical Center, Diagnostic Imaging Department, Providence, Rhode Island

All CT images provided by Roger Williams Medical Center, Diagnostic Imaging Department, Providence, Rhode Island, and Our Lady of Fatima Hospital, Division of St. Joseph's Health Services, North Providence, Rhode Island

Chapter 9:

All MR and CT images provided by Roger Williams Medical Center, Diagnostic Imaging Department, Providence, Rhode Island

Reviewers

Joan M. Berger, BS, RT (R) (M)
Associate Professor
Owens Community College
Toledo, Ohio

Jim Byrne, MEd, RT (R)
Radiography Program Director
Columbus State Community College
Columbus, Ohio

Pamela Anthony Intlekofer, RT (R) (MR)
MRI Program Coordinator
Greenville Technical College
Greenville, South Carolina

Rebecca W. Lam, Med, RT (R)
Associate Professor
Medical College of Georgia
Augusta, Georgia

James Murrell, MSRS, RT (R) (M) (QM) (CT)
Program Director
Northwestern State University
Shreveport, Louisiana

Deborah Osborn, BS, RT (R) (CT) (M)
Consultant
GE Medical Systems
Kenmore, New York

Timothy Troncale, RT (R) (MR), RMRIT
MRI Program Director
American College of Medical Technology
Gardena, California

Jackie Whipple, RT (R)
Clinical Coordinator
Carl Sandburg College
Galesburg, Illinois

Preface

This book aims to serve radiography students, candidates for the computed tomography (CT) and magnetic resonance imaging (MRI) certification exams, and other students interested in acquiring the ability to learn the fundamentals of sectional anatomy. The text can either supplement a lecture series or function alone for independent study. Learning sectional anatomy by viewing CT and MR images can be an intimidating and overwhelming experience if not approached systematically. Therefore, this text uses an approach that is logical and orderly. The first prerequisite is to obtain a solid understanding of anatomy. This promotes learning rather than the process of memorization. Each section, therefore, begins with relevant anatomic information. Anatomy not identified on CT or MR images and functional information are not presented.

The focus is on learning sectional anatomy rather than studying different imaging modalities. Appropriate images are chosen that best serve this purpose. The text presents the information in an organized manner, starting at the vertex of the skull and descending to the symphysis pubis. The vertebral column and major joints of the upper and lower extremities are also included.

An outline is provided at the beginning of each chapter. My experience as an instructor finds that repetition is beneficial, so two complete sets of images are included for each exam. This ensures that virtually all anatomy discussed in each chapter is identified. The images are presented in a sequential order to provide the student with a realistic approach, and are fully labeled to simplify the studying process. Review questions are included at the end of each chapter to allow the student to self-test.

Acknowledgments

Roger Williams Medical Center, Diagnostic Imaging Department, Providence, Rhode Island, and Our Lady of Fatima Hospital, Division of St. Joseph's Health Services, CT Department, North Providence, Rhode Island, graciously provided the images for this book. Without their assistance this endeavor would not have come to fruition. In particular, I would like to thank David DeSante RT (R) (CT) Paul Cunningham RT (R) (T) (MR), and Kathleen St. Pierre RT (R) (CT). Despite their hectic schedules and numerous responsibilities they patiently endured my seemingly endless requests in my search for the perfect CT and MR images.

I would be remiss to not recognize the artist assigned to this project, Joe Chovan. His exceptional talent and ability in accurately demonstrating anatomy is evident in many of the drawings enhancing the material in this book.

About the Author

The academic background of Denise L. Lazo includes training as a radiographer at Mary Fletcher Hospital, Burlington, Vermont, acquiring a BS at Salem College, Salem, West Virginia, and earning an MA from Rhode Island College. A registered radiographer with the American Registry of Radiologic Technologists (ARRT), Ms. Lazo also has an additional certification in mammography. Her extensive clinical experience includes staff and supervisory positions at hospitals in Philadelphia, Pennsylvania and Rhode Island. Currently she is a licensed radiographer in Rhode Island. In 1996 Ms. Lazo accepted a position as an instructor and clinical coordinator for the Radiography Program at the Community College of Rhode Island (CCRI) and in 1999 she was promoted to assistant professor. Courses taught by Ms. Lazo relevant to this book include Radiographic Anatomy and Physiology, Radiographic Sectional Anatomy, and Radiographic Pathology. The CCRI Radiography Program is associated with 10 area hospitals and has an impressive pass rate on the national registry examination. Many of her former students are now practicing in CT and MRI and have successfully passed the ARRT certification exams in their chosen fields.

Introduction

Since Wilhelm Roentgen produced his first radiograph on November 8, 1895, the field of radiology has grown by leaps and bounds. New methods of imaging emerge constantly. It is a natural question for the untrained to ask "Which modality is best?" No one modality is best for each serves a particular function. In many instances, studies previously done in the conventional imaging department now utilize other modalities to provide more diagnostic information. An example is the replacement of cholecystograms (the study of gallbladders with conventional imaging) with ultrasonography of the gallbladder, or, in some instances, a nuclear medicine study. Conventional radiographs of the skull have become almost extinct as most concerns can be addressed with CT. Arthrograms are making the transition from the radiography department to the MRI department. The list continues to change.

All imaging students, at entry level for the study of other modalities, need to have a thorough grounding in sectional anatomy. Knowledge of gross anatomy is no longer sufficient. The intended purpose of this book is to teach sectional anatomy as demonstrated on routine sectional images. The most accurate representations of the body as seen sectionally are CT images and, in some instances, MR images. With CT it is possible to see virtually all body structures in a series of images starting at the vertex of the skull and ending at the symphysis pubis. MRI can provide a similar opportunity in the region of the head and spinal cord, but is less commonly employed in the neck, thorax, and abdomen. For joints of the upper and lower extremities the modality of choice is determined by the area of interest. Thus, CT images are primarily utilized in this text, but the student is introduced to a comparison of CT and MR images in the region of the head. MR images are subsequently incorporated in the chapters on the spine and extremities. It is presumed that the student has previously studied anatomy.

CT

CT involves placing a patient on a couch that slides through a circularly shaped gantry. Within the gantry is an X-ray tube that rotates around the patient. Opposite the X-ray tube are detectors that record the amount of unattenuated radiation (radiation not absorbed by the patient), and convert the information into a signal. The detectors replace the film used as image receptors in conventional imaging. The signal given by the detectors is converted from an analog format to a digital format and sent to a computer where the data are used to construct an image.

Both CT and MRI have distinct advantages. CT is better than MRI at imaging compact bone. (See the section on MRI below for an explanation.) Consequently, CT is the preferred modality for patients with head trauma, as skull and facial bone fractures, as well as brain injuries, are demonstrated. Although metal may cause imaging artifacts on CT images, it is not dangerous. Conversely, a ferromagnetic object within, on, or near the patient can pose serious, potentially fatal, problems in MRI. Thus, a patient on life-support or monitoring equipment could feasibly have a CT, but if any of the equipment has magnetic properties it would not be allowed in the MRI scanning room. If a patient is nontransportable, he or she would be unable to have a CT. As a rule, the scanning time for CT is considerably less than MRI, especially with the newer multislice scanners, so CT is the preferred modality for combative or uncooperative patients. CT offers better tolerance for patient motion. Additionally, CT is less costly than MRI.

Each medical site has a specific examination protocol determining the thickness and number of slices to be obtained. Most CT images are done transaxially, with the cuts generally being perpendicular to the long axis of the body. An exception is brain CT imaging, where the gantry is angled approximately 15 degrees from the long axis of the body to minimize the interface artifacts in the posterior inferior portion of the cranium caused by the intense contrast differences of the dense bone and soft tissue of the brain. (See Figure 1.) Another advantage of the tubal angulation is a reduction in radiation dosage to the eyes. While the X-ray beam is generally perpendicular to the part being imaged in conventional radiography, with CT it is parallel. Occasionally, some images are done in the coronal plane. Sagittal images are rare, as they are difficult to obtain. The computer can reformat the data to produce images in other planes, but the quality, compared to images obtained in the original plane, is poor. With the newest volumetric multislice helical scanners, there is one continuous movement of the X-ray tube around the gantry as the couch moves through the gantry. Multiple rows of detectors measure the unattenuated radiation. As a result the entire section is imaged with one activation of the X-ray tube. Unfortunately, 360 degrees of information is not obtained for each slice, but the data can be used to obtain slices at different levels utilizing the same parameters without re-exposing the patient. The exam time is reduced to seconds and there is improved spatial resolution.

Looking at CT images of the brain is similar to looking at conventional X-ray films with bone appearing white (high attenuation), air appearing black (low attenuation),

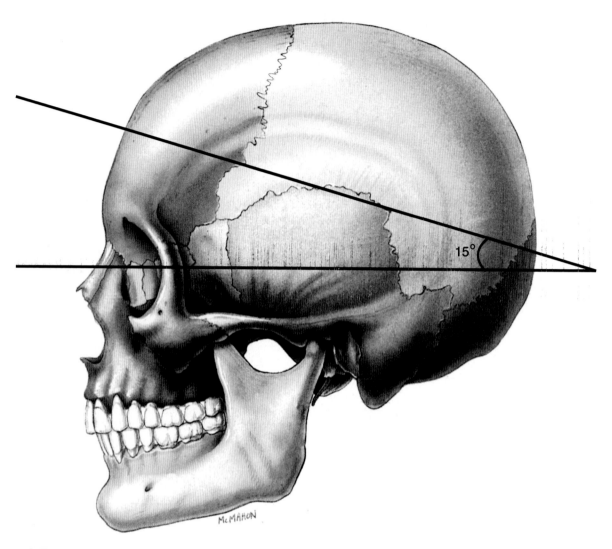

15°

Figure I Typical CT head imaging plane

and fat and other medium density structures appearing in some shade of gray. By varying the window level and window width, the density and contrast can be varied to better visualize certain structures. However, bone still appears white and air still is very dark. Figure 2 A and B are two images produced by a CT computer using the same data and at the same level in the thorax, but 2 A would more clearly demonstrates lung pathology, while 2 B shows the structures in the mediastinum.

Approximately 50% of the time, contrast medium is administered. The contrast medium may be a water-soluble, iodinated medium administered IV. The blood-brain barrier, a mechanism discussed in Chapter 1, should prevent the medium from penetrating the brain tissue. As with all contrast medium injections, the patient is prescreened for contraindications such as a previous history of contrast medium reactions. Many sites use only nonionic contrast medium in CT to minimize the risk of reactions. Often, if a patient has an existing tumor, "ring enhancement" of the tumor is evident, resulting from the contrast medium being visualized in the heavy concentration of blood vessels supplying the tumor. An oral contrast medium may be used for the abdomen, either a low concentration of a barium mixture or a low concentration of a water-soluble, iodinated medium. Similar contrast media may be administered rectally.

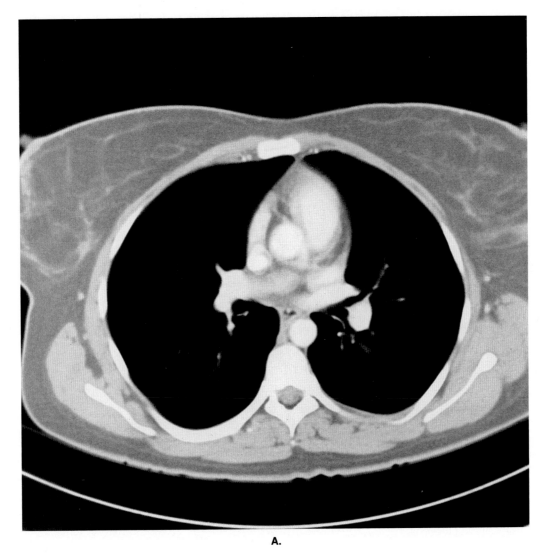

A.

Figure 2 A and B (A) CT image of the thorax selecting window width and level to demonstrate lungs (continues)

MRI

While CT may be the preferred modality for trauma cases as it demonstrates both skull and cranial fractures as well as brain injury, MRI has distinct advantages. Images can be obtained in virtually any plane including transaxial, coronal, sagittal, and oblique. MRI involves no ionizing radiation. When compared to CT, MRI has excellent low-contrast resolution and a superior ability to differentiate soft tissue densities. As the brain and spinal cord are composed of soft tissue, MRI is the preferred modality to demonstrate most central nervous system pathology.

Because the intended purpose of this book is to teach sectional anatomy, anything but a brief synopsis of the

principles of MRI is outside the scope of this text. However, a limited knowledge of the principles of MRI is necessary to understand the capabilities and limitations of MRI. More in-depth information may be obtained from textbooks devoted specifically to studying the physics and principles of MRI, as identified in Appendix B.

Approximately 80% of all atoms in the body are hydrogen. Under normal conditions, protons within the hydrogen atom nuclei are randomly aligned with respect to each other. However, when exposed to strong magnetic fields, the protons act like magnets, which causes them to align with the external magnetic field. The protons also spin about their own axis but in a wobbly motion (precess) and

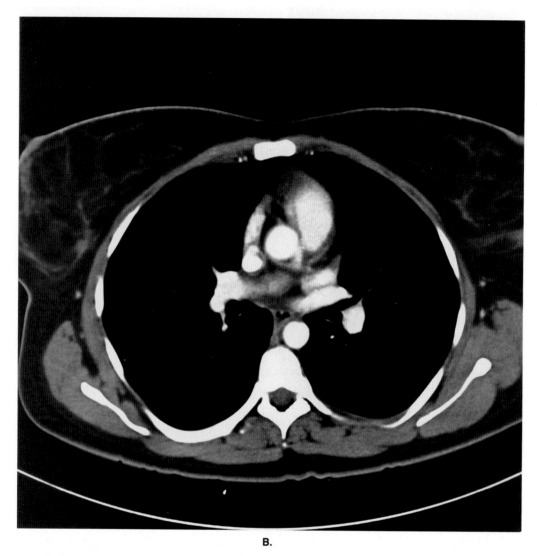

B.

Figure 2 A and B *(continued)* (B) CT image of the thorax selecting window width and level to demonstrate mediastinal structures

not in exact sequence with each other (out-of-phase) when within the magnetic field. MRI utilizes this information about the number and characteristics of hydrogen atoms within the body by placing the patient within a powerful magnetic field. The hydrogen atom protons are then exposed to a radio-frequency pulse, which causes the protons to change their alignment with respect to the existing magnetic field, and to start to precess in phase. The radio-frequency pulsation is discontinued and an antenna is used to record a signal as the protons release the energy absorbed from the radio-frequency pulsation, either through interaction among themselves or into the environment. These data are entered into a computer to produce an image.

This overly simplified explanation of the principles of MRI is necessary to make a single point relevant to MR images in the study of sectional anatomy. Compact bone and air contain few hydrogen atoms so virtually no signal is emitted by either. If compact bone is of interest, MRI is not the imaging modality of choice, nor is it appropriate if the presence of calcium content is an indicator of pathology. However, the absence of bony artifacts can be a distinct advantage, for example, when imaging the posterior inferior brain. MRI also provides excellent information about cancellous bone and joints.

MR images can be "weighted" by one of three methods: PD (proton density), T1 relaxation time (a focus on the release of energy from the radio-frequency application

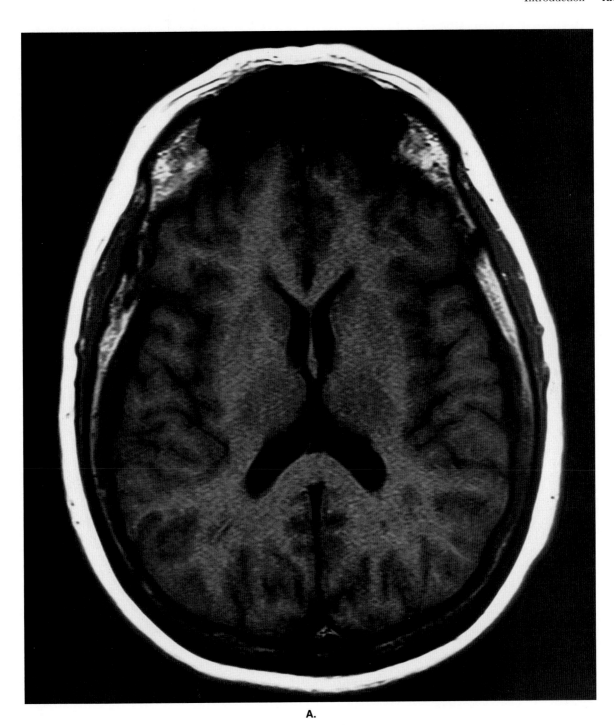

A.

Figure 3 A and B MR images of the same region of the brain with (A) T1 weighted and *(continues)*

by the nuclei to the environment, which causes the protons to return to alignment with the magnetic field), and T2 relaxation time (a focus on the exchange of energy received from the radio-frequency application among the nuclei themselves, which causes them to get out of phase). As a result of the potential variation in how the images are weighted, images on the same plane weighted differently may show the same tissue with different coloration gradations. Figure 3 A and B are two MR images, weighted differently, of the same area of the brain. A familiarity with anatomy allows recognition of the structures imaged.

Motion can present more of a problem with MR imaging than with CT imaging and obtaining quality images in MRI often requires lengthy imaging times. Although some

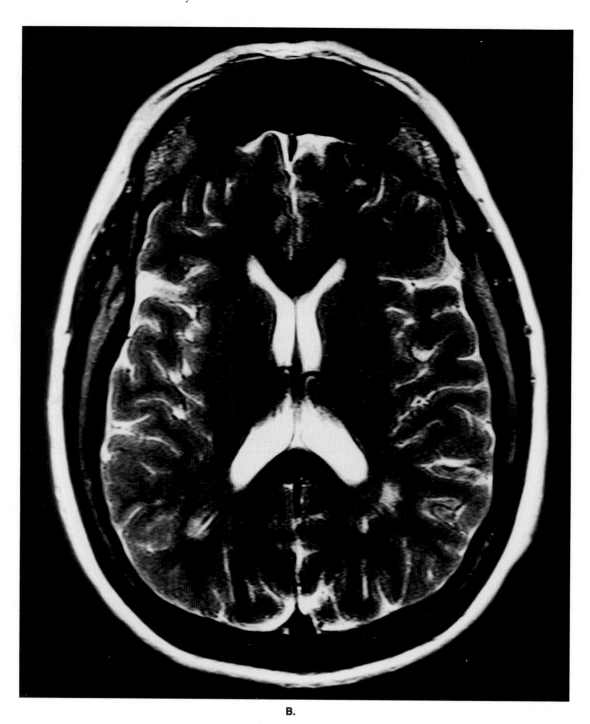

B.

Figure 3 A and B *(continued)* (B) T2 weighted

exams can be completed in less than 10 minutes, other exams may require up to 90 minutes. Fast imaging pulse sequences are used for certain applications but, as a rule, are used to supplement an exam. If the imaging time is decreased, there is a corresponding decrease in the quality of the images. Conversely, if imaging time is increased, image quality is improved but there is a greater potential for patient motion and fewer patients can be imaged. Another motion-related problem is the potential for artifacts caused by cardiac and respiratory motion, most problematic in the thoracic and upper abdominal studies. Cardiac and respiratory gating or triggering can minimize these artifacts, but sacrifice exam time. Gating refers to synchronizing data acquisition to periods of little or no motion, while triggering refers to the synchronization of data acquisition to specific points during motion.

As mentioned, a significant advantage of MRI is that it does not involve any ionizing radiation. This makes it the preferred modality for children and pregnant women. Because of the potential for motion artifacts, children unable to cooperate for the necessary length of time may need to be temporarily sedated. With respect to imaging pregnant women using MRI, it is only recommended if there are no other acceptable alternative procedures available that can provide the required information necessary to manage the case. This cautionary approach is advised because MRI is a relatively new imaging modality. The first significant MRI body image (of a chest cavity) was obtained in 1977; consequently, no longitudinal studies have been completed studying the effects of the combination of magnetic and radio-frequency energy fields at the levels currently used and approved for MRI.

When referring to the effects of ionizing radiation, the ALARA concept (as low as reasonably achievable) prevails because there is no dose of ionizing radiation that is known to be safe. The current research findings on MRI seem to indicate that below certain levels of intensity and length of exposure there are no biological responses. However, safety issues do exist. One definite finding is that above the established low limits there is an increase in temperature produced by the body. The Food and Drug Administration (FDA) also warns all patients with electrically, magnetically, or mechanically activated implanted devices (most importantly cardiac pacemakers), to be carefully screened. Patients should also be questioned about the presence of any other ferromagnetic objects that might have been deliberately or accidentally implanted within their bodies

(such as aneurysm clips), as these can involve serious, if not fatal, risks to the patient. Claustrophobic patients may experience difficulty in the closed magnets, although there are a number of measures that can be taken to minimize the patients' symptoms. Some patients may experience temporary hearing loss caused by the loud banging noises coming from the magnet, but, again, there are steps that can minimize the effects of these loud noises. In addition, any ferromagnetic objects outside the magnet can become hazardous projectile missiles. The last risk involves the use of MRI contrast agents. Roughly 70% of all MRI exams are done utilizing contrast agents. As of this writing, there are a number of FDA-approved contrast agents. The most commonly employed are one of the four gadolinium-based agents, all of which are injectable. There are also two iron oxide-based contrast agents, one that is injected and one that is administered orally. The last agent is magnesium-based and is injected.

All the identified contrast agents are paramagnetic or superparamagnetic. They alter the MRI signal by shortening the T1 and T2 relaxation times, with the superparamagnetic contrast agents effective for T2-weighted images. The contrast agents administered IV are water-soluble agents, which are eliminated from the body primarily through urine output. As a rule, they are unable to cross the blood-brain barrier unless it has been compromised by pathology. Generally, the incidence of reactions to the gadolinium-based contrast agents is less than that of the iodinated contrast agents used for CT. It is suggested that MRI contrast agents be used for pregnant women only when necessary because they can cross through the placenta to the fetus. When excreted by the fetus, the agents re-enter the fetus orally.

Head

CRANIAL BONES

There are eight **cranial bones** that encase the brain. They are the **frontal** bone, two **parietal bones**, **occipital bone**, two **temporal bones**, **sphenoid bone**, and **ethmoid bone**. Many have a unique construction with **diploe** (spongy bone) sandwiched between two layers of compact bone. Figures 1-1, 1-2, and 1-3 show the cranial bones from an external lateral, anterior, and posterior perspective, respectively.

In Chapter 2 numerous landmarks on the cranial bones will become relevant. Included are the **squamous** and

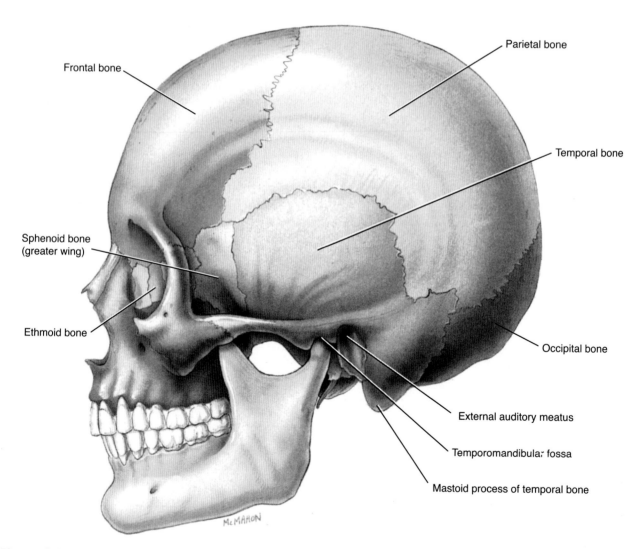

Figure 1-1 External lateral view of cranial bones

horizontal or orbital section of the frontal bone, visible on Figures 1-2 and 1-4, respectively. On Figure 1-4 notice the **foramen magnum**, the part of the occipital bone located posteriorly on the floor of the skull. On the temporal bone, points of interest are the **temporomandibular fossa**, which is involved in forming the temporomandibular joint

(Figure 1-1) and the petrous portion seen on Figure 1-4. The external auditory meatus (EAM) is the external opening into the petrous portion of the temporal bone. Posterior and inferior to the EAM is the mastoid portion of the temporal bone, containing the mastoid air cells.

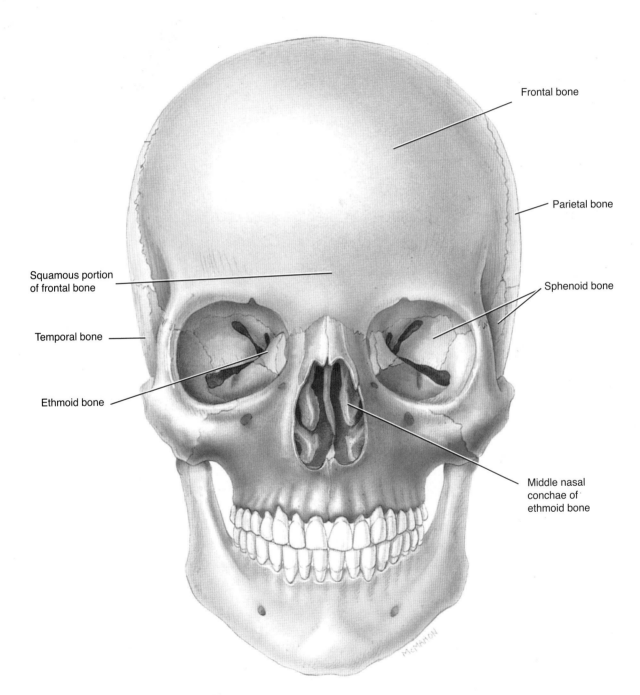

Frontal bone

Parietal bone

Squamous portion of frontal bone

Sphenoid bone

Temporal bone

Ethmoid bone

Middle nasal conchae of ethmoid bone

Figure 1-2 External frontal view of cranial bones

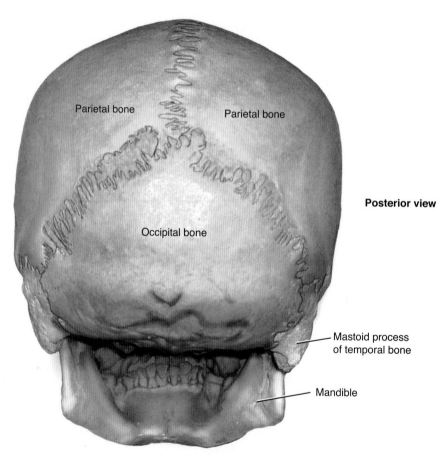

Parietal bone

Parietal bone

Posterior view

Occipital bone

Mastoid process
of temporal bone

Mandible

Figure 1-3 External posterior view of cranial bones

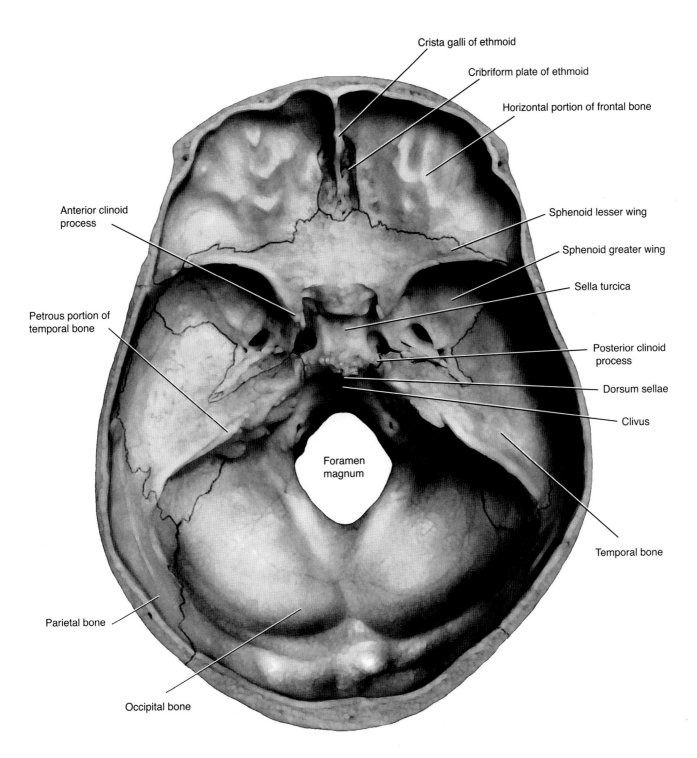

Crista galli of ethmoid

Cribriform plate of ethmoid

Horizontal portion of frontal bone

Anterior clinoid process

Sphenoid lesser wing

Sphenoid greater wing

Sella turcica

Petrous portion of temporal bone

Posterior clinoid process

Dorsum sellae

Clivus

Foramen magnum

Temporal bone

Parietal bone

Occipital bone

Internal base of skull

Figure 1-4 Floor of skull

Figures 1-4 and 1-5 demonstrate the sphenoid bone which sits in the floor of the cranium and acts as an anchor for the other cranial bones. Important landmarks for future reference include the anterior and posterior **clinoids**, the **sella turcica** (a saddlelike depression), the **dorsum sellae** (the back of the sella turcica), the body lying beneath the sella turcica, and the bilateral medial and lateral **pterygoid processes** which extend inferiorly.

Also significant is the ethmoid bone pictured on Figure 1-6 from a frontal or coronal perspective and Figure 1-7, a midsagittal cut. Both line drawings show the cribiform plate and crista galli which sit in the ethmoidal notch of the horizontal or orbital portion of the frontal bone.

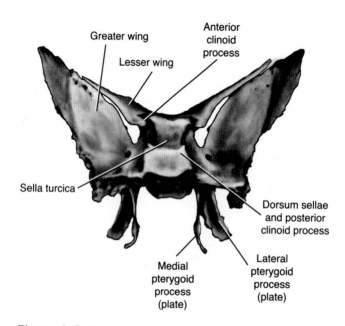

Figure 1-5 Anterior view of sphenoid bone

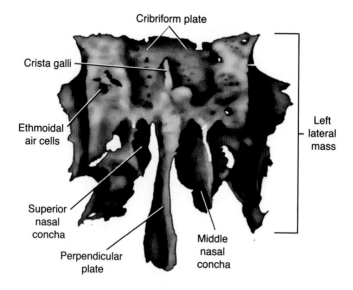

Figure 1-6 Frontal view of ethmoid bone

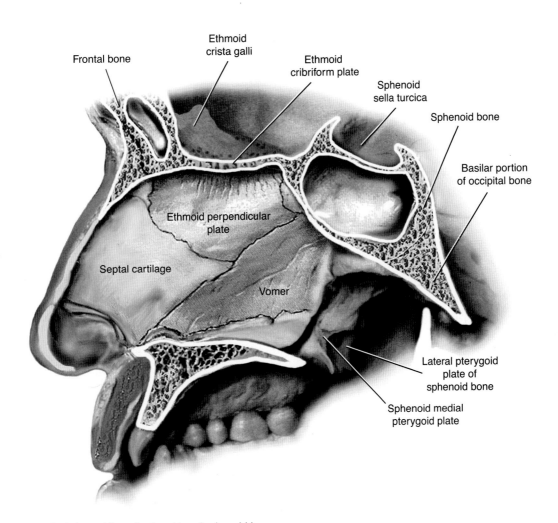

Frontal bone

Ethmoid
crista galli

Ethmoid
cribriform plate

Sphenoid
sella turcica

Sphenoid bone

Basilar portion
of occipital bone

Ethmoid perpendicular
plate

Septal cartilage

Vomer

Lateral pterygoid
plate of
sphenoid bone

Sphenoid medial
pterygoid plate

Figure 1-7 Midsagittal view of frontal, ethmoid, and sphenoid bones

NEURONS

Before you begin the study of the different aspects of the brain on sectional images, you must first understand the basic functional unit of the nervous system, the **neuron**, or nerve cell. There are two different types of neurons, **sensory** and **motor**. **Afferent** neurons, an alternative term for sensory neurons, bring nervous information into the central nervous system from outlying areas of the body. Motor neurons, a type of **efferent** neuron, relay nervous messages coming from the brain to target organs and structures. All neurons have the same components, but these parts appear in a slightly different arrangement. They include the **cell body**, and two types of processes, **dendrites**, carrying messages to the cell body, and **axons**, carrying messages away from the cell body.

Notice on Figure 1-8 A and B, that a typical motor neuron has many dendrites leading into the cell body, whereas the typical sensory neuron has only one. There is never more than one axon. Relay of nervous impulses is always unidirectional, from dendrite to cell body and then out through the axon. Although in both of these drawings a myelin sheath surrounds the axon, all neurons do not have myelin present. In fact, some have no processes at all.

The presence or absence of myelin determines the type of brain tissue. **Gray matter** is composed of unmyelinated neurons or just cell bodies while **white matter** is constructed primarily of neurons with myelinated axons. You will be able to differentiate on computed tomography (CT) and magnetic resonance (MR) images the difference between gray and white matter. Certain types of pathology, such as multiple sclerosis (MS), will destroy this myelin. MR and at times CT images are often able to identify areas of the brain where this destruction has occurred.

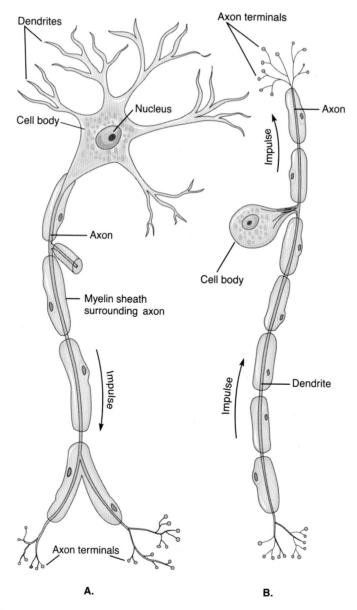

Figure 1-8 A and B (A) Motor and (B) sensory neurons

MENINGES

As we begin our exploration of the brain, we first encounter the coverings of the brain, the **meninges**, which extend down around the spinal cord. There are three layers, starting with the outermost, the **dura mater**. The dura mater, a very tough fibrous membrane, is in direct contact with the cranium. Below the dura mater are the middle and innermost layers, the **arachnoid** and the **pia mater**, respectively. Only the pia mater adheres to and actually follows the contours of the brain. Associated with the meninges are the meningeal spaces. The **epidural space** is located external to the dura mater. The **subdural space** is between the dura mater and the arachnoid and the **subarachnoid space** is between the arachnoid and the pia mater. In the subarachnoid space **cerebrospinal fluid** circulates. The meninges are labeled on Figure 1-9.

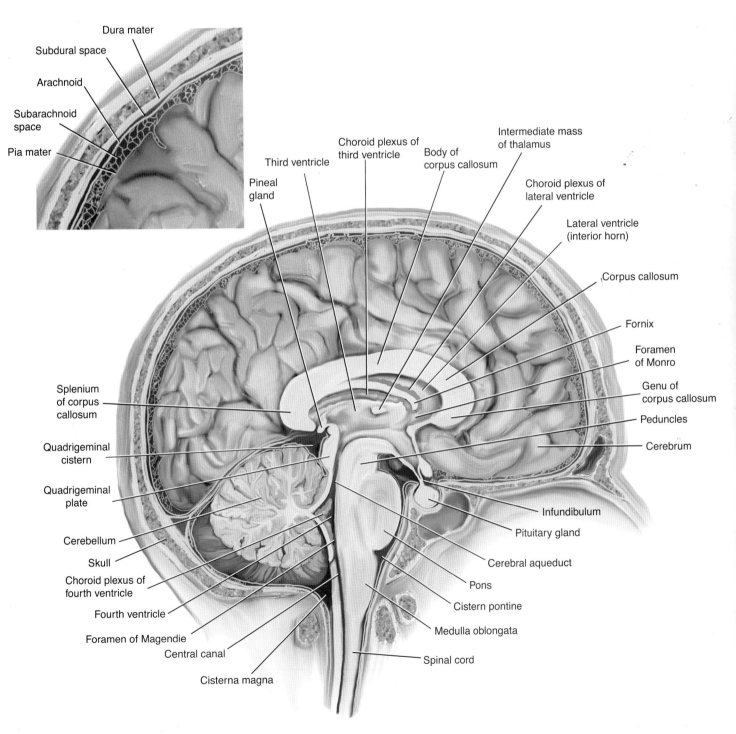

Figure 1-9 Midsagittal view of brain

BRAIN

In the embryo the brain is divided into three main components: the **forebrain**, **midbrain**, and **hindbrain**.

Forebrain

The forebrain can be further subdivided into two parts, the **cerebrum** and the **diencephalon**.

Cerebrum

In examining Figure 1-9, a midsagittal drawing of the brain, you should note that the cerebrum forms the bulk of the brain. The **cortex**, the outer portion of the cerebrum, consists of gray matter. Centrally located in the cerebrum is a region known as the **centrum semiovale**, composed of white matter. Deep in the cerebrum, located inferiorly within the centrum semiovale, are pockets of gray matter called **basal ganglia**.

Hemispheres

The cerebrum is divided into two **hemispheres** or halves, a right and a left. The two hemispheres do not communicate except through the **corpus callosum**, which is composed of white matter. The main part of the corpus callosum is the **body** or **trunk**, the anterior portion is the **genu**, and the posterior portion is the **splenium**, all labeled on Figure 1-9. As the corpus callosum does not coincide with the superior surface of the brain, do not expect to see it in the initial axial cuts.

Lobes

Each of the two hemispheres of the cerebrum is divided into five lobes. Four of these five lobes underlie cranial bones with similar names: the **frontal**, **parietal**, **temporal**, and **occipital** lobes. Figure 1-10, a lateral view of the external surface of the brain, demonstrates them. The **central lobe**, or **insula**, can be found by separating

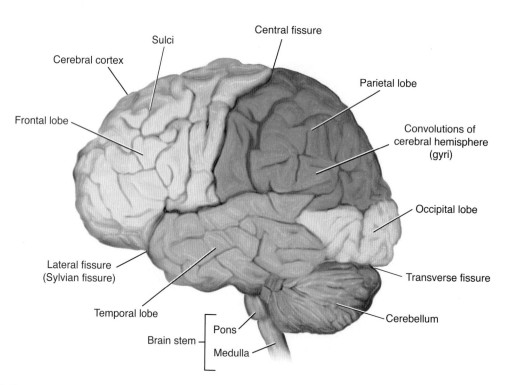

Figure 1-10 External lateral view of brain

the space where the temporal, frontal, and parietal lobes meet. The temporal lobes are seen at the level of the dorsum sellae (see Figure 1-4). The occipital lobes are first seen on axial images at the level of the corpus callosum.

Fissures

The superficial surface of the cerebrum has shallow grooves known as **sulci**. The folds between the grooves are **convolutions** or **gyri**. Deeper grooves separate the two hemispheres, the cerebrum from other parts of the brain, and the frontal, parietal, and temporal lobes from each other. The **longitudinal fissure** divides the right and left hemispheres of the cerebrum as seen on Figure 1-11, a superior view of the brain from an external perspective. The **transverse fissure** separates the occipital lobes of the cerebrum from the **cerebellum**. (We have not yet encountered the cerebellum, but it is readily seen on Figure 1-10 beneath the occipital lobe, along with the fissures being discussed.) The **central fissure** divides the frontal lobe from the parietal lobe. The **Sylvian** or **lateral fissure** separates the frontal, parietal and temporal lobes of the cerebrum. Bending the lips of the Sylvian fissure reveals the central lobe of the cerebrum. insula

The dura mater dips into some of these fissures. The dip of the dura mater into the longitudinal fissure is the **falx cerebri**. The dip of the dura mater into the transverse fissure is the **tentorium cerebelli** while the **falx cerebelli** is the dip of the dura mater between the two hemispheres of the cerebellum.

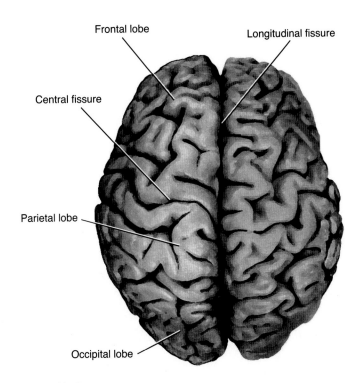

Frontal lobe

Longitudinal fissure

Central fissure

Parietal lobe

Occipital lobe

Figure 1-11 Superior view of brain

Basal Ganglia

The paired basal ganglia are composed of gray matter and are found deep in the cerebrum. The **corpus striatum** is the largest of the basal ganglia. Each of its two components is further divided into two subcomponents, the **caudate nucleus** and the **lentiform nucleus**, both generically called **cerebral nuclei**. If you refer to Figure 1-12 you will see a lateral perspective of the corpus striatum. The caudate nucleus forms a C shape. What you perhaps cannot appreciate from this two-dimensional line drawing is that the paired caudate nuclei are off-centered. Figure 1-13 shows both the caudate nucleus and the lentiform nucleus from a frontal (coronal) perspective. The second part of the corpus striatum, the lentiform nucleus, has two parts to it: the **globus pallidus**, which is located more medially, and the **putamen**, which is lateral to the globus pallidus. On Figure 1-12, they seem to superimpose each other, but on Figure 1-13 you see where they lie with respect to each other. The remaining basal ganglia include the **claustrum**, found lateral to the putamen and the **amygdaloid nucleus**, located at the tail end of the caudate nucleus. When looking at CT and MR images the basal ganglia will appear as gray matter. An internal capsule separates the globus pallidus from the thalamus (to be discussed next) and an external capsule separates the putamen from the claustrum. Both the internal and external capsules are composed of white matter. These lines of demarcation are visible on many sectional images.

Diencephalon

The second part of the forebrain, the diencephalon, has four portions: the epithalamus, the **thalamus**, the metathalamus and the **hypothalamus**. The thalamus and hypothalamus are visible on CT and MR images.

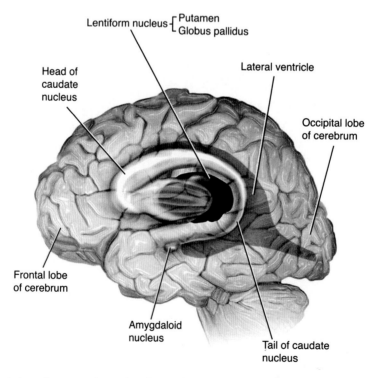

Figure 1-12 External lateral view of corpus striatum (caudate nucleus and lentiform nucleus)

Thalamus

The thalamus is mostly gray matter. By studying Figure 1-13 you should recognize that the thalamus will only appear on sagittal images if the cuts are slightly off-centered. Visible on Figure 1-9 is the **intermediate mass**, a bridge also composed of gray matter which connects parts of the thalamus.

Hypothalamus

The hypothalamus is the second part of the diencephalon visible on CT and MR images. As indicated by the prefix hypo- it is below or under the thalamus. It is also slightly anterior. A stalk called the **infundibulum** attaches the hypothalamus to the **pituitary gland.** The pituitary gland, one of the endocrine glands of the human body, is known as the "master gland." It sits in the sella turcica as seen on Figure 1-4 and manufactures six hormones. Many of these are **tropic** hormones, which stimulate other endocrine glands to secrete their hormones. The pituitary gland has two lobes, anterior and posterior. The posterior lobe does not actually manufacture hormones, but stores and secretes the hormones manufactured by the hypothalamus. The hormones pass through the infundibulum into the pituitary gland. Look back at Figure 1-9 and locate the pituitary gland and infundibulum. Figure 1-13 shows the pituitary gland, infundibulum, and hypothalamus from a coronal perspective.

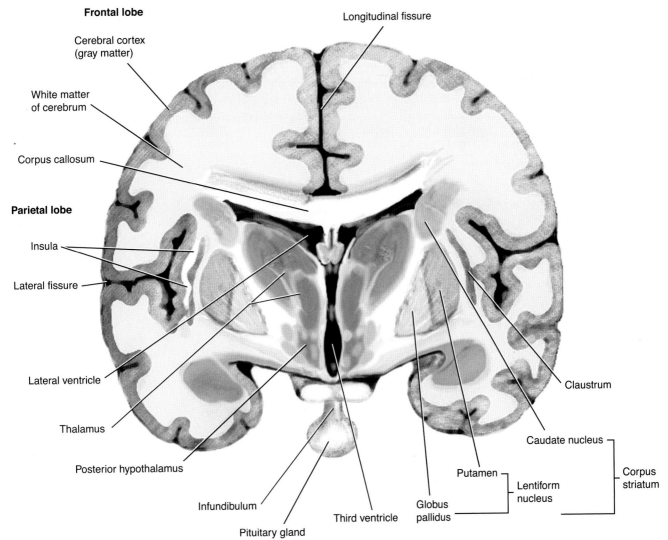

Figure 1-13 Frontal view of basal ganglia

Although not considered part of the forebrain, another structure to identify in line drawings of this area is the **optic chiasma**. **Optic nerves** exit through the back of the orbits and those from the inner half of the retina cross over at the optic chiasma. The fibers travel in optic tracts past this point, and eventually terminate in the thalamus. Figure 1-14 demonstrates this pathway. The optic chiasma appears on some sagittal and coronal images as a short line running perpendicular to the infundibulum.

Midbrain

The midbrain connects the hind brain with the cerebrum.

Peduncles

The two main parts of the midbrain are the **peduncles**, located anteriorly, and the **tectum**, located posteriorly.

Tectum

The tectum is composed of four rounded prominences collectively called the **corpora quadrigemina** or **quadrigeminal plate**. Each of these rounded prominences is a **colliculus**. The colliculi are bilateral, dividing into two superior and two inferior colliculi. The peduncles and quadrigeminal plate can be seen on Figure 1-9.

Hindbrain

The hindbrain has three parts: the **pons**, **medulla oblongata**, and cerebellum.

Pons

By definition pons means "tissue connecting two or more parts." The pons acts as an intermediary between the medulla and the other parts of the brain. Refer back to Figure 1-9 to see that the pons is a rounded prominence located superior to the medulla and anterior to the cerebellum.

Medulla Oblongata

The **medulla**, or medulla oblongata, comprises the most inferior part of the brain. Once it passes through the foramen magnum, the large round hole in the occipital bone at the base of the skull, it becomes the **spinal cord**. All ascending and descending nerve tracts must pass through the medulla to reach the brain. The nerve tracts are white matter. There are some important points to mention about the medulla. Three vital reflex centers are located in it. They are the respiratory center, regulating the rhythm of breathing, the cardiac center, regulating the heart beat and force of contraction, and the vasomotor or vasoconstrictor center, controlling the diameter of the

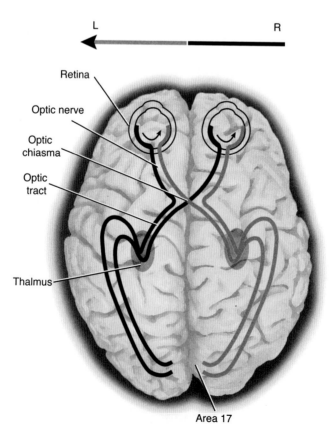

Figure 1-14 Superior view of optic chiasma

blood vessels. Also, of the twelve pairs of cranial nerves, cranial nerves VIII, IX, X, XI and XII arise from the medulla. Finally, in the lower anterior portion of the medulla, a crossing over of some nerve fibers occurs. Because of this crossing over in the **decussation of the pyramids of the medulla** the right half of the brain controls the left half of the body and vice versa. Look at the inferior part of the base of the brain on Figure 1-9 to find the medulla oblongata.

Cerebellum

The cerebellum is the largest part of the hindbrain, and the second largest part of the brain. Like the cerebrum, the cerebellum is broken into two hemispheres, a right and a left. Also, like the cerebrum, these hemispheres are connected, the connecting tissue being the **vermis**. Figure 1-15 shows line drawings of the anterior and posterior surfaces of the cerebellum. Notice its butterfly shape. Figure 1-10 shows the cerebellum from an external lateral perspective and Figure 1-9 displays its location with respect to the cerebrum, pons, and medulla. It is inferior to the posterior aspect of the cerebrum and posterior to the pons. You should recollect that the transverse fissure

separates the cerebellum from the cerebrum and that the tentorium cerebelli is the dip of the dura mater in the transverse fissure. Look again at Figure 1-15, and notice the two notches, the **anterior cerebellar notch** and the **posterior cerebellar notch**. The posterior cerebellar notch accommodates the falx cerebelli. Remember that the falx cerebelli is the dip of the dura mater between the two hemispheres of the cerebellum inferiorly. *[handwritten: not important]*

There are three pairs of peduncles, or bundles of nerve fibers, that are associated with the cerebellum. They are named according to their location, the inferior, the middle, and the superior. The inferior peduncles connect the cerebellum to the medulla. The middle peduncles connect the cerebellum to the pons and the superior peduncles connect the cerebellum to the midbrain. *[handwritten: know]*

Although not considered part of the hindbrain, the **pineal gland** is mentioned here. One of the endocrine glands, it is located superiorly to the cerebellum, beneath the splenium of the corpus callosum. (Using these landmarks, find it on Figure 1-9.) It often calcifies early in life and should not be confused with a cross-section of a contrast-filled blood vessel when seen on axial CT images. It is found exactly midsagittally, and posteriorly on axial cuts. *[handwritten: know]*

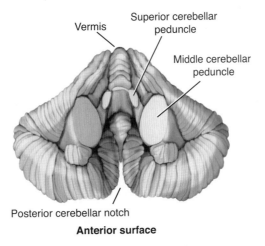

Vermis Superior cerebellar peduncle

Middle cerebellar peduncle

Posterior cerebellar notch

Anterior surface

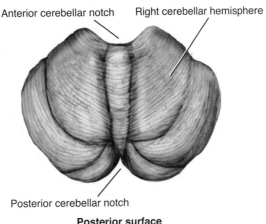

Anterior cerebellar notch   Right cerebellar hemisphere

Posterior cerebellar notch

Posterior surface

Figure 1-15 Anterior and posterior view of cerebellum

Brain Stem

The **brain stem** connects the hemispheres of the cerebrum with the spinal cord. It is made of the midbrain, pons, and medulla. Ten of the twelve cranial nerves arise from the brain stem. Knowing the critical reflex centers located in the medulla oblongata and that all nerve tracts, ascending and descending, must pass through the medulla, pons, and midbrain, you should understand the severity of brain stem injuries.

VENTRICLES

The **ventricles** are cavities in the brain filled with cerebrospinal fluid. They communicate with each other, with the central canal of the spinal cord, and with the subarachnoid space. There are two lateral ventricles, and the third and fourth ventricles that lie midline.

Choroid Plexus

The **choroid plexus** is an infolding of a cluster of capillaries in the pia mater that lines certain parts of all the ventricles. It manufactures cerebrospinal fluid by filtration and secretion. The unique construction of the choroid plexus helps form the **blood-brain barrier**, prohibiting certain substances from passing into the brain and ventricles. In some cases this protective mechanism makes it difficult to treat pathology chemically. The **collateral trigone** is an area of the lateral ventricles where there is a heavy concentration of choroid plexus. It is evident on sectional images when contrast is administered into the circulatory system. Refer to Figure 1-9 to see the choroid plexus.

Lateral Ventricles

The lateral ventricles are the largest of the ventricles. Figure 1-16 shows a lateral perspective of the ventricles while Figure 1-17 A and B show the ventricles from a coronal and superior perspective.

Body

The central and most superior aspect of the lateral ventricles is the body. The corpus callosum, connecting tissue of the two cerebral hemispheres, sits over the lateral ventricles. Once the corpus callosum is encountered on axial images, you should expect to next see the body of the lateral ventricles.

Frontal/Anterior Horn

The bilateral **frontal** or **anterior horns** sit within the frontal lobes of the two hemispheres of the cerebrum. The anterior horns are the only sections of the lateral ventricles that approach the midsagittal plane and thus the only sections of the lateral ventricles shown on Figure 1-9, a midsagittal drawing of the brain. Under the anterior horns, using axial cuts, is the head of the caudate nucleus. (It may be helpful to review the section on the basal ganglia at this time, in particular, the caudate nucleus which sits within and follows the shape of the lateral ventricles.)

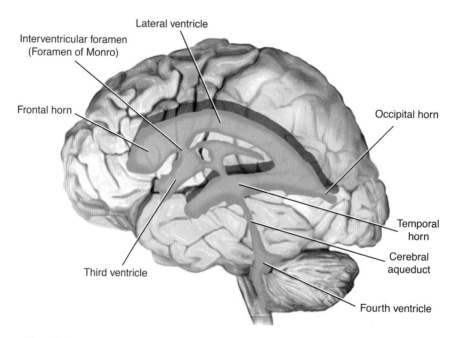

Interventricular foramen (Foramen of Monro)

Lateral ventricle

Frontal horn

Occipital horn

Temporal horn

Cerebral aqueduct

Third ventricle

Fourth ventricle

Figure 1-16 External lateral view of ventricles of the brain

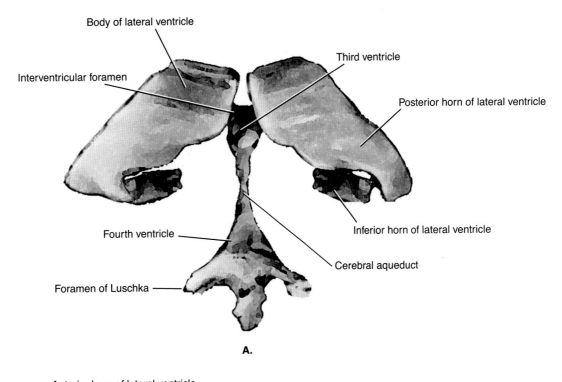

Body of lateral ventricle

Third ventricle

Interventricular foramen

Posterior horn of lateral ventricle

Inferior horn of lateral ventricle

Fourth ventricle

Cerebral aqueduct

Foramen of Luschka

A.

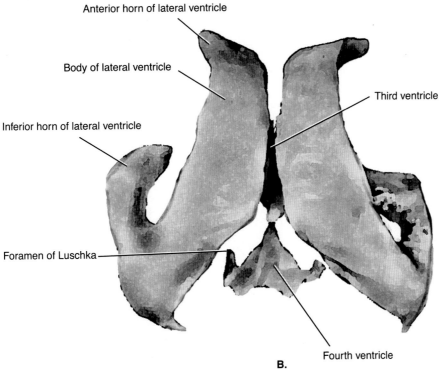

Anterior horn of lateral ventricle

Body of lateral ventricle

Third ventricle

Inferior horn of lateral ventricle

Foramen of Luschka

Fourth ventricle

B.

Figure 1-17 A and B Posterior and superior view of ventricles

Occipital/Posterior Horn

The bilateral **occipital** or **posterior horns**, are found in the occipital lobes of the two hemispheres of the cerebrum.

Inferior/Temporal Horn

The bilateral **temporal** or **inferior horns** are found in the temporal lobes of the two hemispheres of the cerebrum.

Collateral Trigone

The collateral trigone, previously defined as an area of the lateral ventricles with a heavy concentration of choroid plexus, is at the junction of the occipital and temporal horns.

Septum Pellucidum

The **septum pellucidum** separates the two lateral ventricles and is seen on axial cuts midline. Because the corpus callosum is curved and sits over the lateral ventricles, the genu and splenium of the corpus callosum are seen at the same level as the septum pellucidum on axial CT and MR images.

Fornix

The **fornix**, best seen on MR sagittal images, is composed of white matter and forms the floor of the lateral ventricles. This arch-shaped structure extends anteriorly from the splenium of the corpus callosum and constructs the inferior margin of the septum pellucidum. You may observe the fornix by looking anterior to the splenium of the corpus callosum on Figure 1-9.

Interventricular Foramen

The two lateral ventricles communicate and drain into the third ventricle through the **interventricular foramen** or **foramen of Monro**. They can be located on Figures 1-16 and 1-17 A.

Third Ventricle

The third ventricle can be seen on Figures 1-16 and 1-17 A and B inferior to the body of the lateral ventricles,

but at the same level as the anterior and posterior horns. Similarly, all three are seen on axial sectional images. The third ventricle is midline. The pineal gland can be found posterior to the third ventricle. The lateral walls of the third ventricle are formed by the thalamus, while the ventral wall is formed by the hypothalamus (see Figure 1-13). Figure 1-9 clearly shows the third ventricle, along with the intermediate mass, the bridge between the thalamus. The pineal gland, also seen on Figure 1-9, is posterior to the third ventricle.

Cerebral Aqueduct

The third ventricle communicates with the fourth ventricle through the **cerebral** or **Sylvian aqueduct** (aqueduct of Sylvius), which passes through the midbrain. It can be seen on Figures 1-9, 1-16, and 1-17 A.

Fourth Ventricle

The fourth ventricle is the most inferior and posterior of the ventricles. It sits anterior to the cerebellum in the anterior cerebellar notch and posterior to the pons. Landmarks on axial sectional images indicating the level of the fourth ventricle are the petrous portions of the temporal bones. You can see the fourth ventricle on Figures 1-9, 1-16, and 1-17 A and B. The fourth ventricle has three anterior openings through which it drains.

Foramen of Magendie

The **foramen of Magendie**, or **median aperture**, is an opening found along the anterior median section of the fourth ventricle. It drains into the central canal of the spinal cord, the **cisterna magna**, and the subarachnoid space. Figure 1-9 demonstrates the foramen of Magendie; Figures 1-16 and 1-17 B show the foramina in general.

Foramina of Luschka

The **foramina of Luschka**, or **lateral apertures**, seen on Figure 1-17 A and B, are two lateral openings also draining the fourth ventricle. Through these two openings cerebrospinal fluid enters the subarachnoid space.

Hydrocephalus

As the choroid plexus is constantly secreting cerebrospinal fluid, there is a mechanism to absorb the excess fluid. The cerebrospinal fluid, along with venous blood from the head, drains into the **dural sinuses**, located between the two layers of the dura mater. Figure 1-18 shows a sagittal oblique view of the dural sinuses. If there is an overaccumulation of fluid in the ventricles, (**hydrocephalus**), the ventricles would appear grossly enlarged on sectional images and would cause increased intracranial pressure along with the associated symptoms. Any mass lesion would alter the normally symmetric appearance of the ventricles within the brain.

CISTERNS

Cisterns are pooling areas for cerebrospinal fluid in the brain that result from a widening of the subarachnoid space. They are named according to their locations. Three in particular can be easily identified on sectional images and are listed below.

Cisterna Magna

The cisterna magna, as indicated by its nomenclature, is the largest. It is located between the medulla oblongata and the inferior cerebellar hemispheres.

Quadrigeminal Cistern

The **quadrigeminal cistern** is located immediately posterior to the quadrigeminal plate, the posterior aspect of the midbrain.

Cistern Pontine

The **cistern pontine** is anterior and inferior to the pons. Examine Figure 1-9 to find the location of these three important cisterns.

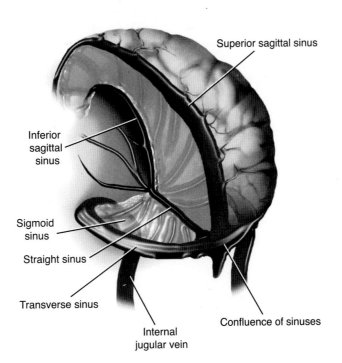

Figure 1-18 Sagittal oblique view of dural sinuses

VASCULAR SYSTEM

Blood is supplied to the head through arteries which drain first into the dural sinuses and then out through veins. Unlike much of the body, all arteries in the head do not have parallel veins with similar names. Primary interest in studying sectional anatomy of the brain as seen on CT and MR images is to identify the arteries.

Arteries

In order to understand the arterial system supplying the head you must first be familiar with the point of origination, the **arch of the aorta** arising from the heart, located in the **mediastinum**. Figure 1-19 shows the arch of the aorta. Three major vessels arise from it. The one on the right is the **brachiocephalic** or **innominate artery**.

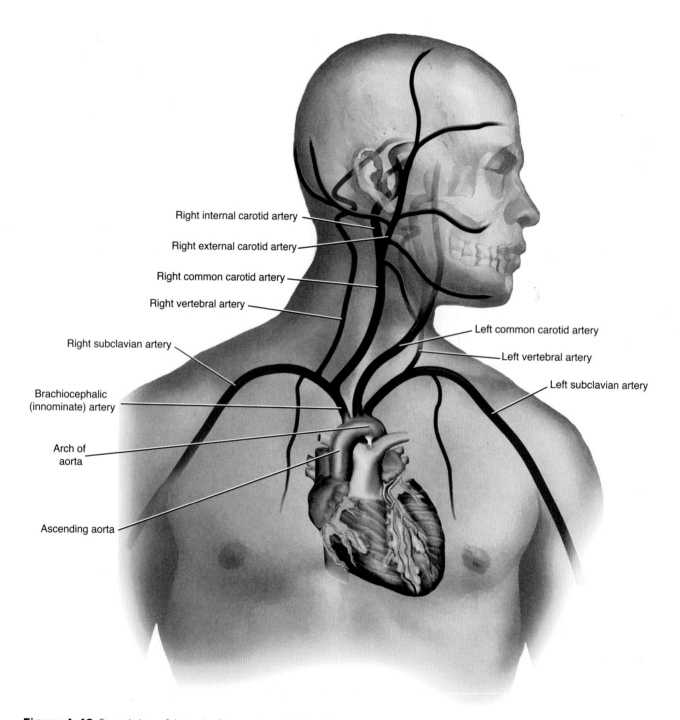

Figure 1-19 Frontal view of the arch of the aorta and its branches

The central vessel is the **left common carotid artery**, and the one on the left is the **left subclavian artery**. At this point there is no symmetry. However, if you follow the right brachiocephalic artery on Figure 1-19, you will notice that it has a branch heading off in a superior direction, the **right common carotid artery**, with the brachiocephalic artery assuming a new name after that point, the **right subclavian artery**. At this point a right and left common carotid and a right and left subclavian artery exist. Now let us continue to study the common carotid arteries. Around C3/C4 the common carotids bifurcate into the **internal** and **external carotid arteries**. The external carotids are not of much interest here as they supply the face, scalp, and most of the neck and throat with blood, however, the branches off the internal carotids are seen on sectional images. The internal carotid arteries eventually bifurcate into **anterior** and **middle cerebral arteries**, bilaterally. If you look at the angiographic images, Figure 1-20, coronal and sagittal images, you can see that the anterior cerebral artery supplies the anterior and medial aspect of the brain with freshly oxygenated blood and, similarly, the middle cerebral artery supplies the lateral portion of the brain.

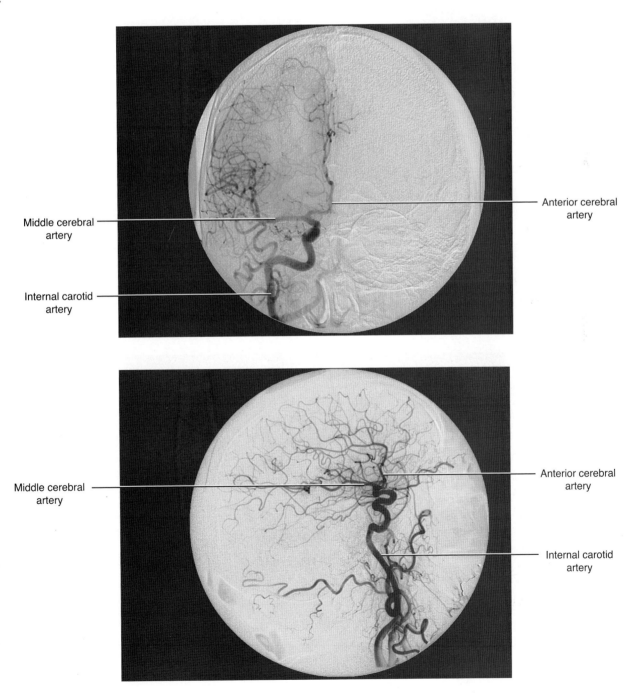

Figure 1-20 Coronal and sagittal arteriograms of carotid artery

What should be apparent is that there seems to be no blood supply to the posterior brain. These images were obtained injecting only one internal carotid artery. To understand how the posterior portion of the brain receives blood we must go back to Figure 1-19 and look more closely at the right and left subclavian arteries. You should see two vessels arising from them in a superior direction, the right and left **vertebral arteries**, which will eventu-

ally supply the posterior aspect of the brain with blood. After entering the cranium through the foramen magnum the two vertebral arteries merge together at approximately the level of the lower pons and form the **basilar artery**, seen on the same axial cuts as the dorsum sellae. The basilar artery soon redivides and forms two major vessels, the right and left **posterior cerebral arteries**. Figure 1-21, shows an injection of a single vertebral artery with the

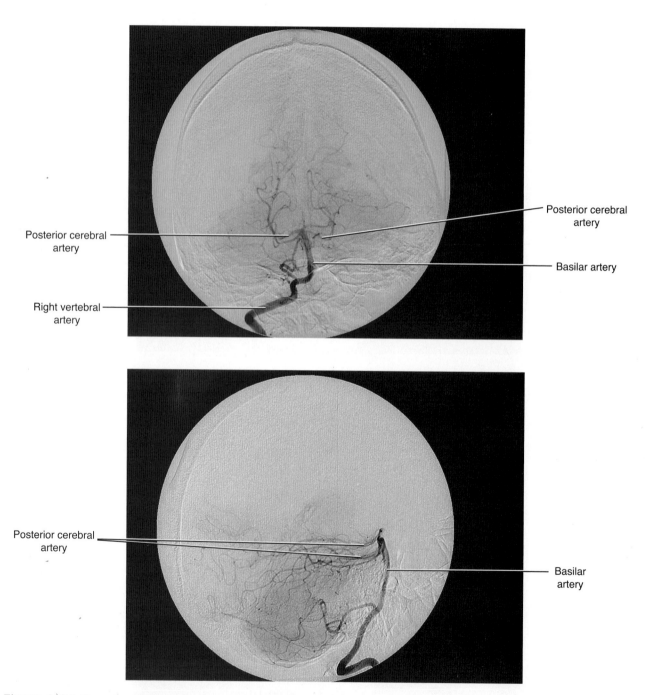

Figure 1-21 Coronal and sagittal arteriograms of vertebral artery

subsequent flow of blood into the basilar artery which then splits into the right and left posterior cerebral arteries. The posterior cerebral arteries supply the posterior aspect of the brain with blood. A schematic diagram of the flow of blood leading to the brain, starting at the arch of the aorta, is shown on Figure 1-22.

Circle of Willis

Because the blood supply to the brain is so critical the body has an ingenious device to equalize blood pressure within the brain and to provide alternative sources of blood should one of the main vessels be compromised. It is accomplished through a structure commonly known as

Scheme of Distribution

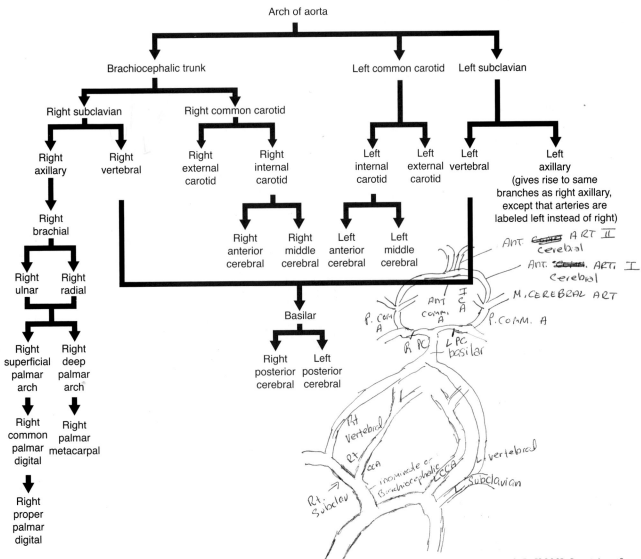

Figure 1-22 Schematic diagram of superior blood flow off the arch of the aorta (Tortora, G. and Grabowski, S. R. [2000]. *Principles of Anatomy & Physiology* [9th ed]. New York: John Wiley & Sons, Inc. This material is used by permission of John Wiley & Sons, Inc.)

the **circle of Willis**, located at the base of the brain. Study Figure 1-23 and you will see a cross-section of the internal carotid arteries and their branches, the middle and anterior cerebral arteries. Also find the basilar artery with its two branches, the two posterior cerebral arteries. Notice the presence of three vessels not previously mentioned, the two **posterior communicating arteries**, joining the posterior cerebral arteries with the internal carotid arteries, and the single **anterior communicating artery**, joining together the two anterior cerebral arteries. Collectively the vessels have assumed a circular shape (the circle of Willis), thereby providing optional sources of blood should a problem exist with one of the vessels involved in supplying the brain with blood.

Dural Sinuses

The arterial blood eventually drains into the dural sinuses, mentioned earlier in the section on hydrocephalus. Into the dural sinuses drains the arterial blood and the cerebrospinal fluid with the dural sinuses eventually draining into the veins. These veins are discussed in more depth when studying sectional images of the neck. In the region of the head the superior sagittal sinus (see Figure 1-18) is seen in cross-section at the anterior and posterior edges of the longitudinal fissure.

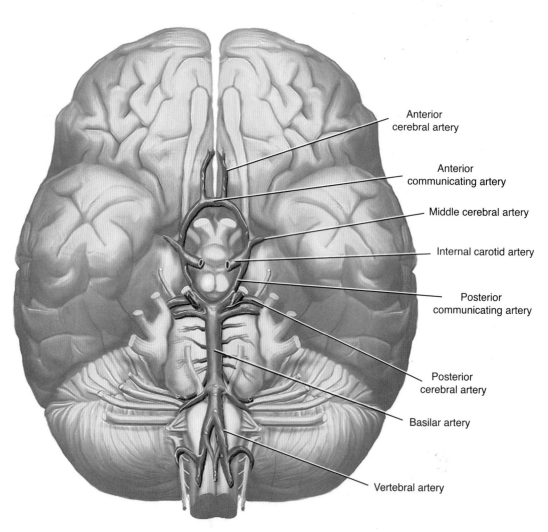

Anterior cerebral artery

Anterior communicating artery

Middle cerebral artery

Internal carotid artery

Posterior communicating artery

Posterior cerebral artery

Basilar artery

Vertebral artery

Figure 1-23 Circle of Willis

CT IMAGES

We begin our study of sectional images by looking at CT images of the head. Of interest is the fact that white matter contains more fatty tissue than does gray matter and so appears darker than the cortex or cerebral nuclei. Studies done with contrast medium demonstrate blood vessels and the choroid plexus, especially in the trigone where there is a heavy concentration. The blood-brain barrier should prevent the contrast medium from penetrating into the actual brain tissue or the ventricles of the brain.

To properly orient yourself to look at sectional images it is important that you imagine yourself looking at the images as though looking up from the level of the feet rather than looking down from the level of the head.

Exam 1

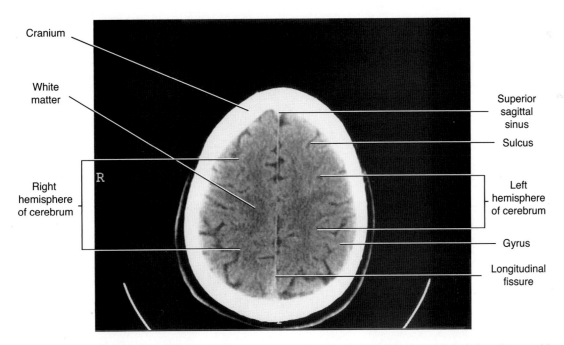

Figure 1-24 Figure 1-24 is the first of the CT images. Cuts above this level are not included as they would primarily demonstrate cranium, rather than brain. The cut at this level is moving into the region of the centrum semi-ovale, which is apparent because of the presence of white matter.

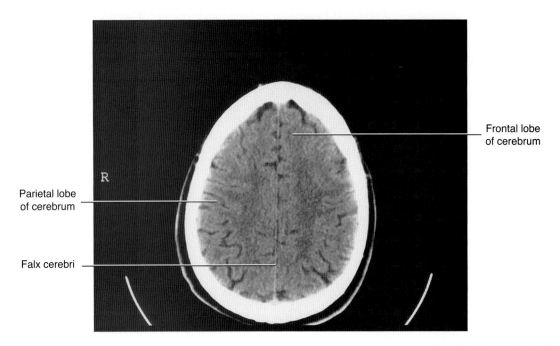

Figure 1-25 On Figure 1-24, the line dividing the right and left cerebral hemispheres is labeled the longitudinal fissure. Figure 1-25 alternatively labels it the falx cerebri, which is the dip of the dura mater into the longitudinal fissure.

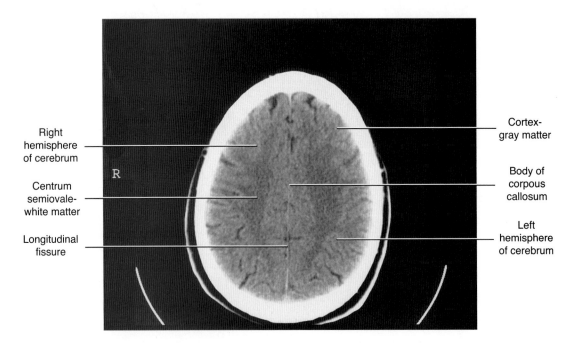

Figure 1-26 On Figure 1-26, the longitudinal fissure starts to disappear and is replaced by the body of the corpus callosum. The corpus callosum is the tissue through which the right and left hemispheres of the cerebrum communicate. The presence of more white matter is an indication that this cut is less superficial.

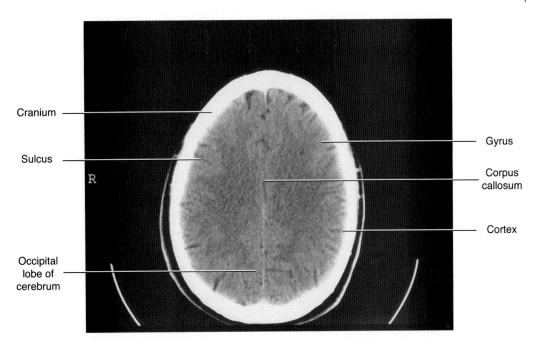

Cranium

Sulcus

R

Occipital
lobe of
cerebrum

Gyrus

Corpus
callosum

Cortex

Figure 1-27 Figure 1-27 shows sulci and gyri only along the peripheral edges, the only remainder of cortex. As the corpus callosum, which forms the roof of the lateral ventricles, is evident, we expect to see the lateral ventricles in the next few cuts. The posterior portion of the cerebrum is now labeled the occipital lobe, originating at the level of the corpus callosum.

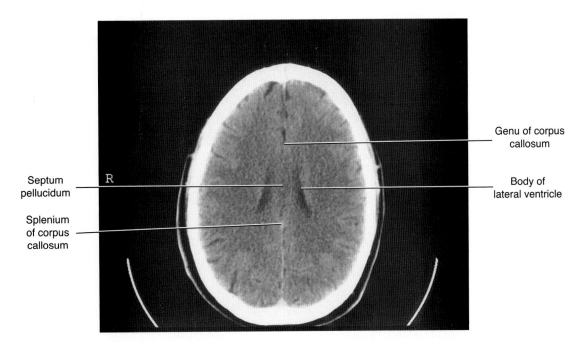

Septum
pellucidum

R

Splenium
of corpus
callosum

Genu of corpus
callosum

Body of
lateral ventricle

Figure 1-28 As expected, on Figure 1-28, the body of the lateral ventricles present themselves. As the corpus callosum is arch-shaped, the genu and the splenium are visible anteriorly and posteriorly to the body of the lateral ventricles.

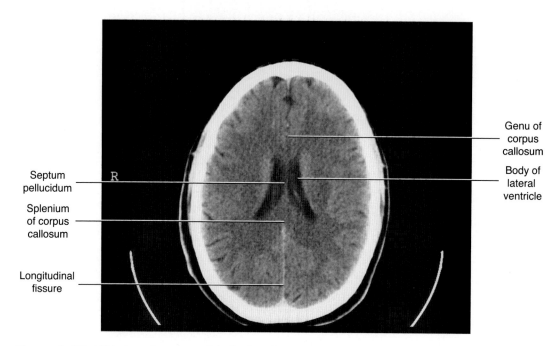

Genu of
corpus
callosum

Body of
lateral
ventricle

Septum
pellucidum

Splenium
of corpus
callosum

Longitudinal
fissure

R

Figure 1-29 With the enlargement of the bodies of the lateral ventricles on Figure 1-29, the anterior or frontal and posterior or occipital horns of the lateral ventricles should soon appear.

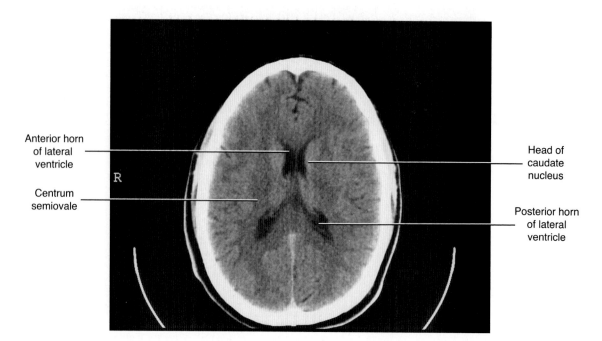

Anterior horn
of lateral
ventricle

Centrum
semiovale

Head of
caudate
nucleus

Posterior horn
of lateral
ventricle

R

Figure 1-30 Look closely at the centrum semiovale on Figure 1-30 to see pockets of gray matter, the basal ganglia. Immediately posterior to the frontal horn of the lateral ventricles is the head of the caudate nucleus.

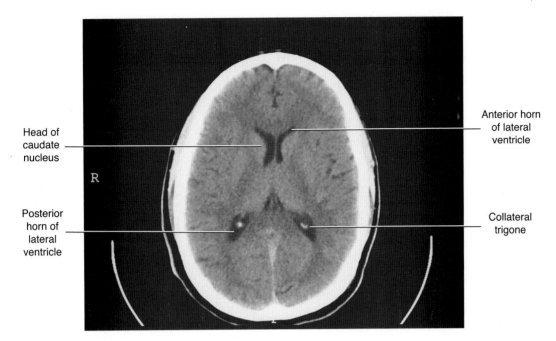

Head of
caudate
nucleus

Posterior
horn of
lateral
ventricle

Anterior horn
of lateral
ventricle

Collateral
trigone

R

Figure 1-31 On Figure 1-31, the areas of opacity found in the posterior horns of the lateral ventricles are a heavy concentration of the choroid plexus. This region is the collateral trigone, where the posterior or occipital horns meet the temporal horns of the lateral ventricles. With administration of contrast medium, the concentrated plexus can be visualized. A function of the choroid plexus is to secrete cerebrospinal fluid.

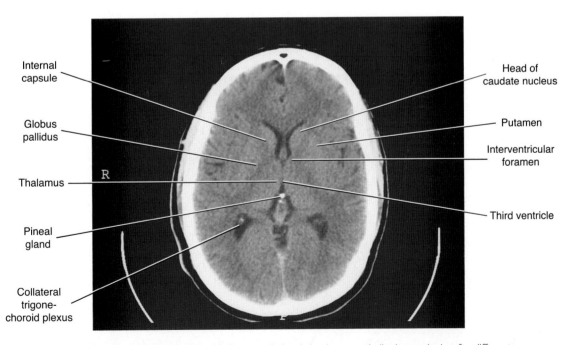

Internal
capsule

Globus
pallidus

Thalamus

Pineal
gland

Collateral
trigone-
choroid plexus

Head of
caudate nucleus

Putamen

Interventricular
foramen

Third ventricle

R

Figure 1-32 On Figure 1-32, the choroid plexus and pineal gland appear similar in opacity but for different reasons. The choroid plexus is opaque because of the presence of contrast medium while the pineal gland has calcified. Also seen is the interventricular foramen, the point where the two lateral ventricles drain into the third ventricle. Forming the wall of the third ventricle is the thalamus. Lateral to the thalamus are the globus pallidus and putamen, two of the components of the lentiform nucleus. The lentiform nuclei are basal ganglia and are separated from the thalamus by the internal capsule.

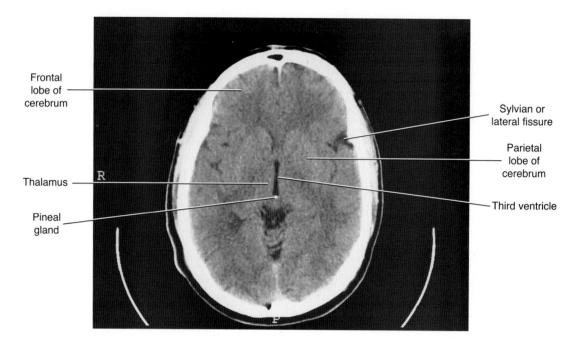

Frontal lobe of cerebrum

Sylvian or lateral fissure

Parietal lobe of cerebrum

Thalamus

Third ventricle

Pineal gland

Figure I-33 On Figure I-33, the Sylvian or lateral fissure, which separates the frontal, temporal, and parietal lobes, starts to appear.

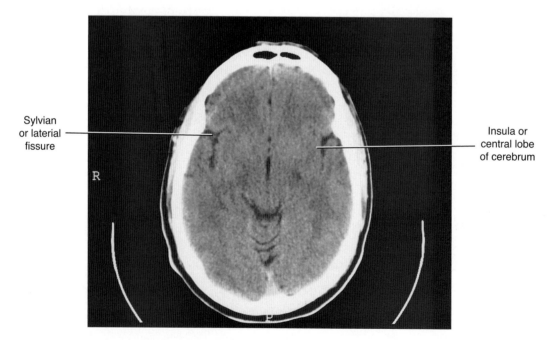

Sylvian or laterial fissure

Insula or central lobe of cerebrum

Figure I-34 The lateral fissure is now fully visible on Figure I-34. The insula or central lobe of the cerebrum is found along the medial edges of the lateral fissure.

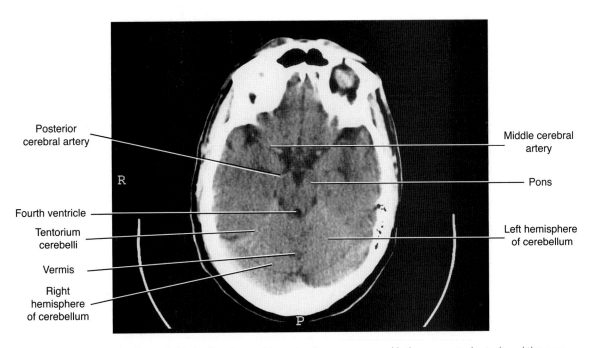

Peduncle

Quadrigeminal
cistern

R

Quadrigeminal
plate

Aqueduct of
Sylvius

P

Figure 1-35 Figure 1-35 clearly shows the aqueduct of Sylvius which drains the third ventricle into the fourth ventricle. The Sylvian aqueduct, as it is also called, passes through the midbrain with the peduncles found anterior to the aqueduct and the quadrigeminal plate, composed of the four colliculi, posterior to the aqueduct. Also seen is the quadrigeminal cistern, a pooling area for cerebrospinal fluid, immediately posterior to the quadrigeminal plate.

Posterior
cerebral artery

R

Fourth ventricle

Tentorium
cerebelli

Vermis

Right
hemisphere
of cerebellum

Middle cerebral
artery

Pons

Left hemisphere
of cerebellum

P

Figure 1-36 On Figure 1-36, the fourth ventricle makes its appearance, with the pons anterior to it and the cerebellum posterior. The cerebellum, like the cerebrum, is divided into two hemispheres, right and left. The hemispheres communicate with each other through a bridge of tissue, the vermis.

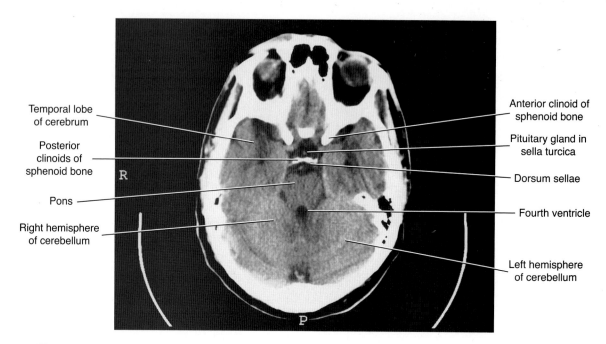

Temporal lobe
of cerebrum

Posterior
clinoids of
sphenoid bone

Pons

Right hemisphere
of cerebellum

Anterior clinoid of
sphenoid bone

Pituitary gland in
sella turcica

Dorsum sellae

Fourth ventricle

Left hemisphere
of cerebellum

Figure 1-37 Figure 1-37 demonstrates the upper edges of the sella turcica, formed by the anterior and posterior clinoids of the sphenoid bone. The sella turcica houses the pituitary gland. The posterior aspect of the sella turcia is the dorsum sellae. Once the dorsum sellae is visible, the temporal lobes of the cerebrum can be identified.

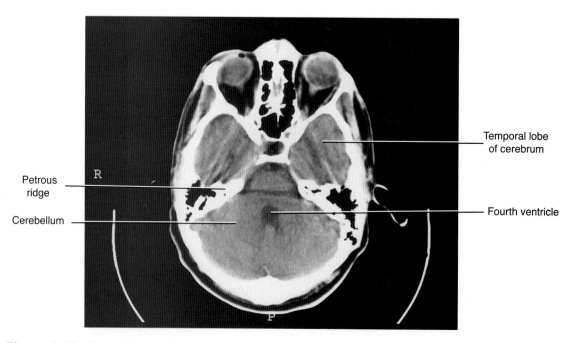

Petrous
ridge

Cerebellum

Temporal lobe
of cerebrum

Fourth ventricle

Figure 1-38 Figure 1-38, the final image in this series, demonstrates the petrous ridges of the temporal bones. Any cuts below this level may include numerous artifacts caused by the contrast differences between the dense bone and softer brain tissue.

Exam 2

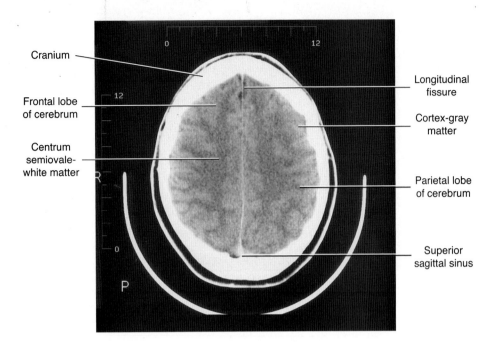

Cranium

Frontal lobe
of cerebrum

Centrum
semiovale-
white matter

Longitudinal
fissure

Cortex-gray
matter

Parietal lobe
of cerebrum

Superior
sagittal sinus

R

P

Figure 1-39 On Figure 1-39, the white matter seen in each hemisphere of the cerebrum is the centrum semiovale.

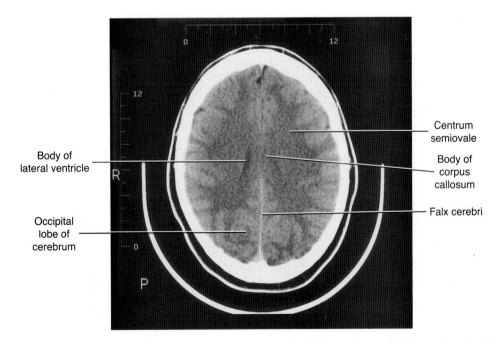

Body of
lateral ventricle

Occipital
lobe of
cerebrum

Centrum
semiovale

Body of
corpus
callosum

Falx cerebri

R

P

Figure 1-40 The bodies of the lateral ventricles are barely visible on Figure 1-40, suggesting that the tissue between is probably still the body of the corpus callosum.

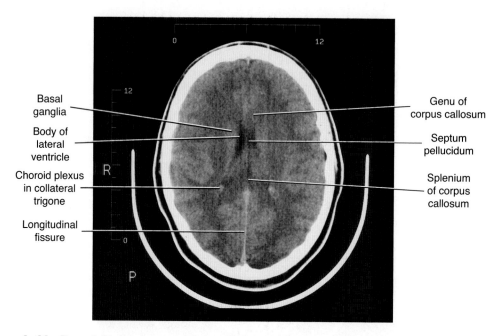

Figure 1-41 Figure 1-41 demonstrates the choroid plexus in the region of the collateral trigone bilaterally. The lateral ventricles are separated by the septum pellucidum with the genu and splenium of the corpus callosum seen anterior and posterior to the septum. The basal ganglia, pockets of gray matter, are now evident.

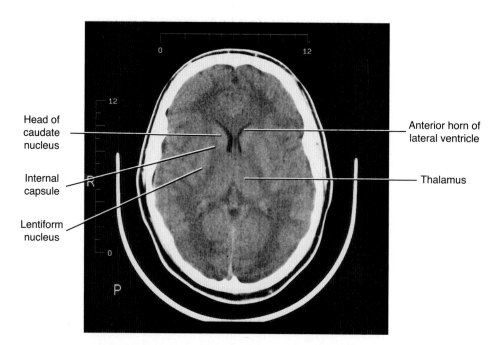

Figure 1-42 The heads of the caudate nuclei are seen immediately posterior to the anterior horns of the lateral ventricles on Figure 1-42.

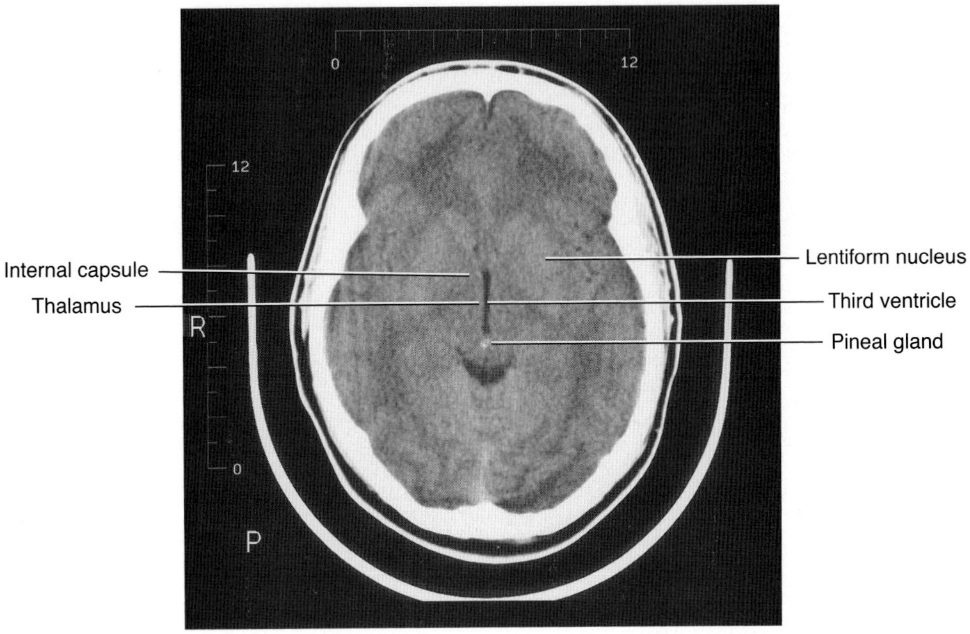

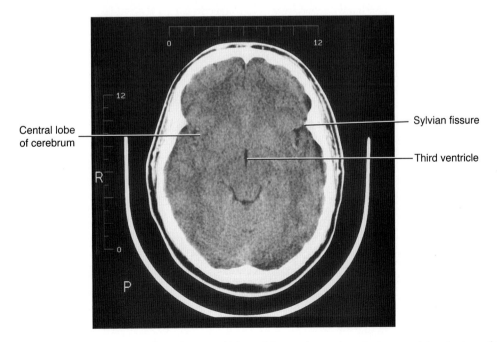

Figure 1-43 On Figure 1-43, the thalamus is seen on either side of the third ventricle. Adjacent to the thalamus is the internal capsule separating the thalamus and head of the caudate nucleus from the lentiform nucleus (composed of the putamen and globus pallidus).

Internal capsule

Thalamus

R

P

Lentiform nucleus

Third ventricle

Pineal gland

Central lobe
of cerebrum

R

P

Sylvian fissure

Third ventricle

Figure 1-44 Visible on Figure 1-44 are the central lobes of the cerebrum along the inner peripheral edges of the Sylvian fissure.

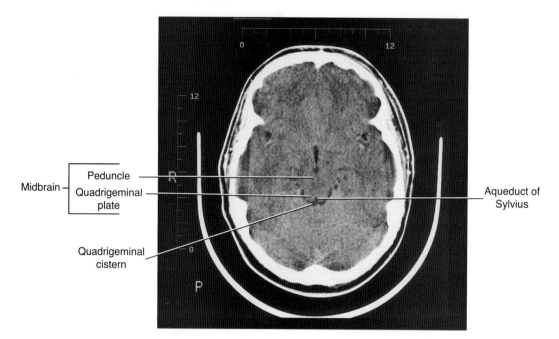

Figure 1-45 Structures found on Figure 1-45 include the cerebral aqueduct which drains the third ventricle into the fourth ventricle, the peduncles which are anterior to the aqueduct, and the quadrigeminal plate which is posterior to it. Behind the quadrigeminal plate is the quadrigeminal cistern.

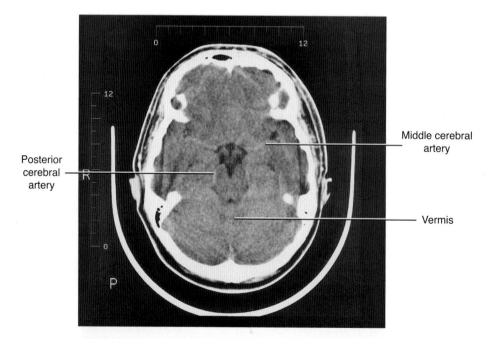

Figure 1-46 On Figure 1-46, the vermis (the bridge of tissue connecting the right and left hemispheres of the cerebellum) is seen along with the posterior and middle cerebral arteries. The circle of Willis involves these arteries along with the anterior cerebral arteries.

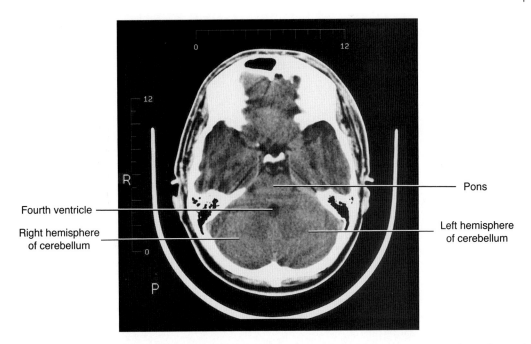

Figure 1-47 Figure 1-47 marks the appearance of the fourth ventricle, and those structures anterior and posterior to it, the pons and cerebellum.

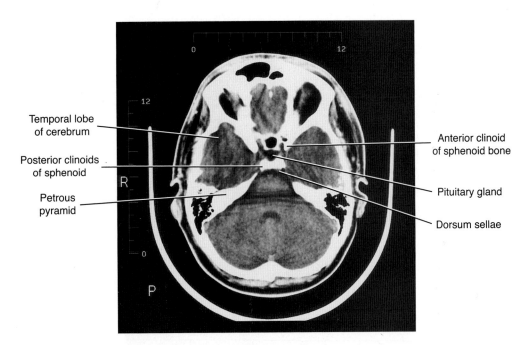

Figure 1-48 The final image in this series, Figure 1-48, shows the petrous pyramids and the pituitary gland sitting in the sella turcica. As this image is at the level of the dorsum sellae, the posterior aspect of the sella turcica, the temporal lobes of the cerebrum can be identified bilaterally.

MR IMAGES

Exam 1

Axial Images

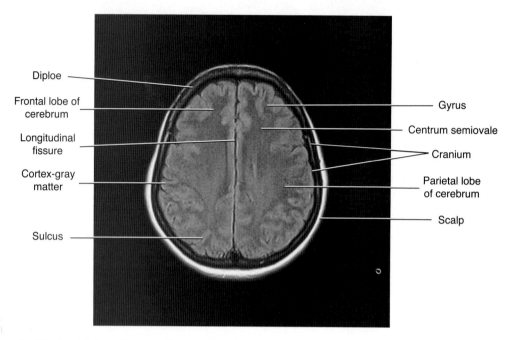

Figure 1-49 On this first MR image, Figure 1-49, notice that the cranium appears black. Compact bone contains little or no hydrogen and thus will not give off a signal. Compared to CT, the gray and white matter are more easily identified as MRI has a better ability to differentiate soft tissue densities.

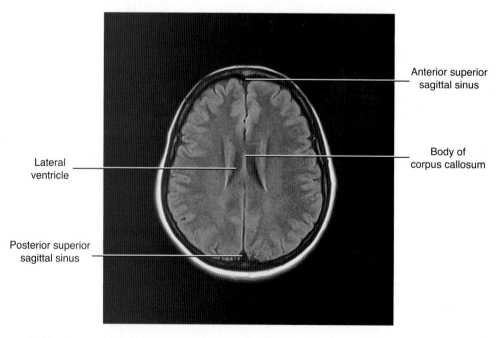

Figure 1-50 Figure 1-50 shows the cerebrospinal fluid in the lateral ventricles appearing black because of the way the images were weighted; therefore, they may seem similar to CT images.

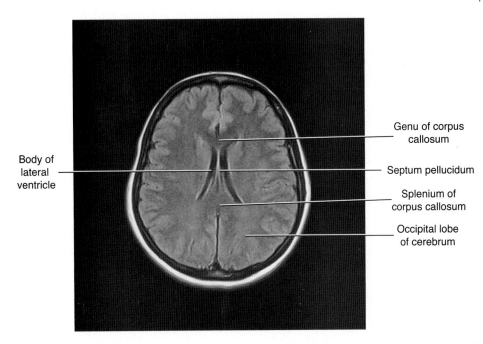

Genu of corpus callosum

Body of lateral ventricle

Septum pellucidum

Splenium of corpus callosum

Occipital lobe of cerebrum

Figure 1-51 The bodies of the lateral ventricles are seen on Figure 1-51, as are the genu and splenium of the corpus callosum. The corpus callosum is the arch-shaped structure forming the roof of the lateral ventricles.

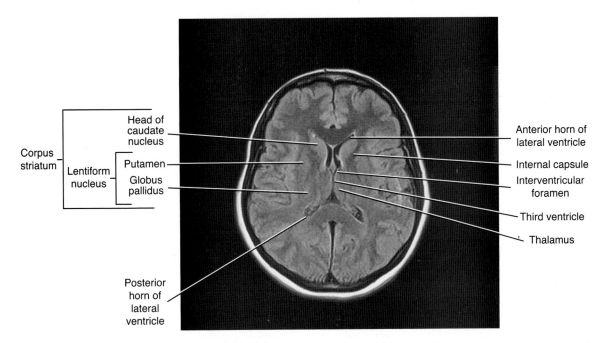

Corpus striatum

Lentiform nucleus

Head of caudate nucleus

Putamen

Globus pallidus

Anterior horn of lateral ventricle

Internal capsule

Interventricular foramen

Third ventricle

Thalamus

Posterior horn of lateral ventricle

Figure 1-52 On Figure 1-52, the basal ganglia are easily identified, particularly the head of the caudate nucleus and the lentiform nucleus. Also shown are the interventricular foramina draining the lateral ventricles into the third ventricle. The internal capsule separates the lentiform nucleus from the caudate nucleus and the thalamus.

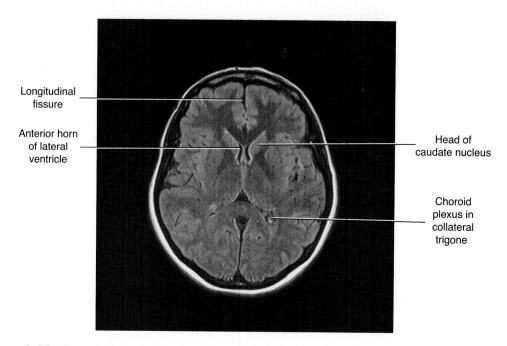

Longitudinal fissure

Anterior horn of lateral ventricle

Head of caudate nucleus

Choroid plexus in collateral trigone

Figure 1-53 Figure 1-53 clearly demonstrates the collateral trigone, which contains a heavy concentration of choroid plexus.

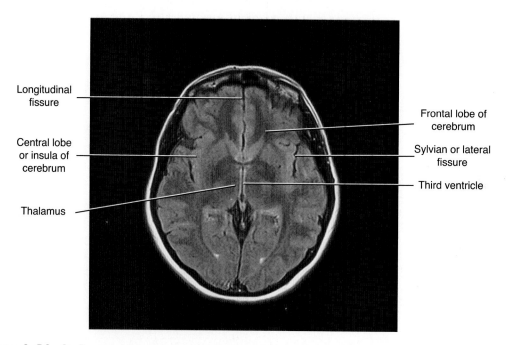

Longitudinal fissure

Central lobe or insula of cerebrum

Thalamus

Frontal lobe of cerebrum

Sylvian or lateral fissure

Third ventricle

Figure 1-54 On Figure 1-54, the third ventricle is shown with the thalamus forming the lateral walls. The Sylvian fissure, separating the frontal, temporal, and parietal lobes of the cerebrum is seen, as is the insula or central lobe along its medial edge.

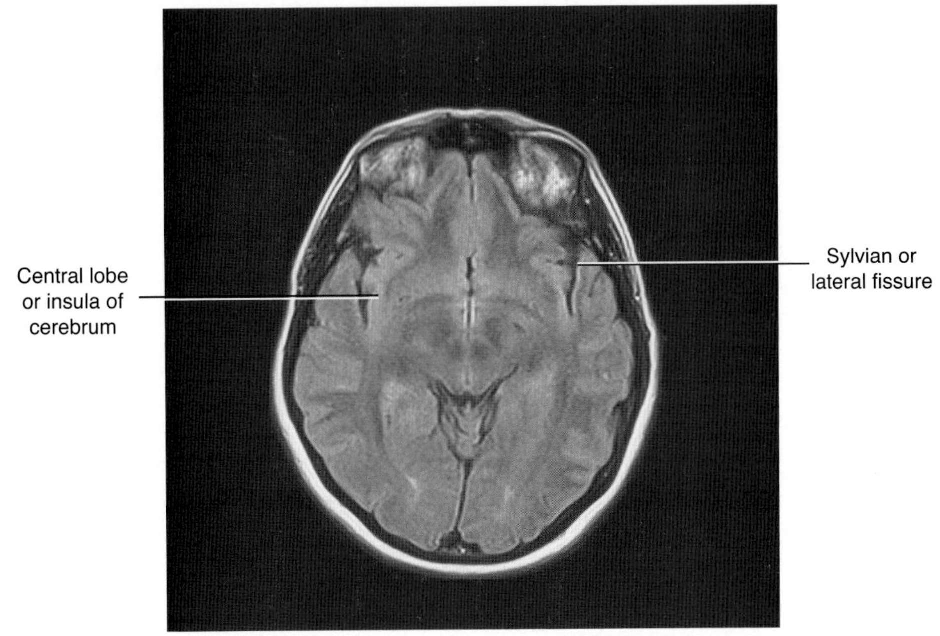

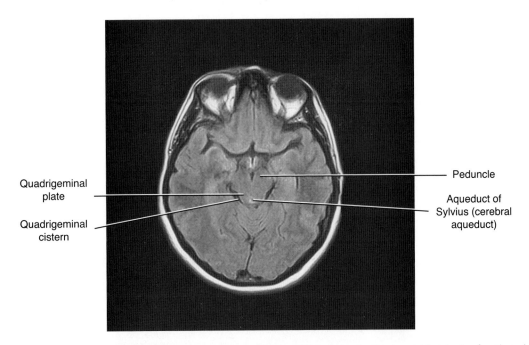

Central lobe
or insula of
cerebrum

Sylvian or
lateral fissure

Figure 1-55 Figure 1-55 allows another look at the Sylvian fissure and central lobe.

Quadrigeminal
plate

Quadrigeminal
cistern

Peduncle

Aqueduct of
Sylvius (cerebral
aqueduct)

Figure 1-56 Seen on Figure 1-56 are the aqueduct of Sylvius which drains the third ventricle into the fourth, and the parts of the midbrain, the peduncles and quadrigeminal plate. The quadrigeminal cistern is seen posterior to the quadrigeminal plate.

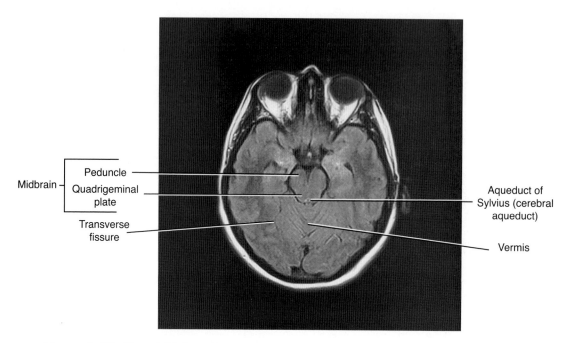

Figure 1-57 Figure 1-57 shows the vermis connecting the right and left hemispheres of the cerebellum and the transverse fissure, which separates the cerebellum from the cerebrum.

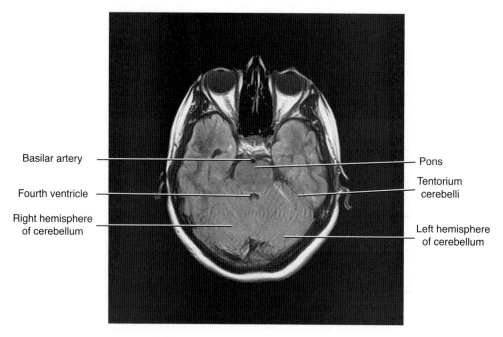

Figure 1-58 The fourth ventricle is seen bound by the pons anteriorly and the cerebellum posteriorly on Figure 1-58.

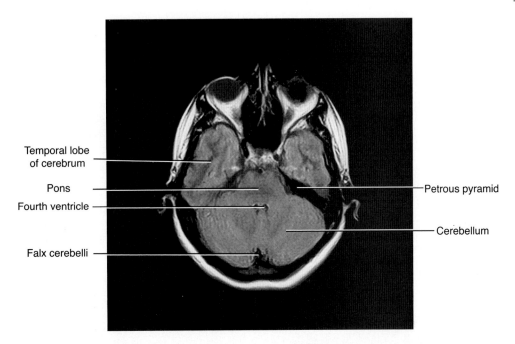

Temporal lobe
of cerebrum

Pons

Fourth ventricle

Falx cerebelli

Petrous pyramid

Cerebellum

Figure 1-59 On Figure 1-59, the petrous pyramids, which are composed of dense bone giving off no signal, appear black. Anterior to the pyramids are the temporal lobes of the cerebrum. Still visible are the fourth ventricle, pons, and cerebellum. Also labeled is the falx cerebelli, the dip of the dura mater into the space separating the right and left hemispheres of the cerebellum.

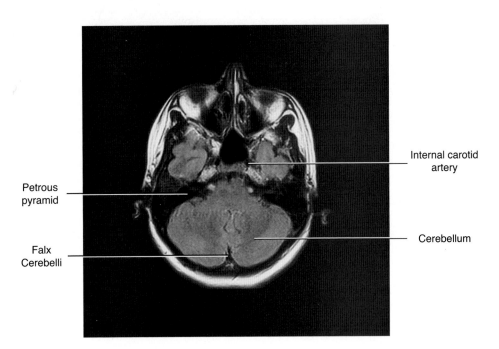

Internal carotid
artery

Petrous
pyramid

Falx
Cerebelli

Cerebellum

Figure 1-60 On this final axial MR image of this set, Figure 1-60, note the lack of artifacts often seen in CT images at this level. As bone gives off no signal, it does not cause the artifacts seen with CT.

Sagittal Image

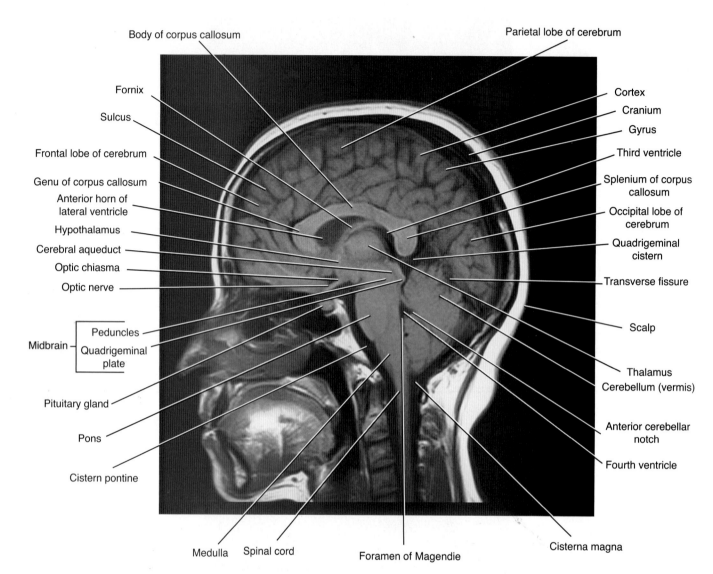

Body of corpus callosum

Parietal lobe of cerebrum

Fornix

Sulcus

Frontal lobe of cerebrum

Genu of corpus callosum

Anterior horn of
lateral ventricle

Hypothalamus

Cerebral aqueduct

Optic chiasma

Optic nerve

Midbrain — Peduncles

Quadrigeminal
plate

Pituitary gland

Pons

Cistern pontine

Cortex

Cranium

Gyrus

Third ventricle

Splenium of corpus
callosum

Occipital lobe of
cerebrum

Quadrigeminal
cistern

Transverse fissure

Scalp

Thalamus
Cerebellum (vermis)

Anterior cerebellar
notch

Fourth ventricle

Medulla   Spinal cord   Foramen of Magendie   Cisterna magna

Figure 1-61   Like the drawing Figure 1-9, this MR sagittal image, Figure 1-61, has much to observe. The only point of communication between the two hemispheres of the cerebrum is seen in the corpus callosum. Similarly, the vermis, which connects the two hemispheres of the cerebellum, is also identified. Not shown on previous CT and MRI axial cuts is the fornix, arising from the splenium of the corpus callosum and forming the floor of the lateral ventricles. It can be identified on this image. The thalamus, helping to form the walls of the third ventricle, is labeled for your examination. The hypothalamus is seen as described in the text, inferior and slightly anterior to the thalamus. It forms the ventral wall of the third ventricle. Passing through the midbrain, composed of the peduncles and quadrigeminal plate, is the cerebral aqueduct. If you look very closely at the quadrigeminal plate you can differentiate the superior and inferior colliculi on one side of the brain. Located behind the quadrigeminal plate, or tectum, is the quadrigeminal cistern. Other structures visualized are: the transverse fissure separating the cerebrum from the cerebellum, the foramen of Magendie (the medial opening of the fourth ventricle) which is draining into the subarachnoid space, the central canal of the spinal cord, and the cisterna magna.

Coronal Images

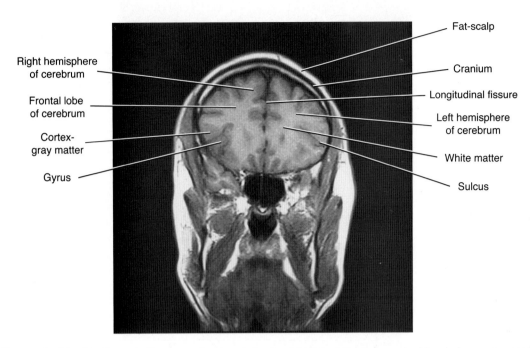

Fat-scalp

Right hemisphere
of cerebrum

Cranium

Frontal lobe
of cerebrum

Longitudinal fissure

Left hemisphere
of cerebrum

Cortex-
gray matter

White matter

Gyrus

Sulcus

Figure 1-62 On Figure 1-62, you are looking at the frontal lobe of the two cerebral hemispheres separated by the longitudinal fissure. The falx cerebri sits in that fissure. As the first few slices of this exam are not included, the cortex is visible along the peripheral edges with white matter being seen centrally.

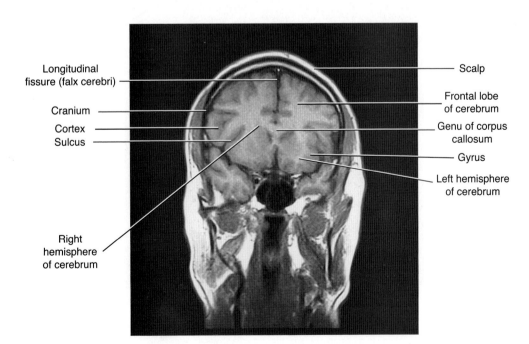

Longitudinal
fissure (falx cerebri)

Scalp

Frontal lobe
of cerebrum

Cranium

Genu of corpus
callosum

Cortex

Sulcus

Gyrus

Left hemisphere
of cerebrum

Right
hemisphere
of cerebrum

Figure 1-63 There is a break in the longitudinal fissure on Figure 1-63. This is the genu of the corpus callosum. The two hemispheres of the cerebrum communicate only through the corpus callosum.

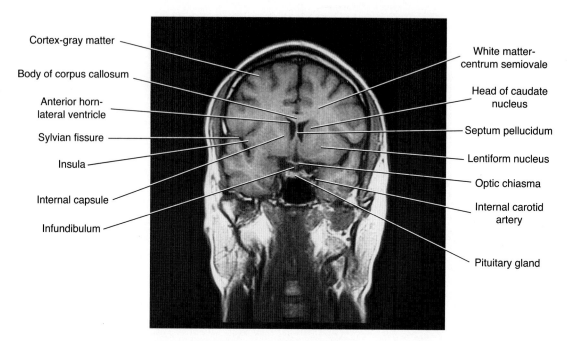

Cortex-gray matter

Body of corpus callosum

Anterior horn-lateral ventricle

Sylvian fissure

Insula

Internal capsule

Infundibulum

White matter-centrum semiovale

Head of caudate nucleus

Septum pellucidum

Lentiform nucleus

Optic chiasma

Internal carotid artery

Pituitary gland

Figure 1-64 On Figure 1-64, the anterior horns of the lateral ventricles are seen separated by the septum pellucidum. Immediately inferior to each anterior horn is the head of the caudate nucleus. Other pockets of gray matter located in the centrum semiovale are identified as the lentiform nucleus, which is composed of the globus pallidus and putamen. The internal capsule separates the caudate nucleus from the lentiform nucleus. (Dividing the lentiform nucleus and claustrum is the external capsule.) The central or Sylvian fissure has been labeled, allowing you to locate the central lobe or insula of the cerebrum. Also of interest is the pituitary gland and its point of connection with the hypothalamus, the infundibulum. The structure seen tranverse to the infundibulum is the optic chiasma (the point where the optic nerves cross over after exiting the posterior orbit). The portion of the corpus callosum visualized is the body.

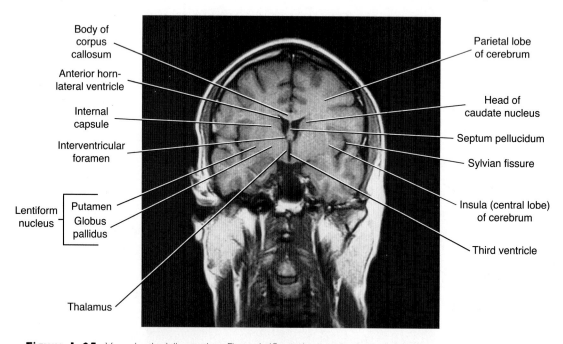

Body of corpus callosum

Anterior horn-lateral ventricle

Internal capsule

Interventricular foramen

Lentiform nucleus { Putamen Globus pallidus

Thalamus

Parietal lobe of cerebrum

Head of caudate nucleus

Septum pellucidum

Sylvian fissure

Insula (central lobe) of cerebrum

Third ventricle

Figure 1-65 Very clearly delineated on Figure 1-65 are the anterior horns of the lateral ventricles with the head of the caudate nuclei inferior to them. The caudate nuclei follow the same curvatures as the lateral ventricles. Draining the lateral ventricles into the third ventricle are the interventricular foramina. On either side of the third ventricle is the thalamus. The septum pellucidum divides the two lateral ventricles. As this cut is posterior, you are seeing the parietal lobes of the cerebrum. This particular image allows you to differentiate the two subcomponents of the lentiform nucleus, the globus pallidus and putamen.

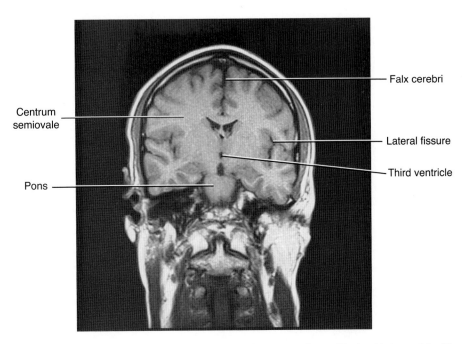

Centrum semiovale

Falx cerebri

Lateral fissure

Third ventricle

Pons

Figure 1-66 Seen on Figure 1-66 is the anterior aspect of the pons along with the third ventricle, falx cerebri, and centrum semiovale.

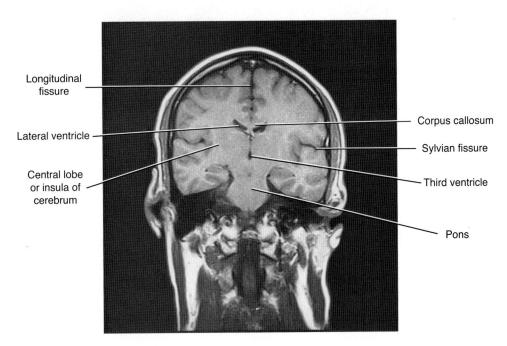

Longitudinal fissure

Lateral ventricle

Central lobe or insula of cerebrum

Corpus callosum

Sylvian fissure

Third ventricle

Pons

Figure 1-67 The Sylvian fissure is still evident on Figure 1-67, thereby allowing you to realize the dimensions of the central lobe. The corpus callosum is seen forming the roof of the lateral ventricles.

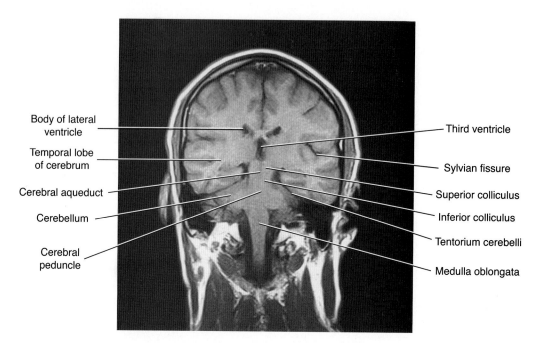

Body of lateral ventricle

Temporal lobe of cerebrum

Cerebral aqueduct

Cerebellum

Cerebral peduncle

Third ventricle

Sylvian fissure

Superior colliculus

Inferior colliculus

Tentorium cerebelli

Medulla oblongata

Figure 1-68 Figure 1-68 demonstrates the cerebral aqueduct passing through the midbrain. The midbrain is composed of the peduncles anteriorly and the four colliculi (or tectum) posteriorly. With some imagination, you can differentiate the superior and inferior colliculi bilaterally. Extending down is the medulla oblongata. Portions of the cerebellum are just becoming visible. Also labeled are the cerebral peduncles, the temporal lobes, and the body of the lateral ventricles.

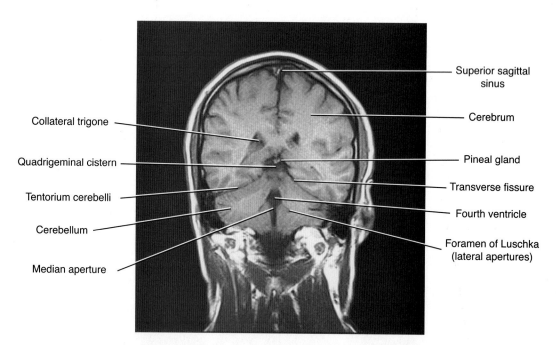

Collateral trigone

Quadrigeminal cistern

Tentorium cerebelli

Cerebellum

Median aperture

Superior sagittal sinus

Cerebrum

Pineal gland

Transverse fissure

Fourth ventricle

Foramen of Luschka (lateral apertures)

Figure 1-69 Figure 1-69 clearly demonstrates the transverse fissure separating the cerebrum from the cerebellum. The tentorium cerebelli lies within the transverse fissure. Nicely demonstrated is the fourth ventricle and its three anterior openings, the median aperture or foramen of Magendie and the foramina of Luschka, draining cerebrospinal fluid into the central canal of the spinal cord, the subarachnoid space, and the cisterna magna. As this cut is posterior to the quadrigeminal plate, notice the quadrigeminal cistern with the pineal gland situated above it. The collateral trigone is labeled, the region where the posterior and inferior horns of the lateral ventricles meet. The superior sagittal sinus is also visualized.

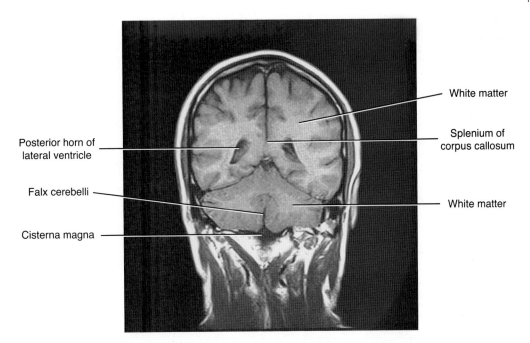

White matter

Splenium of
corpus callosum

White matter

Posterior horn of
lateral ventricle

Falx cerebelli

Cisterna magna

Figure 1-70 On Figure 1-70, there is still communication between the two halves of the cerebrum via the posterior aspect of the corpus callosum, the splenium. Shown are the posterior horns of the lateral ventricles as well as the falx cerebelli dipping into the space between the two hemispheres of the cerebellum. White matter is seen in both the cerebrum and cerebellum. There is a distinct pooling of the cerebrospinal fluid in the cisterna magna.

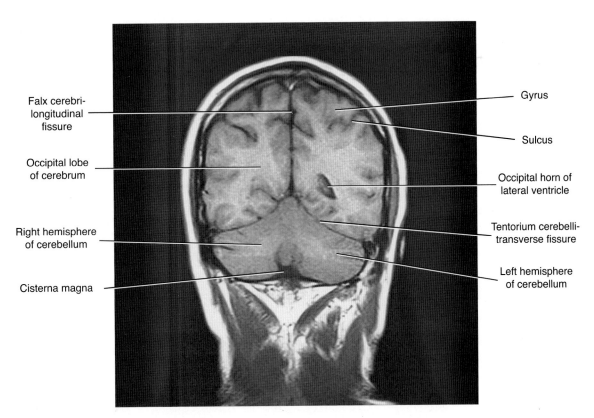

Falx cerebri-
longitudinal
fissure

Occipital lobe
of cerebrum

Right hemisphere
of cerebellum

Cisterna magna

Gyrus

Sulcus

Occipital horn of
lateral ventricle

Tentorium cerebelli-
transverse fissure

Left hemisphere
of cerebellum

Figure 1-71 On the left side of Figure 1-71 is the occipital or posterior horn of the lateral ventricle. Shown without interruption are the transverse and longitudinal fissures containing the tentorium cerebelli and falx cerebri, respectively. The cisterna magna is seen at the base of the brain.

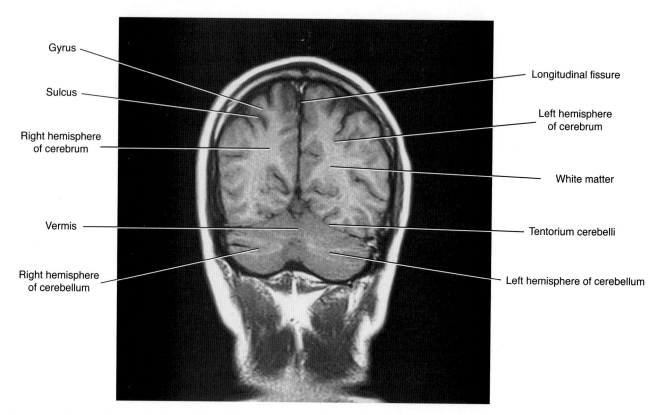

Gyrus

Sulcus

Right hemisphere
of cerebrum

Vermis

Right hemisphere
of cerebellum

Longitudinal fissure

Left hemisphere
of cerebrum

White matter

Tentorium cerebelli

Left hemisphere of cerebellum

Figure 1-72 On Figure 1-72 the vermis can be seen connecting the right and left hemispheres of the cerebellum.

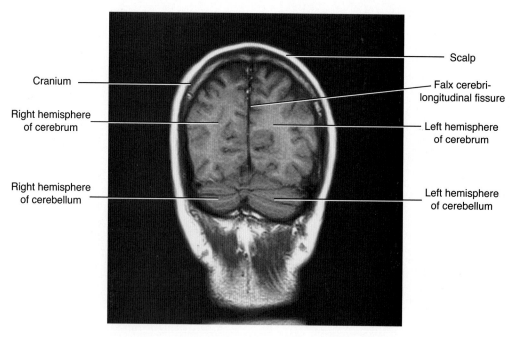

Cranium

Right hemisphere
of cerebrum

Right hemisphere
of cerebellum

Scalp

Falx cerebri-
longitudinal fissure

Left hemisphere
of cerebrum

Left hemisphere
of cerebellum

Figure 1-73 The falx cerebri can be found in the longitudinal fissure separating the two hemispheres of the cerebrum on Figure 1-73. Also identified are the cranium, scalp, and the two hemispheres of the cerebellum.

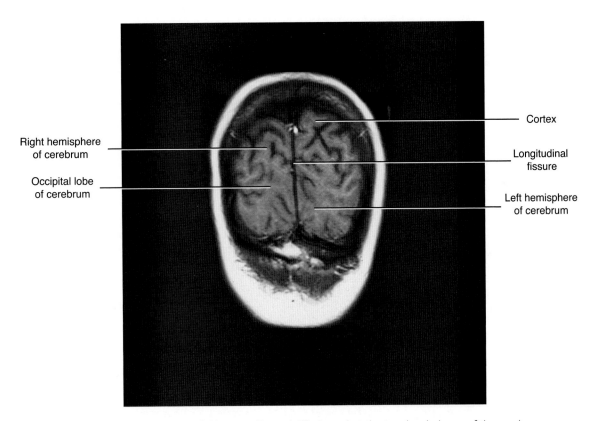

Figure 1-74   Figure 1-74 is located fairly posteriorly so little white matter is evident and the images are moving out of the vicinity of the cerebellum.

Figure 1-75   The last image of this exam, Figure 1-75, shows just the two hemispheres of the cerebrum separated by the longitudinal fissure. Only the gray matter of the cortex remains. This image shows the occipital lobes of the cerebrum.

Exam 2

Axial Images

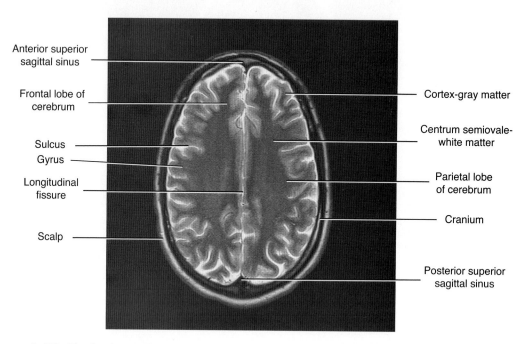

Anterior superior
sagittal sinus

Frontal lobe of
cerebrum

Sulcus

Gyrus

Longitudinal
fissure

Scalp

Cortex-gray matter

Centrum semiovale-
white matter

Parietal lobe
of cerebrum

Cranium

Posterior superior
sagittal sinus

Figure 1-76 The first image of this set, Figure 1-76, shows cortex along the peripheral edges and the centrum semiovale located centrally. Once again, notice the superior ability of MRI to differentiate white matter from gray matter.

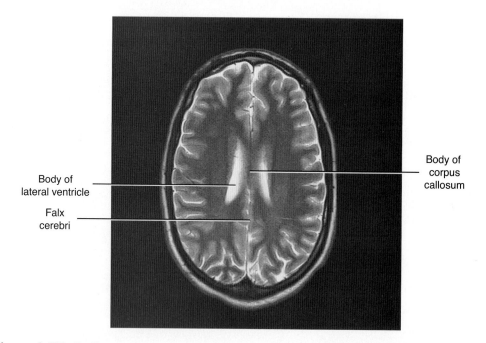

Body of
lateral ventricle

Falx
cerebri

Body of
corpus
callosum

Figure 1-77 On Figure 1-77 it is obvious that this set of images is weighted differently compared to the first axial set of MR images (Exam 1). The cerebrospinal fluid in the ventricles is opaque rather than translucent, but familiarity with the location and shape of structures allows for recognition. In most instances, both T1- and T2-weighted images are done of the head. This book includes either one or the other per exam.

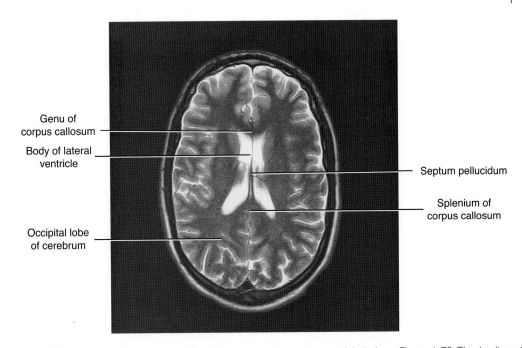

Figure 1-78   At this point, you should easily recognize the structures labeled on Figure 1-78. The bodies of the lateral ventricles are separated by the septum pellucidum, and the genu and the splenium of the corpus callosum are seen.

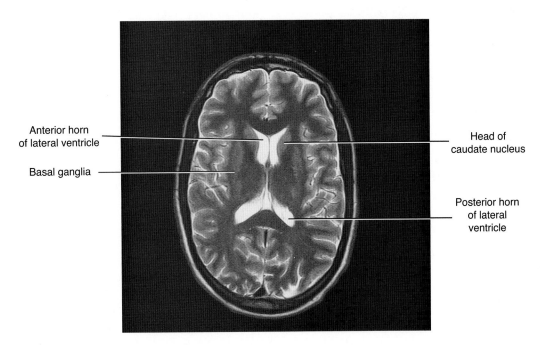

Figure 1-79   Figure 1-79 shows the anterior and posterior horns of the lateral ventricles along with the basal ganglia, the pockets of gray matter situated in the centrum semiovale.

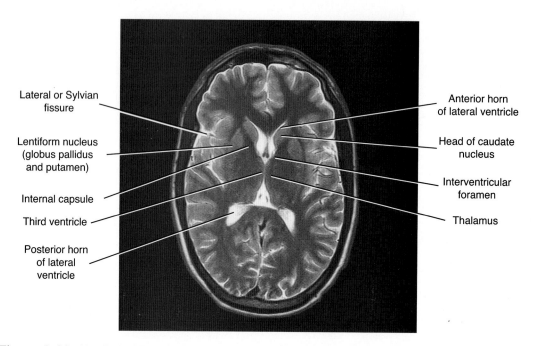

Lateral or Sylvian fissure

Lentiform nucleus (globus pallidus and putamen)

Internal capsule

Third ventricle

Posterior horn of lateral ventricle

Anterior horn of lateral ventricle

Head of caudate nucleus

Interventricular foramen

Thalamus

Figure 1-80   Identified on Figure 1-80 are the interventricular foramina draining the two lateral ventricles bilaterally into the third ventricle. The head of the caudate nucleus is seen posterior to the anterior horn of the lateral ventricles, bilaterally. The lateral fissure, separating the frontal, parietal, and temporal lobes has appeared.

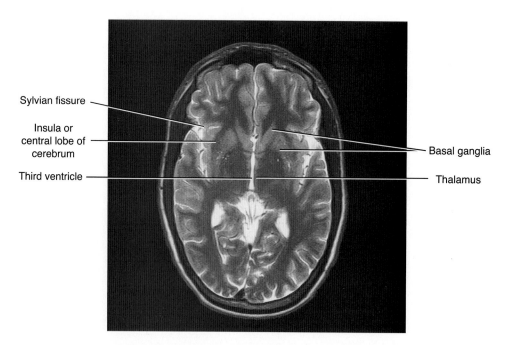

Sylvian fissure

Insula or central lobe of cerebrum

Third ventricle

Basal ganglia

Thalamus

Figure 1-81   On Figure 1-81, the third ventricle is shown midline. On either side is found the thalamus, forming the walls of the third ventricle.

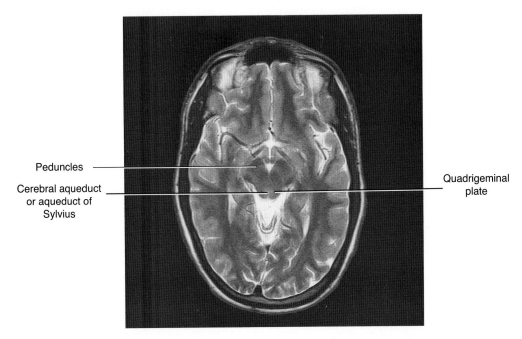

Peduncles

Cerebral aqueduct
or aqueduct of
Sylvius

Quadrigeminal
plate

Figure 1-82 The cerebral aqueduct appears on Figure 1-82, draining the third ventricle into the fourth. The aqueduct of Sylvius, the alternative name for the cerebral aqueduct, passes through the midbrain, composed of the peduncles and quadrigeminal plate.

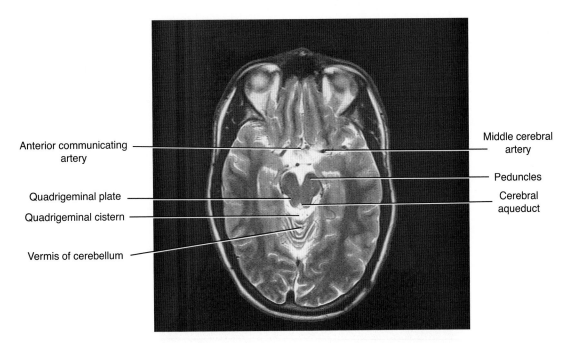

Anterior communicating
artery

Quadrigeminal plate

Quadrigeminal cistern

Vermis of cerebellum

Middle cerebral
artery

Peduncles

Cerebral
aqueduct

Figure 1-83 The peduncles, anterior to the cerebral aqueduct, are found on Figure 1-83. On either side of the aqueduct and slightly posterior is the quadrigeminal plate. Behind the quadrigeminal plate lies the quadrigeminal cistern. The vermis is seen on this image.

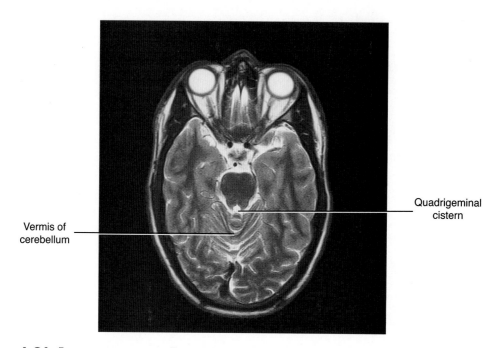

Figure 1-84   Even more apparent on Figure 1-84 is the vermis, the connecting tissue of the two hemispheres of the cerebellum. Also shown are the remnants of the quadrigeminal cistern.

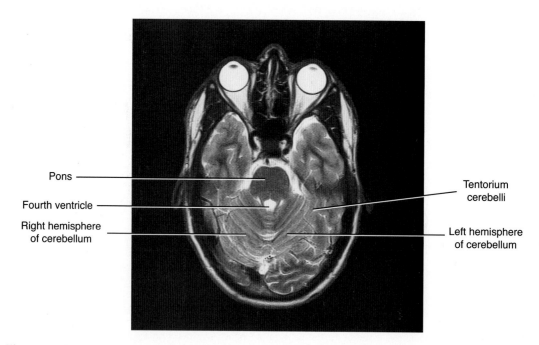

Figure 1-85   Figure 1-85 is at the level of the fourth ventricle, found between the pons, which is anterior, and the cerebellum, which is posterior.

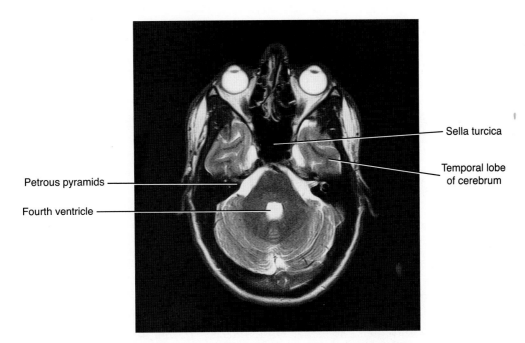

Sella turcica

Temporal lobe
of cerebrum

Petrous pyramids

Fourth ventricle

Figure 1-86 The last image in this series, Figure 1-86, shows the temporal lobes of the cerebrum anterior to the petrous pyramids. As the petrous pyramids and sella turcica are composed of dense bone, they give off no signal and appear black.

Sagittal Image

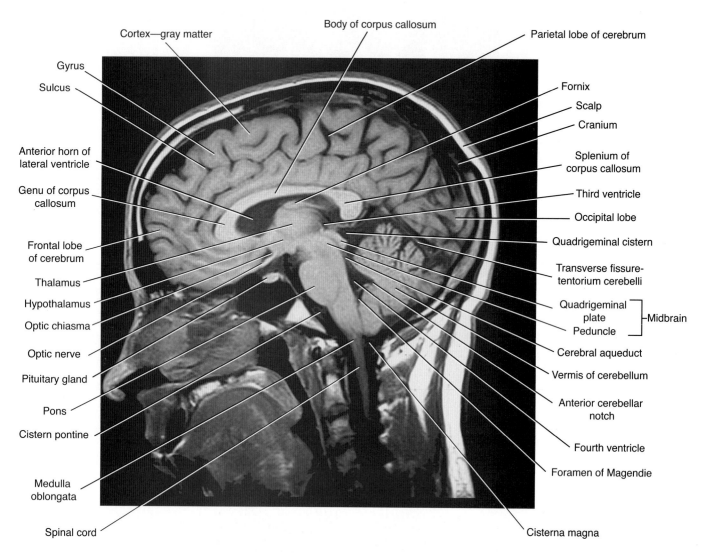

Cortex—gray matter

Body of corpus callosum

Parietal lobe of cerebrum

Gyrus

Sulcus

Fornix

Scalp

Cranium

Anterior horn of
lateral ventricle

Splenium of
corpus callosum

Genu of corpus
callosum

Third ventricle

Occipital lobe

Frontal lobe
of cerebrum

Quadrigeminal cistern

Thalamus

Transverse fissure-
tentorium cerebelli

Hypothalamus

Quadrigeminal
plate — Midbrain
Peduncle

Optic chiasma

Optic nerve

Cerebral aqueduct

Pituitary gland

Vermis of cerebellum

Pons

Anterior cerebellar
notch

Cistern pontine

Fourth ventricle

Foramen of Magendie

Medulla
oblongata

Spinal cord

Cisterna magna

Figure 1-87 Figure 1-87 demonstrates many of the same structures seen on the sagittal cut from the first MRI study (Exam 1), including the anterior horns of the lateral ventricles, the third, and fourth ventricles. The tentorium cerebelli is distinct. The inability to clearly see the spinal cord is an indication that this image is slightly off center.

Coronal Images

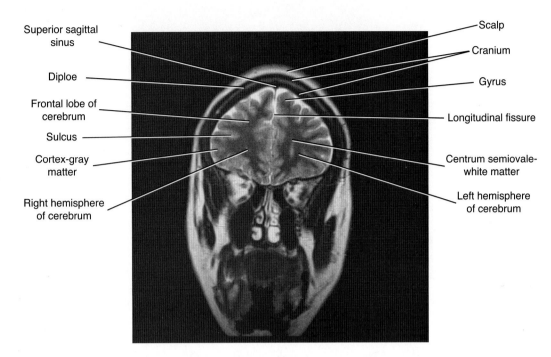

Superior sagittal sinus

Scalp

Cranium

Diploe

Gyrus

Frontal lobe of cerebrum

Longitudinal fissure

Sulcus

Cortex-gray matter

Centrum semiovale-white matter

Right hemisphere of cerebrum

Left hemisphere of cerebrum

Figure 1-88 On this first image of this series, Figure 1-88, the frontal lobes of the right and left hemispheres of the cerebrum are shown separated by the longitudinal fissure. Both gray matter (in the cortex) and white matter (in the centrum semiovale) are evident.

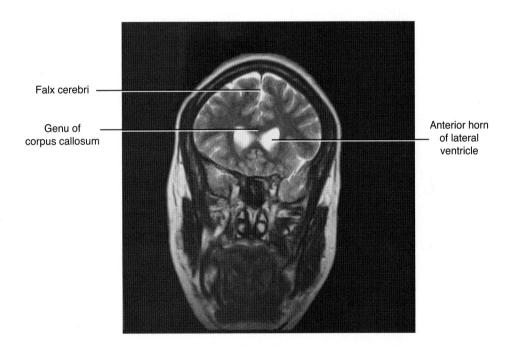

Falx cerebri

Genu of corpus callosum

Anterior horn of lateral ventricle

Figure 1-89 Figure 1-89 allows you to visualize the anterior horns of the lateral ventricles, with the corpus callosum forming the roof of the ventricles.

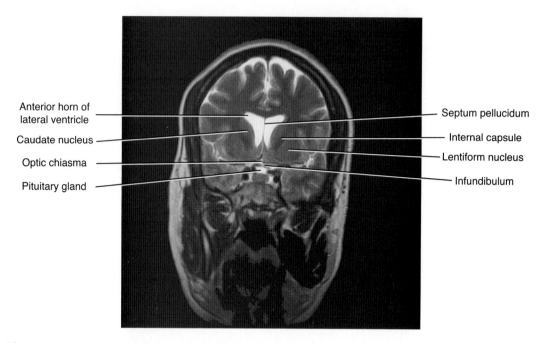

Anterior horn of lateral ventricle

Caudate nucleus

Optic chiasma

Pituitary gland

Septum pellucidum

Internal capsule

Lentiform nucleus

Infundibulum

Figure 1-90 The septum pellucidum, separating the two lateral ventricles, is seen on Figure 1-90. Inferior to the lateral ventricle on each side is the head of the caudate nucleus.

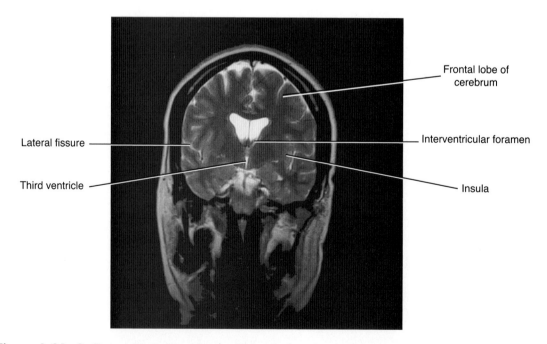

Lateral fissure

Third ventricle

Frontal lobe of cerebrum

Interventricular foramen

Insula

Figure 1-91 On Figure 1-91, the lateral fissures, dividing the frontal, parietal, and temporal lobes of the cerebrum, are apparent. The insula or central lobe of the cerebrum borders the medial edge of each central fissure.

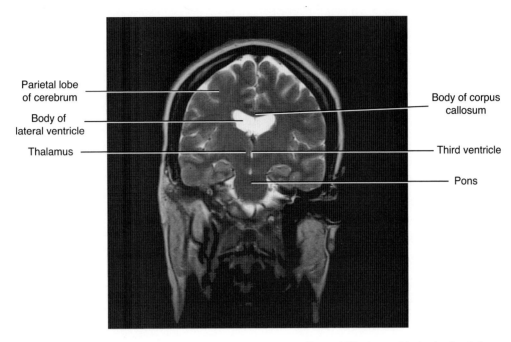

Parietal lobe of cerebrum

Body of lateral ventricle

Thalamus

Body of corpus callosum

Third ventricle

Pons

Figure 1-92 The bodies of the lateral ventricles are seen on Figure 1-92, along with the body of the corpus callosum superior to them. The third ventricle is inferior to the lateral ventricles, midline. The anterior surface of the pons has appeared.

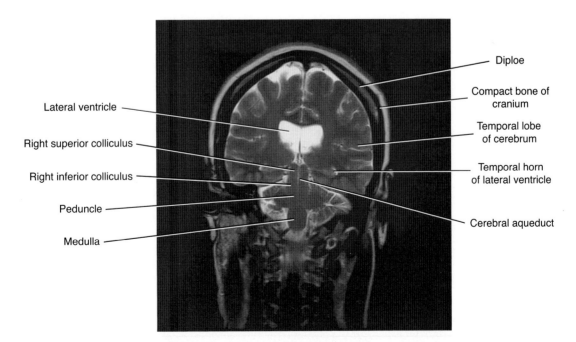

Lateral ventricle

Right superior colliculus

Right inferior colliculus

Peduncle

Medulla

Diploe

Compact bone of cranium

Temporal lobe of cerebrum

Temporal horn of lateral ventricle

Cerebral aqueduct

Figure 1-93 On Figure 1-93, the cerebral aqueduct, draining the third ventricle into the fourth, is seen passing through the midbrain. In the same plane are the temporal horns of the lateral ventricles and the temporal lobes of the cerebrum.

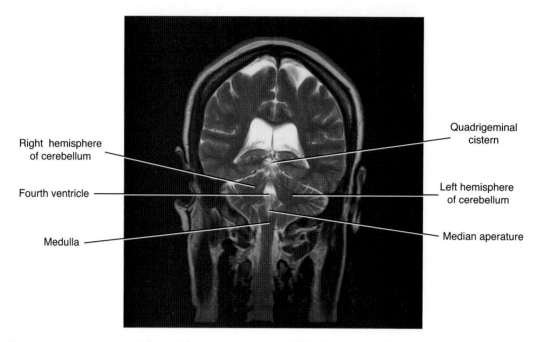

Right hemisphere of cerebellum

Fourth ventricle

Medulla

Quadrigeminal cistern

Left hemisphere of cerebellum

Median aperature

Figure 1-94 Although Figure 1-94 is a thinner interslice gap than the preceding images, it is included because it is the only image showing the quadrigeminal cistern, located posterior to the quadrigeminal plate, and the fourth ventricle, sitting in the anterior cerebellar notch of the cerebellum.

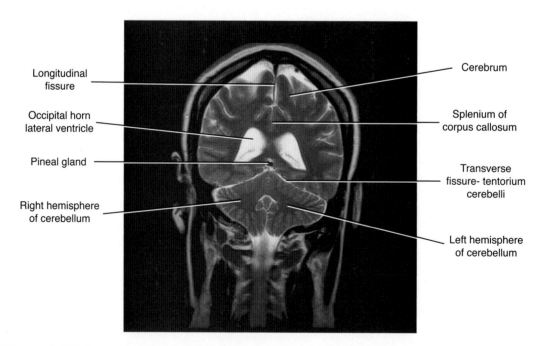

Longitudinal fissure

Occipital horn lateral ventricle

Pineal gland

Right hemisphere of cerebellum

Cerebrum

Splenium of corpus callosum

Transverse fissure- tentorium cerebelli

Left hemisphere of cerebellum

Figure 1-95 Figure 1-95 is in the region of the trigone (where the occipital horns of the lateral ventricles meet the temporal horns). The transverse fissure is shown separating the cerebrum from the cerebellum.

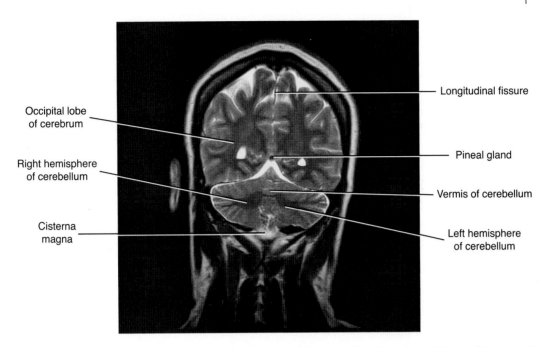

Occipital lobe
of cerebrum

Right hemisphere
of cerebellum

Cisterna
magna

Longitudinal fissure

Pineal gland

Vermis of cerebellum

Left hemisphere
of cerebellum

Figure 1-96 The vermis, connecting the two hemispheres of the cerebellum, is labeled on Figure 1-96, along with the occipital lobes of the cerebrum and the longitudinal fissure separating the two hemispheres.

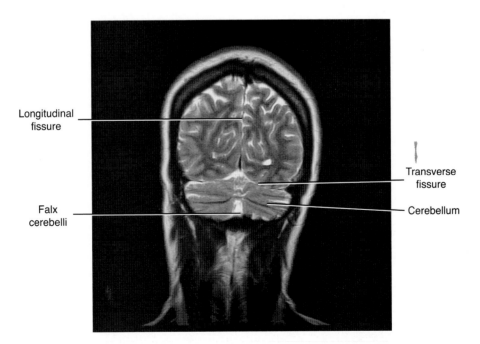

Longitudinal
fissure

Falx
cerebelli

Transverse
fissure

Cerebellum

Figure 1-97 The falx cerebelli can be identified on Figure 1-97 along the inferior medial aspect of the cerebellum. The falx cerebelli dips between the two hemispheres of the cerebellum. Both the longitudinal and transverse fissures are seen.

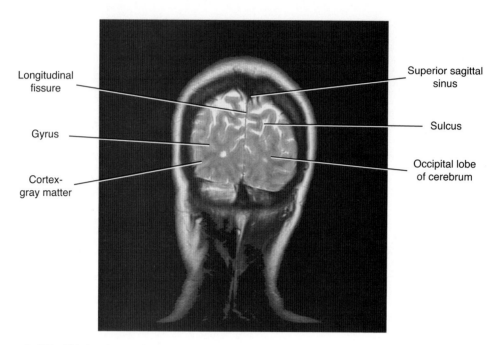

Longitudinal fissure

Gyrus

Cortex-gray matter

Superior sagittal sinus

Sulcus

Occipital lobe of cerebrum

Figure 1-98 This last image, Figure 1-98, has primarily only the cortex of the cerebrum remaining. You can identify the sulci and gyri, along with the superior sagittal sinus.

REVIEW QUESTIONS

1. The number of cranial bones is ___8___ .

2. Which cranial bone(s) act(s) as an anchor for all the cranial bones?
   a. Ethmoid
   b. Sphenoid
   c. Occipital
   d. Parietal bones

3. White brain matter is composed of neurons without myelinated axons.
   a. True
   b. False

4. Which of the following meningeal layers adheres to the surface of the brain?
   a. Dura mater
   b. Arachnoid
   c. Pia mater
   d. They all do
   e. None of the above.

5. Between which two layers of the meninges would you find cerebrospinal fluid?
   a. Dura mater and arachnoid
   b. Arachnoid and pia mater
   c. Pia mater and dura mater
   d. It is found in the epidural space.
   e. None of the above.

6. The appearance of the corpus callosum on axial images arranged in a descending order immediately precedes the appearance of the
   a. longitudinal fissure.
   b. body of the lateral ventricles.
   c. frontal lobes of the cerebrum.
   d. cerebellum.

7. Which lobe of the cerebrum is medial to the Sylvian fissure?
   a. Parietal
   b. Temporal
   c. Frontal
   d. Occipital
   e. Central

8. The temporal lobes are seen on axial images at the level of the
   a. dorsum sellae.
   b. corpus callosum.
   c. frontal lobes.
   d. parietal lobes.

9. The occipital lobes of the cerebrum are first seen on axial images at the level of the
   a. longitudinal fissure.
   b. third ventricle.
   c. corpus callosum.
   d. vermis.

10. Which of the following is a dip of the dura mater into the transverse fissure?
    a. Falx cerebri
    b. Falx cerebelli
    c. Tentorium cerebelli
    d. None of the above.

11. Which fissure separates the frontal, parietal, and temporal lobes?
    a. Longitudinal
    b. Sylvian
    c. Transverse
    d. Central

12. The name for the white matter located centrally in the brain is the
    a. corpus striatum.
    b. basal ganglia.
    c. cerebral nuclei.
    d. centrum semiovale.

13. Which of the following is not considered part of the lentiform nucleus?
    a. Putamen
    b. Globus pallidus
    c. Claustrum
    d. They all are.

14. The diencephalon is part of the
    a. forebrain.
    b. midbrain.
    c. hindbrain.
    d. none of the above—it is a separate entity.

15. On a sagittal image the optic chiasma would appear in the vicinity of the
    a. infundibulum.
    b. pineal gland.
    c. quadrigeminal plate.
    d. fornix.

16. The cerebral aqueduct runs through the
    a. forebrain.
    b. midbrain.
    c. hindbrain.
    d. none of the above.

17. On an axial image, the colliculi are posterior to the peduncles and anterior to the
    a. cerebral aqueduct.
    b. quadrigeminal cistern.
    c. frontal lobes.
    d. pons.

18. The connecting tissue of the two hemispheres of the cerebellum is the
    a. corpus striatum.
    b. centrum semiovale.
    c. corpus callosum.
    d. vermis.

19. Identify a significant brain activity found in the vicinity of the medulla oblongata.

    _____

    _____

20. The pineal gland is located superior to the cerebellum and inferior to the splenium of the corpus callosum.
    a. True
    b. False

21. Included in the brain stem are the
    I. pons
    II. medulla
    III. cerebellum
    a. I and II
    b. II and III
    c. I and III
    d. I, II, and III
    e. None of the above.

22. Which of the following statements is true with reference to the choroid plexus?
    a. They manufacture cerebrospinal fluid.
    b. The heaviest concentration would be in the collateral trigone.
    c. They are active in the blood-brain barrier.
    d. They originate in the pia mater.
    e. They are all true.

23. The collateral trigone is a triangular area found where which two parts of the lateral ventricles unite?
    a. Frontal horn and body
    b. Frontal horn and occipital horn
    c. Frontal horn and temporal horn
    d. Occipital horn and temporal horn

Match the following:

___a___ 24. Foramen of Monro

___b___ 25. Foramen of Magendie

___d___ 26. Foramina of Luschka

___c___ 27. Cerebral aqueduct

    a. Connects lateral ventricles with third ventricle
    b. Connects fourth ventricle with spinal cord
    c. Connects third ventricle with fourth
    d. Connects fourth ventricle with meningeal space

28. The two lateral ventricles are separated by the
    a. septum pellucidum.
    b. fornix.
    c. corpus striatum.
    d. choroid plexus.

29. As seen on coronal images the lateral walls of the third ventricle are formed by
    a. hypothalamus.
    b. claustrum.
    c. thalamus.
    d. fornix.

30. As seen on a midsagittal MR image the fourth ventricle is bordered anteriorly and posteriorly by the
    I. anterior cerebellar notch
    II. posterior cerebellar notch
    III. pons
    IV. midbrain
    a. I and II
    b. II and IV
    c. I and III
    d. I and IV

31. The largest cistern in the brain is the
    a. cisterna magna.
    b. cistern pontine.
    c. quadrigeminal cistern.
    d. none of the above.

32. The vertebral arteries join together to form the
    a. posterior communicating artery.
    b. posterior cerebral artery.
    c. common carotid artery.
    d. basilar artery.

33. The internal carotid arteries are branches of the
    a. common carotid arteries.
    b. subclavian arteries.
    c. vertebral arteries.
    d. basilar arteries.

34. Identify the functions of the circle of Willis.

    _____

    _____

35. On an axial CT image cross-sections of the superior sagittal sinuses are seen immediately anterior and posterior to the
    a. transverse fissure.
    b. body of lateral ventricles.
    c. parietal lobes of the cerebrum.
    d. longitudinal fissure.

Face

OUTLINE

FACIAL BONES

Chapter 1 presented the eight cranial bones: the frontal, two parietals, occipital, two temporals, sphenoid, and ethmoid. In examining CT images for **facial bones** you again encounter some of these same bones as well as the 14 facial bones themselves. The list of facial bones includes the two maxillae, two zygomatic bones, two lacrimal bones, two nasal bones, two nasal conchae, two palatine bones, one vomer, and one mandible.

Maxillary Bones

The two **maxillary bones** are the largest immovable bones of the face and are solidly united midline inferiorly. They are involved in forming three cavities: the oral, nasal, and orbital. The upper teeth are imbedded in the inferior margin, the **alveolar process** or **alveolar ridge**. Figure 2-1 demonstrates the maxillary bones from an anterior perspective, including the **frontal processes** articulating with the frontal bone. Figure 2-2 shows the inferior horizontal portion of the maxillary bone, the **palatine process**. It forms the anterior part of the **hard palate**, or roof of the mouth.

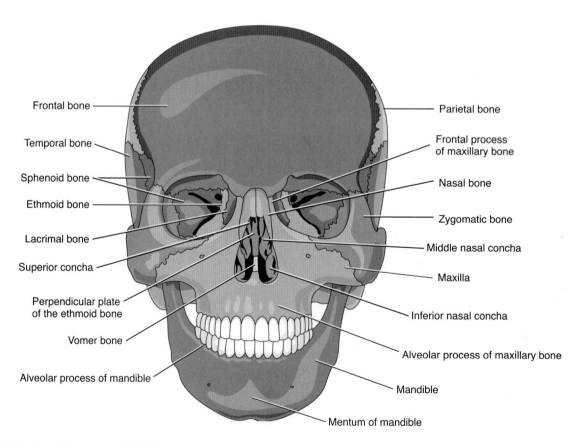

Figure 2-1 External frontal view of facial bones

Zygomatic Bones

The two **zygomatic** or **malar bones** form the prominent part of our "cheek bones" and are seen on Figure 2-1. The zygomatic bones have three points of attachment: anteriorly with the maxillary bone, superiorly with the frontal bone, and posteriorly with the temporal bone. Trauma may cause them to become free-floating, an injury called a "tripod" fracture.

Lacrimal Bones

The two **lacrimal bones**, also seen on Figure 2-1, are very tiny bones that help form the medial wall of the orbits. They are difficult to distinguish on CT images because of their size.

Nasal Bones

The two **nasal bones** are fused midline and form the bridge of the nose as seen on Figure 2-1.

Inferior Nasal Conchae

Also demonstrated on Figure 2-1 are the two inferior nasal **conchae**, or **turbinates**, which are separate facial bones.

Palatine Bones

Forming the posterior part of the hard palate are the two **palatine bones**. On Figure 2-2, they are seen posterior to the palatine processes of the maxilla. The palatine bones have vertical portions that extend superiorly and are minimally involved in forming the orbit.

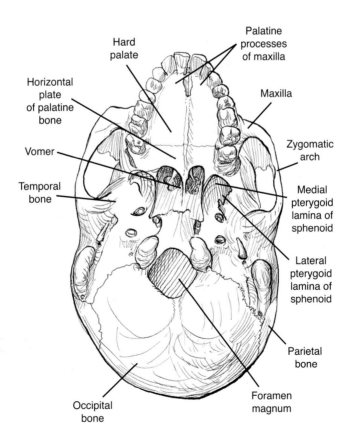

Figure 2-2 External view of inferior skull

Vomer

The **vomer** forms the inferior part of the bony nasal septum while the perpendicular plate of the ethmoid bone forms the superior segment. Their relationship is shown on Figures 2-1 and 2-3.

Mandible

The **mandible** is the largest facial bone and the only movable bone in the adult skull. Figure 2-1 demonstrates the mandible from an anterior perspective and Figure 2-4 demonstrates it from a lateral perspective. The lower teeth are rooted in the alveolar ridge or process of the mandible. The inferior tip of the mandible is the chin or **mentum** and is identified on Figures 2-1 and 2-4. Also seen on Figure 2-4 is one of the bilateral **condyloid processes** of the mandible. These processes articulate with the temperomandibular fossae of the temporal bones to form the **temporomandibular joints**.

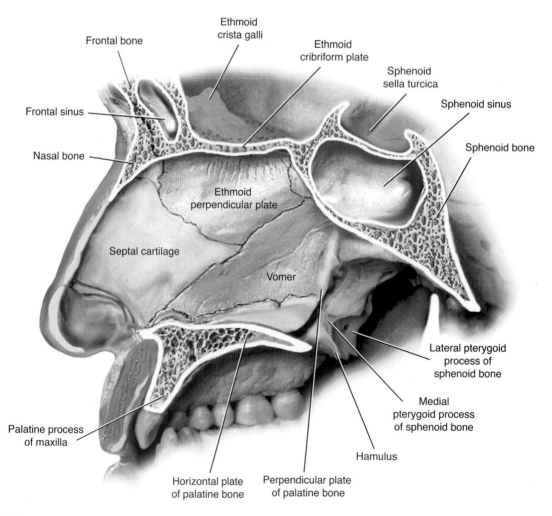

Figure 2-3 Midsagittal view of bony nasal septum

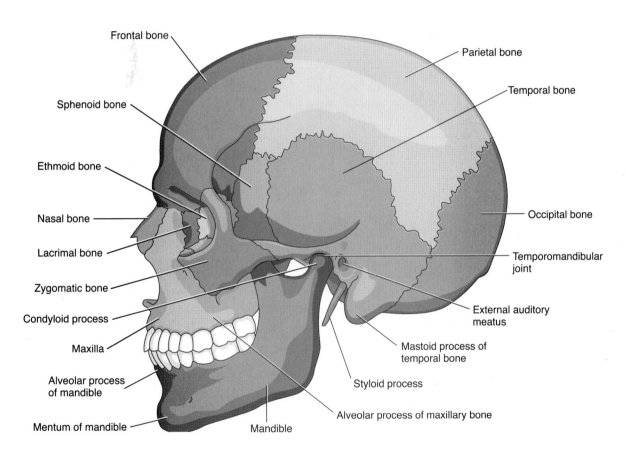

Figure 2-4 External lateral view of facial bones

BONY NASAL SEPTUM

The **nasal septum**, the partition separating the two **nasal fossae**, is cartilaginous anteriorly and bony posteriorly. The bony nasal septum is actually composed of two separate pieces of bone. Superiorly it is formed by the **perpendicular plate of the ethmoid bone**, as pictured from an anterior perspective on Figure 2-5. Figure 2-6 places the ethmoid bone with respect to the orbits and nasal cavity. The inferior portion of the bony nasal septum is a separate facial bone, the vomer. Look back at Figure 2-3, a mid-sagittal line drawing of the nasal septum, and you see both the perpendicular plate of the ethmoid bone and the vomer. When studying coronal CT images, the perpendicular plate of the ethmoid bone is easily differentiated from the vomer. The separate components of the bony nasal septum are more difficult to identify on axial CT images. Also easily identified on CT coronal images are the **cribiform plate**, the horizontal superior portion of the ethmoid bone, and the **crista galli**, the small superior extension off the cribiform plate. Figures 2-3, 2-5, and 2-6 show these structures.

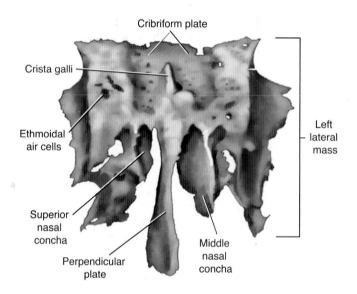

Figure 2-5 Frontal view of ethmoid bone

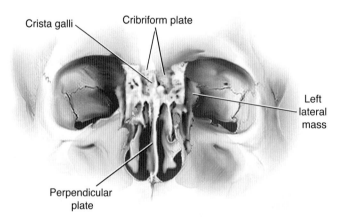

Figure 2-6 Ethmoid bone in place

NASAL FOSSAE

The nasal fossae, cavities found on either side of the nasal septum, are broken into compartments by smaller scroll-like bones called conchae or turbinates. There are three pairs of conchae or turbinates, the superior, middle, and inferior. The superior and middle conchae are medial extensions off the two lateral masses of the ethmoid bone. The inferior conchae are separate facial bones. The function of the conchae is to separate the nasal cavity into smaller compartments. When air is inhaled, it is forced to travel through the compartments, and is warmed, filtered by the cilia, and moistened by the mucous membranes lining the nasal cavity. From a coronal perspective, the inferior and middle conchae are visible on CT images. The superior conchae are much smaller and may not always be identifiable. Figure 2-1 labels the conchae.

ORBIT

There are seven bones involved in forming the **orbit**. The roof of the orbit is formed by the horizontal portion of the frontal bone. The floor is formed by the maxillary bone along the medial aspect and the zygomatic bone along the lateral aspect. The medial wall is formed by the ethmoid and lacrimal bones. The lateral wall is formed by the zygomatic bone and posterolaterally by the sphenoid bone. Minimally involved is the vertical portion of the palatine

bone. All are visible on Figure 2-7. The orbit is conical in shape, as shown on Figure 2-8, with the widest portion, the base, being located anteriorly. When doing coronal CT images, it becomes increasingly smaller as one cuts posteriorly. If someone receives a direct hit in the region of the orbit, the orbit will give in the weakest region, the floor. This would be termed a "blow-out" fracture.

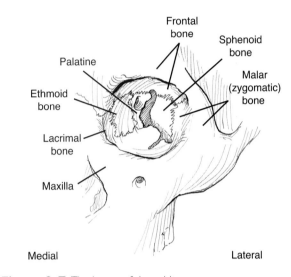

Figure 2-7 The bones of the orbit

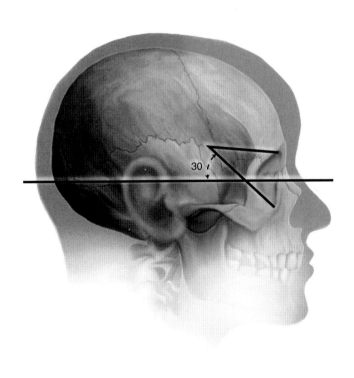

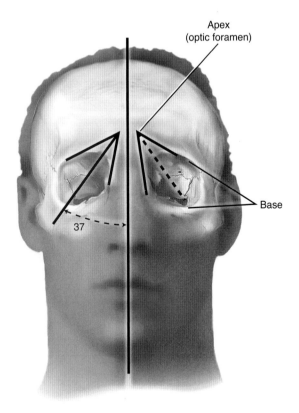

Figure 2-8 The orbits

EYE

Certain muscles are involved in moving the eye. Those evident on CT images are the superior, inferior, medial (or internal), and lateral (or external) **rectus muscles**. From a coronal perspective you see all four; from an axial perspective you see the medial and lateral muscles; and from a sagittal perspective you see the superior and inferior. The **retina** is the innermost layer in the posterior eye that contains the **rods** and **cones**, the nerve cells responsible for vision. The optic nerve exits through the optic foramen in the posterior orbit carrying the sensory information received by the retina. The optic nerve is seen on coronal CT images as an area of opacity in the center of the eye. Looking at axial images, it is visible as a linear area of opac-

ity exiting the back of the eye. The **lens** of the eye is also visible on sagittal and axial CT images, but should not be confused with the optic nerve on coronal images, as it is not visible. It is transparent and convex, allowing light to reach the retina, but at the same time causing refraction of light. Figure 2-9 demonstrates the medial and lateral rectus muscles, optic nerve, retina, and lens while Figure 2-10 shows three of the four rectus muscles.

PARANASAL SINUSES

The **paranasal** or **accessory nasal sinuses** are air-filled cavities located in some cranial and facial bones. They communicate with the nasal cavity and with each other.

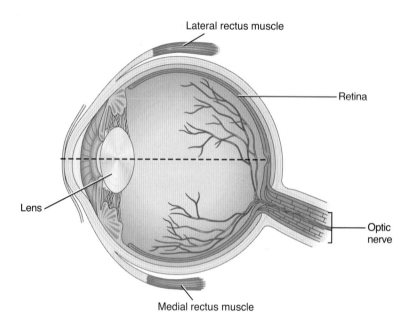

Figure 2-9 Transverse view of the eye

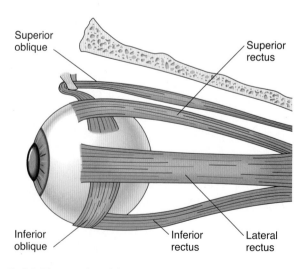

Figure 2-10 The muscles of the eye

Their function is to lighten the head and add resonance to the voice. They are lined with mucous membranes and with pathology can become filled with fluid. Named for the bones in which they are located, they are the **maxillary**, **frontal**, **ethmoid**, and **sphenoid**. Only the maxillary sinuses are present at birth. The frontal and sphenoids form around the age of 6 or 7, and the last to develop, in the late teens, are the ethmoids. The largest are the maxillary sinuses, with one being located in the body of each of the two maxillary bones. The frontal sinuses are in the vertical portion of the frontal bone. There may be either one or two, with a **septum** or wall dividing them if two exist. Rarely are they symmetric. The many ethmoid sinuses are located within the two lateral masses of the ethmoid bone, found along the medial wall of each orbit.

The sphenoid sinuses are beneath the sella turcica, in the body of the sphenoid bone. A septum separates the sphenoid sinus from the ethmoid sinuses and an additional septum exists if there is more than one sphenoid sinus. The sphenoid sinuses are located posterior to the ethmoid sinuses, as drawn on Figure 2-11. The frontal sinuses are the most superior and the maxillary sinuses the most inferior. Coronal CT images demonstrate that the frontal sinuses are the most anterior and the sphenoid sinuses the most posterior. If the orbits are visible on coronal cuts, the sinuses you are visualizing are probably the ethmoids rather than sphenoids. Figure 2-12 demonstrates all four paranasal sinuses from a coronal perspective. The sinuses appear translucent on CT images unless pathology exists.

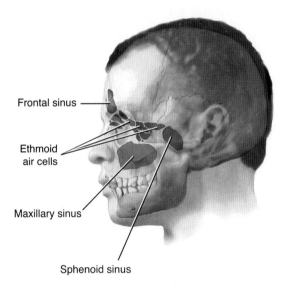

Figure 2-11 Lateral view of paranasal sinuses

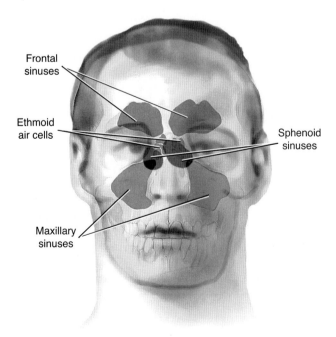

Figure 2-12 Frontal view of paranasal sinuses

CT IMAGES

Exam 1

Coronal Images

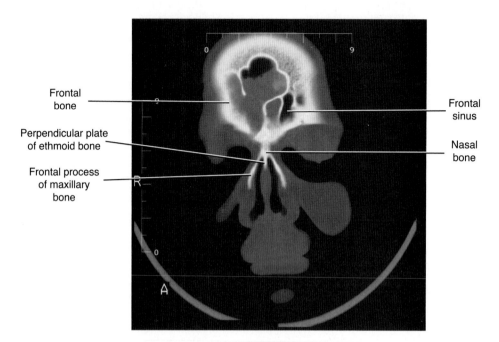

Frontal bone

Perpendicular plate of ethmoid bone

Frontal process of maxillary bone

Frontal sinus

Nasal bone

Figure 2-13 Although Figure 2-13 is not the first image of this exam, it is anterior enough to demonstrate the unusually large but typical asymmetric frontal sinuses. The nasal bones are seen along with the portions of the maxillary bones involved in forming the medial walls of the orbits, the frontal processes. Just starting to appear is the perpendicular plate of the ethmoid bone which forms the superior portion of the bony nasal septum.

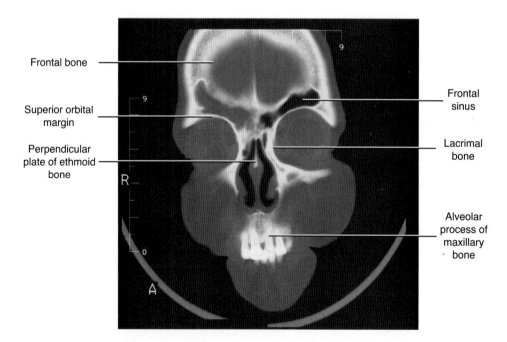

Frontal bone

Superior orbital margin

Perpendicular plate of ethmoid bone

Frontal sinus

Lacrimal bone

Alveolar process of maxillary bone

Figure 2-14 The superior orbital margin, formed by the frontal bone, is evident on Figure 2-14. More of the perpendicular plate of the ethmoid bone has appeared. The lower edge of the maxillary bone, the alveolar process, is shown. It is here that the upper teeth attach. The lacrimal bones, which help to make up the medial walls of the orbits, are labeled.

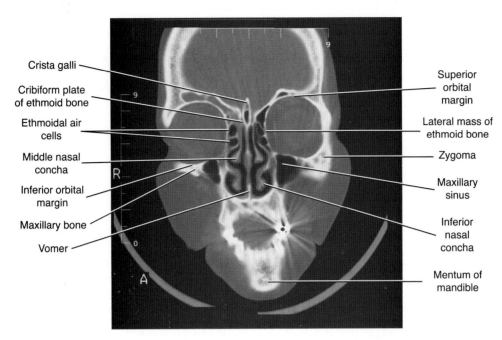

Crista galli

Cribiform plate of ethmoid bone

Ethmoidal air cells

Middle nasal concha

Inferior orbital margin

Maxillary bone

Vomer

Superior orbital margin

Lateral mass of ethmoid bone

Zygoma

Maxillary sinus

Inferior nasal concha

Mentum of mandible

Figure 2-15 Clearly seen on Figure 2-15 is the crista galli extending superiorly from the cribiform plate of the ethmoid bone. Some of the many ethmoidal air cells, found in the lateral mass of the ethmoid bone, have become visible. In addition to the lacrimal bones, the lateral masses of the ethmoid bone help form the medial walls of the orbits. Just starting to appear are the largest of the sinuses, the maxillary sinuses, in the bodies of the maxillary bones. Figure 2-15 also shows the midpoint of the mandible, the mentum, as well as the inferior and middle conchae or turbinates. The inferior conchae, separate facial bones, and the superior and middle conchae extending medially from the lateral masses of the ethmoid bone divide the nasal cavities into compartments. The vomer is seen forming the inferior part of the bony nasal septum. Notice the role the nasal maxillary bones assume in forming the inferior orbital margin.

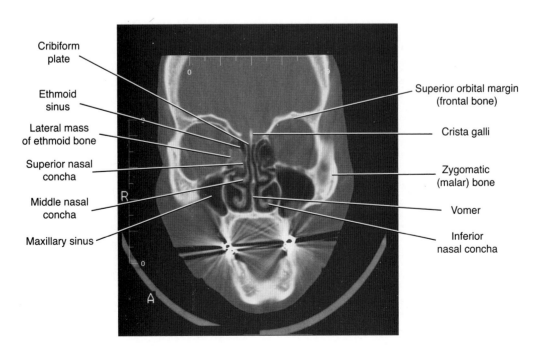

Cribiform plate

Ethmoid sinus

Lateral mass of ethmoid bone

Superior nasal concha

Middle nasal concha

Maxillary sinus

Superior orbital margin (frontal bone)

Crista galli

Zygomatic (malar) bone

Vomer

Inferior nasal concha

Figure 2-16 Figure 2-16 demonstrates the cribiform plate of the ethmoid bone along with the crista galli. The zygomatic or malar bones are prominent and their involvement in forming the lateral walls of the orbits can be appreciated.

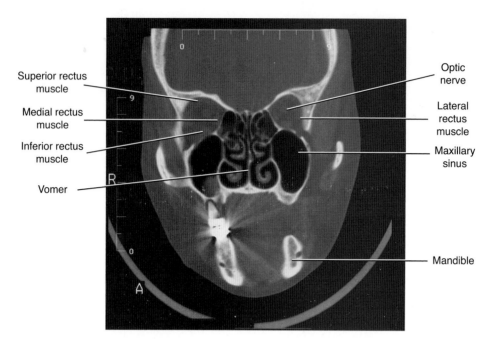

Figure 2-17 On Figure 2-17, the maxillary sinuses are fully demonstrated, for the most part nonpathologic except for a small area of opacity in the lower right maxillary sinus. A small part of the upper mandible is just starting to appear. Also seen on this coronal image are the four rectus muscles (superior, inferior, lateral, and medial), along with the optic nerve.

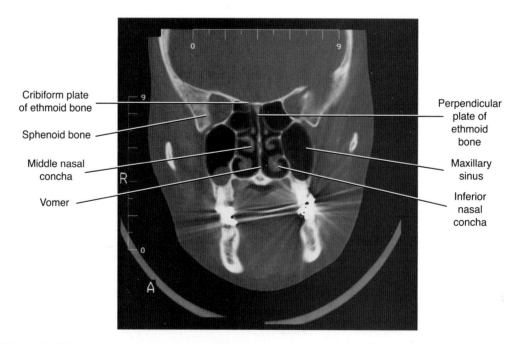

Figure 2-18 Notice the diminished size of the orbits on Figure 2-18, an indication that the image is posterior. The sphenoid bone is seen making up the posterolateral walls of the orbits.

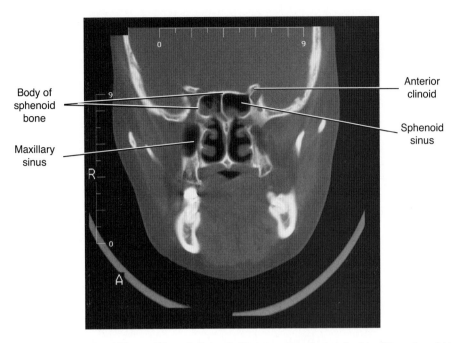

Figure 2-19 This last coronal image of Exam 1, Figure 2-19, shows the anterior clinoids of the sphenoid bone along with the sphenoid sinuses, found in the body of the sphenoid bone. Little of the maxillary sinuses remain to be seen this far posteriorly.

Axial Images

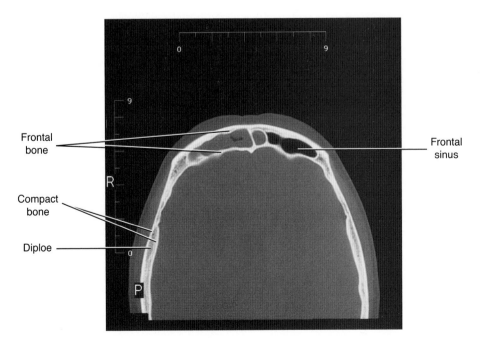

Figure 2-20 This first axial image of Exam 1, Figure 2-20, demonstrates the frontal sinuses within the frontal bone. It also shows the unique construction of the cranial bones with diploe sandwiched between two layers of compact bone.

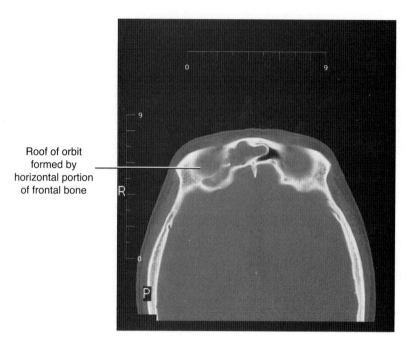

Roof of orbit
formed by
horizontal portion
of frontal bone

Figure 2-21 Figure 2-21 shows how the roof of the orbits is formed by the horizontal portion of the frontal bone.

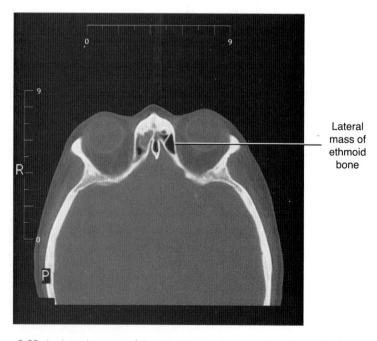

Lateral
mass of
ethmoid
bone

Figure 2-22 On Figure 2-22, the lateral masses of the ethmoid bone are involved in forming the medial walls of the orbits.

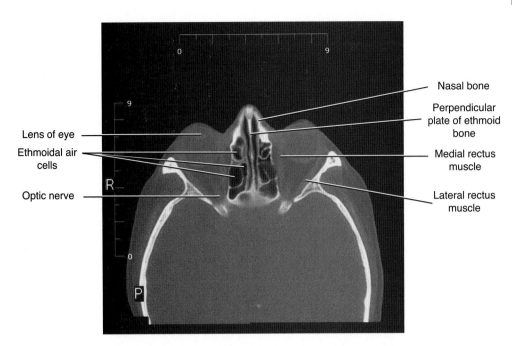

Figure 2-23 Seen on Figure 2-23 are the small, numerous, ethmoidal air cells found in the lateral masses or labrynths of the ethmoid bone. Identified are the nasal bones, as well as the perpendicular plate of the ethmoid bone forming the superior portion of the bony nasal septum. Although faintly visible, you can distinguish the medial and lateral rectus muscles, optic nerve, and lens of the eye.

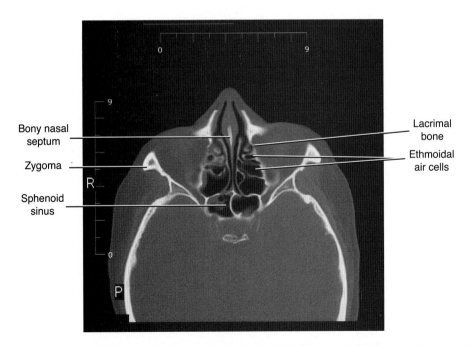

Figure 2-24 The bony nasal septum separates the two nasal fossae on Figure 2-24. Between the two orbits are the ethmoidal sinuses. Helping to form the medial walls of the orbits are the two lacrimal bones. The zygoma, involved in forming the lateral walls of the orbits, is shown.

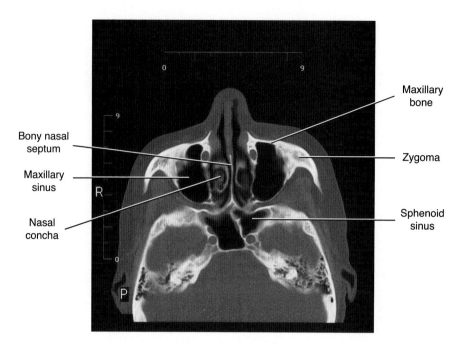

Figure 2-25 Appearing for the first time in this series of images on Figure 2-25 are the maxillary sinuses and the maxillary bones. Also distinguishable are the sphenoidal sinuses, located in the body of the sphenoid bone beneath the sella turcica. On either side of the bony nasal septum are the conchae or turbinates. The prominent zygoma is seen in profile.

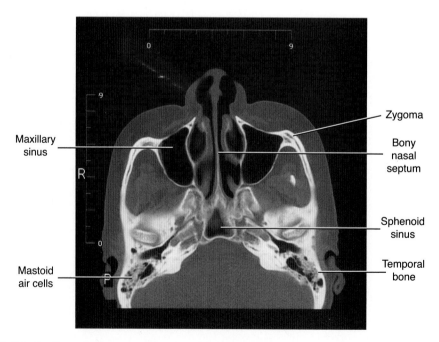

Figure 2-26 On Figure 2-26, compare the size of the maxillary sinuses, the largest and the only ones present at birth, to the frontal, ethmoidal, and sphenoidal sinuses. In the mastoid region of the temporal bones are the mastoid air cells.

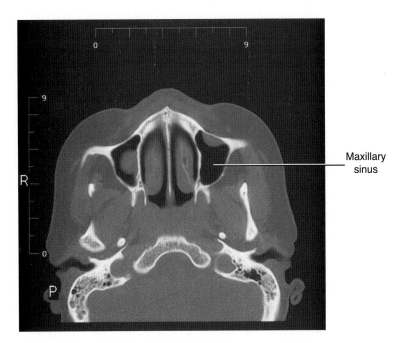

Maxillary sinus

Figure 2-27 Figure 2-27 is at a lower level of the maxillary sinuses.

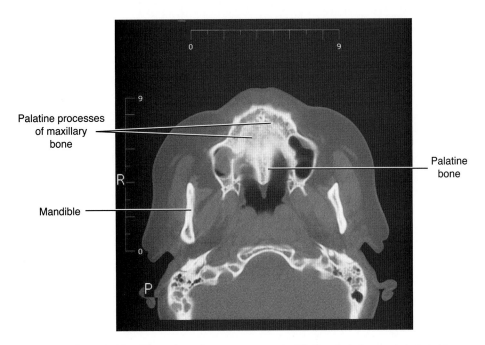

Palatine processes of maxillary bone

Palatine bone

Mandible

Figure 2-28 Figure 2-28, a thinner interslice gap compared to the previous images, is included because it demonstrates the hard palate. The hard palate or roof of the mouth is composed of the palatine processes (the horizontal portion of the maxillary bone) anteriorly and the two palatine bones posteriorly. Both should be united midline.

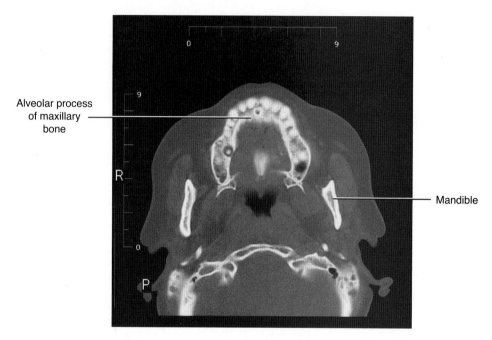

Alveolar process of maxillary bone

Mandible

Figure 2-29 This last slice of Exam 1, Figure 2-29, shows the mandible, along with the alveolar process of the maxillary bones where the teeth insert.

Exam 2

Coronal Images

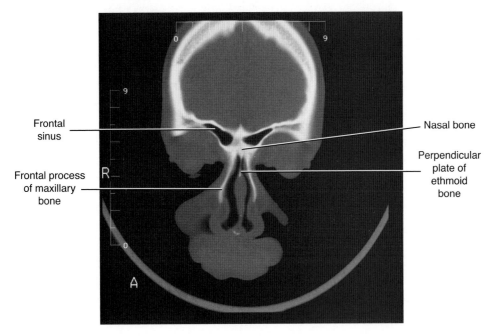

Figure 2-30 Seen on Figure 2-30 are the frontal sinuses within the frontal bone, the union of the frontal bone with the frontal processes of the maxillary bones, the nasal bones, and the perpendicular plate of the ethmoid bone.

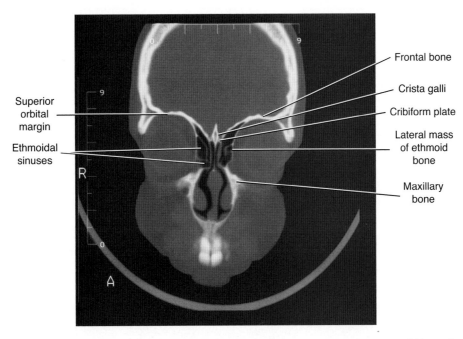

Figure 2-31 On Figure 2-31, the lateral masses of the ethmoid bone descending from the cribiform plate form the medial walls of the orbits. Extending superiorly from the cribiform plate is the crista galli and within the lateral masses are the ethmoid sinuses. The maxillary bones are just becoming visible. The superior orbital margin is formed by the frontal bone.

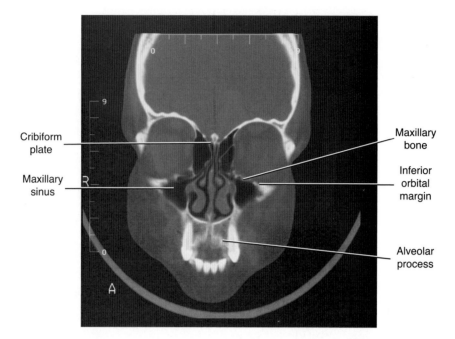

Figure 2-32 The inferior orbital margins are shown on Figure 2-32 formed by the maxillary bones medially and the two zygomatic bones laterally. The upper teeth are imbedded in the alveolar process of the maxillary bone. Just starting to appear are the maxillary sinuses.

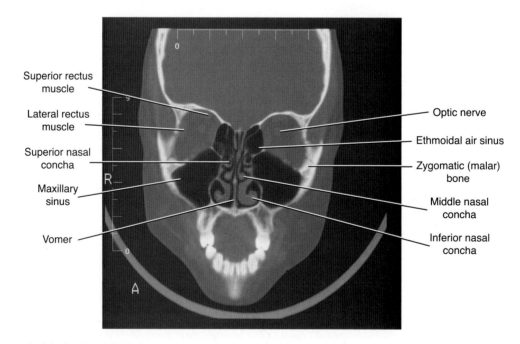

Figure 2-33 On Figure 2-33 the conchae are seen dividing the nasal fossae into compartments. The size of the maxillary sinuses is appreciated. The vomer, making up the lower bony nasal septum, is identified as is the zygomatic prominence forming the cheeks bilaterally. Lastly, notice the rectus muscles and optic nerve.

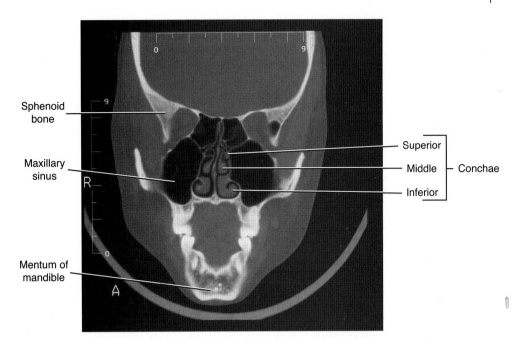

Figure 2-34 Figure 2-34 has labeled the mentum or midpoint of the chin.

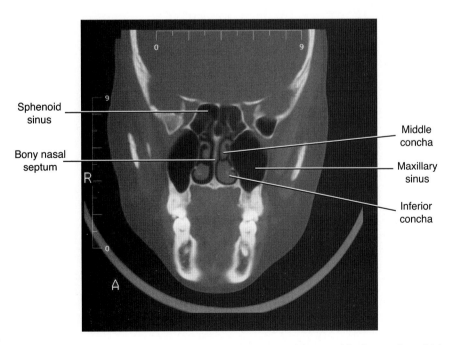

Figure 2-35 On Figure 2-35, the nasal septum separates the two nasal fossae while the conchae divide them into compartments.

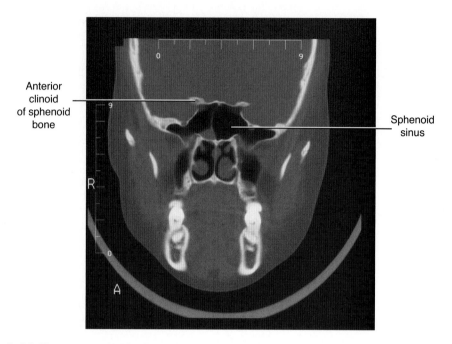

Figure 2-36 The anterior clinoids of the sphenoid bone are seen on Figure 2-36 along with the sphenoid sinuses in the body of the sphenoid bone beneath the sella turcica.

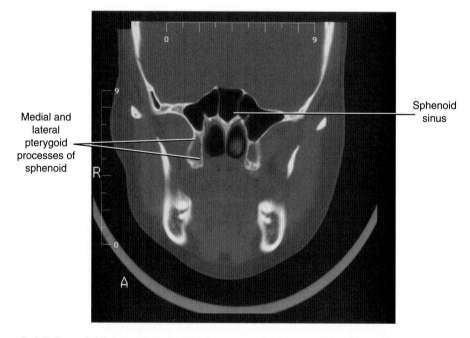

Figure 2-37 Figure 2-37 shows the sphenoid sinuses as well as the medial and lateral pterygoid processes of the sphenoid bone.

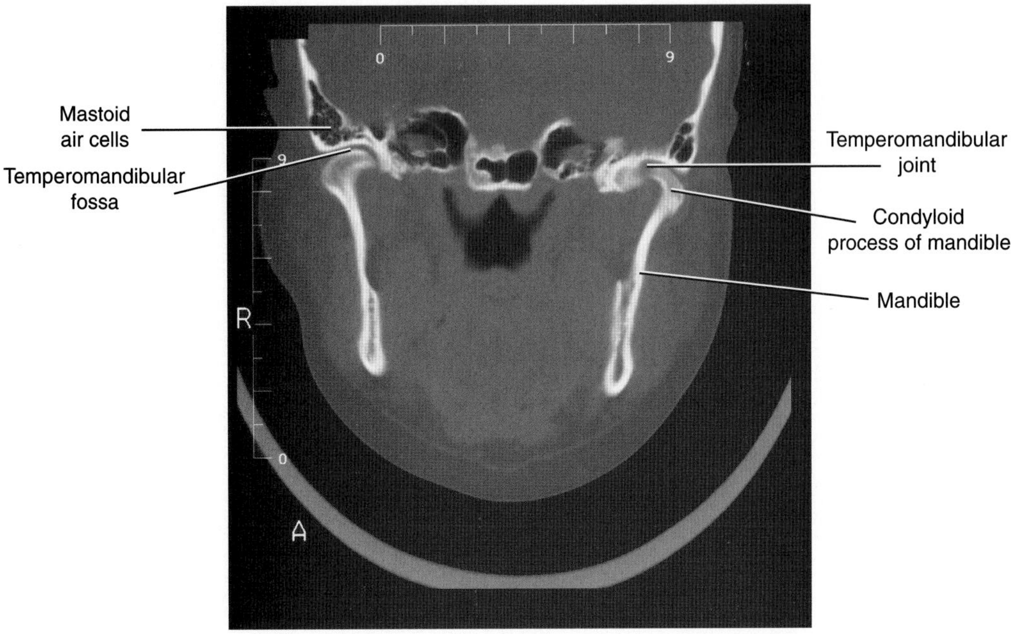

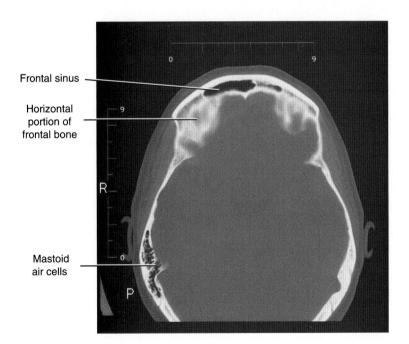

Mastoid air cells

Temperomandibular fossa

Temperomandibular joint

Condyloid process of mandible

Mandible

Figure 2-38 Figure 2-38, the last image in this series, is a larger interslice gap compared to the previous images but is included to demonstrate the condyloid processes of the mandible articulating with the temporomandibular fossae of the temporal bones comprising the temporomandibular joints.

Axial Images

Frontal sinus

Horizontal portion of frontal bone

Mastoid air cells

Figure 2-39 On Figure 2-39 you see the horizontal portion of the frontal bone forming the roof of the orbits. The frontal sinuses within the squamous portion of the frontal bone are also identified.

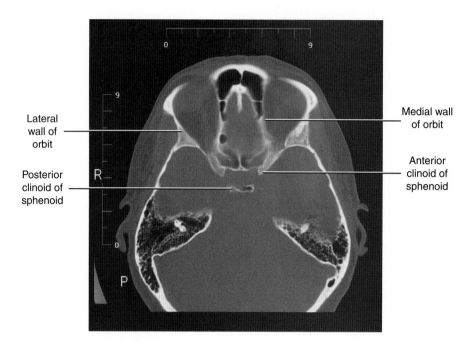

Lateral wall of orbit

Posterior clinoid of sphenoid

Medial wall of orbit

Anterior clinoid of sphenoid

Figure 2-40 Figure 2-40 demonstrates the medial and lateral walls of the orbits taking shape. The anterior and posterior clinoids of the sphenoid bone are shown.

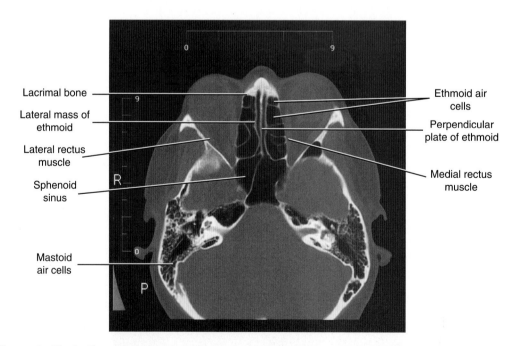

Lacrimal bone

Lateral mass of ethmoid

Lateral rectus muscle

Sphenoid sinus

Mastoid air cells

Ethmoid air cells

Perpendicular plate of ethmoid

Medial rectus muscle

Figure 2-41 On Figure 2-41, the ethmoid and sphenoid sinuses are seen. Also identified is the medial wall of the orbit, formed by the lateral masses of the ethmoid bone and by the lacrimal bones. Labeled is the perpendicular plate of the ethmoid bone forming the superior portion of the bony nasal septum. Notice the medial and lateral rectus muscles and the mastoid air cells.

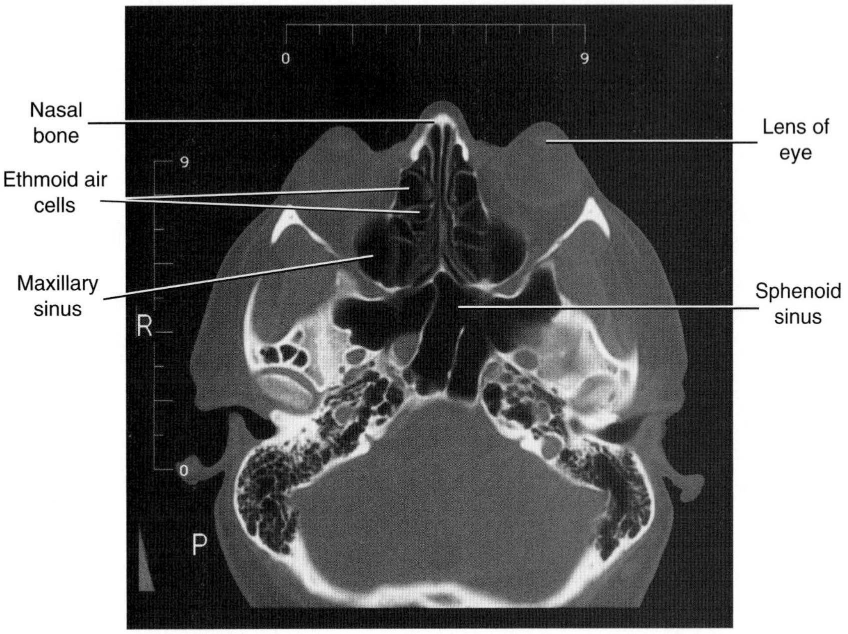

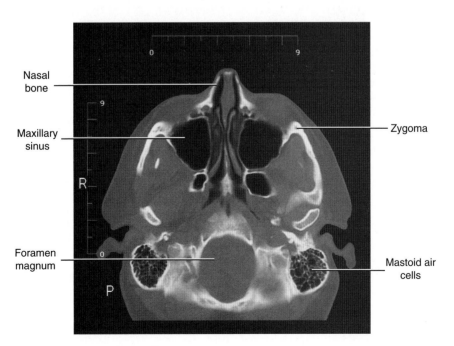

Nasal bone

Ethmoid air cells

Maxillary sinus

Lens of eye

Sphenoid sinus

Figure 2-42 Three of the four sinuses are seen on Figure 2-42: the maxillary, sphenoid, and ethmoid. All communicate with the nasal cavity. Also seen are the lens of the eyes and the nasal bones.

Nasal bone

Maxillary sinus

Foramen magnum

Zygoma

Mastoid air cells

Figure 2-43 Still apparent on Figure 2-43 are the nasal bones but more obvious now is the zygoma. The foramen magnum is seen along with the mastoid region of the temporal bones containing the mastoid air cells.

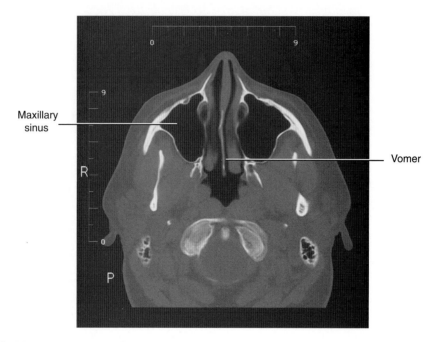

Figure 2-44 Demonstrated on Figure 2-44 is the inferior bony nasal septum formed by the vomer. The fully formed maxillary sinuses are also seen.

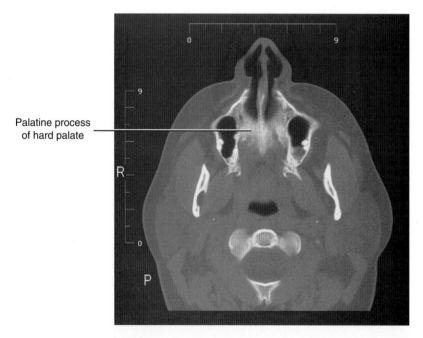

Figure 2-45 Figure 2-45, the last image shown in this exam, is a bigger interslice gap than the preceding images but is included to demonstrate the palatine process of the hard palate.

REVIEW QUESTIONS

1. The superior, middle, and inferior turbinates are part of the lateral masses of the ethmoid bone.
   a. True
   b. False

2. Which bone ends up disassociated in a tripod fracture?
   a. Frontal
   b. Zygoma
   c. Temporal
   d. Maxilla

3. Which bone forms the superior portion of the bony nasal septum?
   a. Ethmoid
   b. Sphenoid
   c. Vomer
   d. Frontal bone

4. What is the function of the conchae or turbinates in the nasal cavity?

   _____

   _____

Match the different portions of the orbit with the bones composing them.

____ 5. Roof   a. Maxillary, zygoma

____ 6. Floor   b. Ethmoid, lacrimal

____ 7. Medial wall   c. Zygoma, sphenoid

____ 8. Lateral wall   d. Frontal bone

9. Which part of the orbit is involved in a blowout fracture?
   a. Roof
   b. Lateral wall
   c. Medial wall
   d. Floor

10. Which of the following imaging planes will *not* demonstrate the lens of the eye?
    a. Coronal
    b. Axial
    c. Sagittal
    d. They all will demonstrate the lens of the eye.

11. On which imaging plane would you be able to see all four rectus muscles of the eye?
    a. Sagittal
    b. Coronal
    c. Axial
    d. All would be visible on all imaging planes.

12. Which paranasal sinus would appear first on CT images of the face done in a coronal plane arranged from anterior to posterior?
    a. Ethmoid
    b. Maxillary
    c. Frontal
    d. Sphenoid

13. The largest of the paranasal sinuses are the
    a. frontal.
    b. ethmoid.
    c. sphenoid.
    d. maxillary.

14. The first paranasal sinuses to develop are the
    a. frontal.
    b. ethmoid.
    c. maxillary.
    d. sphenoid.

15. The function of the paranasal sinuses is

    _____

    _____ .

Neck

OUTLINE

PHARYNX

The **pharynx** is the common passageway for food and liquid going to the stomach and air going to the lungs. Figure 3-1 shows the three sections of the pharynx, named according to the adjacent organs: the nasopharynx, oropharynx, and laryngopharynx. On CT axial images it is seen as an air-filled structure located anteriorly in the upper neck.

LARYNX

The distal portion of the pharynx is called the **laryngopharynx**. The relationship of the **larynx** to the pharynx is demonstrated on Figure 3-1. Contained within the larynx are the vocal cords, hence the lay term "voicebox." The larynx is composed of nine pieces of cartilage, enclosing and protecting the pharynx. With appropriate windowing, the dense cartilage almost takes on the appearance of bone on CT images. There are three single pieces, the **epiglottis**, **thyroid cartilage**, and **cricoid** and three pairs, the **arytenoids**, **corniculates**, and **cuneiforms**. Figure 3-2 A

and B identifies all but the cuneiforms. Because the cuneiforms are so tiny they are not seen on CT images either.

Epiglottis

In descending order the first laryngeal cartilage you encounter on sectional images is the epiglottis, which closes the airway when food or drink is being swallowed. It is seen at the same level as the **hyoid bone** (a U-shaped bone in the anterior neck with the opening facing posteriorly) and the mandible. The epiglottis is demonstrated on axial CT images as a transverse, linear, opaque object in the pharynx. Although the hyoid bone is included on Figure 3-2 A and B, it is not part of the larynx. The inferior aspect of the epiglottis attaches to the thyroid cartilage.

Thyroid Cartilage

Inferior to the epiglottis is the *thyroid cartilage*, italicized to differentiate it from the thyroid gland, discussed later in this chapter. The thyroid cartilage is open posteriorly and has a V-shaped indentation along the superior

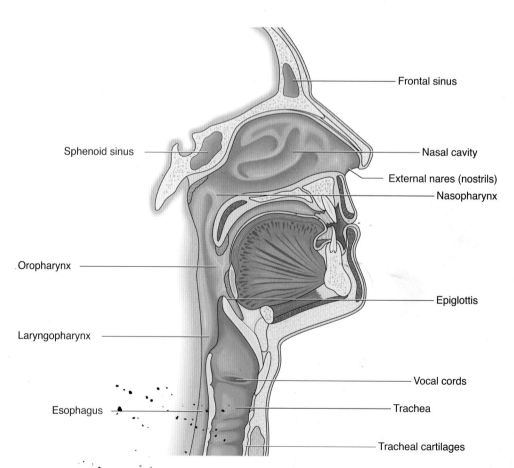

Figure 3-1 Sagittal view of pharynx

anterior aspect, accounting for the anterior opening when you first encounter the thyroid on axial CT images. Although somewhat similar in shape, the fully formed thyroid cartilage cannot be confused with the hyoid bone if you remember that the hyoid bone is seen at the level of the mandible. It is the thyroid cartilage that forms the "Adam's apple."

Cricoid Cartilage

Shaped like a signet ring, the cricoid is the last singular piece of the larynx. The fully formed cricoid can easily be identified because it is the only piece of laryngeal cartilage to completely surround the pharynx. Because of its unique shape, the initial axial images demonstrating the cricoid cartilage find the pharynx surrounded by the back of the cricoid cartilage along the posterior edge and the thyroid cartilage along the anterior edge. The cricoid cartilage is significant because the inferior aspect marks the point where the pharynx divides at approximately C5/C6 into the **trachea** anteriorly, and the **esophagus** posteriorly. The

point where this occurs is obvious on CT axial images because the round or oval shape of the pharynx becomes blunted posteriorly once the trachea originates.

Arytenoids

Figure 3-2 shows the remaining pair of cartilage pertinent to sectional imaging, the arytenoids. They sit on both sides of the superior posterior aspect of the cricoid and are seen on CT axial cuts at the level of the lower thyroid cartilage, just prior to the appearance of the posterior aspect of the cricoid cartilage.

Vocal Cords

The **vocal cords** are found within the larynx and consist of two ligaments covered with a mucous membrane. They attach anteriorly to the thyroid cartilage and posteriorly to the arytenoids. Movement of the vocal cords controls the amount of air passing through the larynx, allowing for sound production. They are also shown on Figure 3-1.

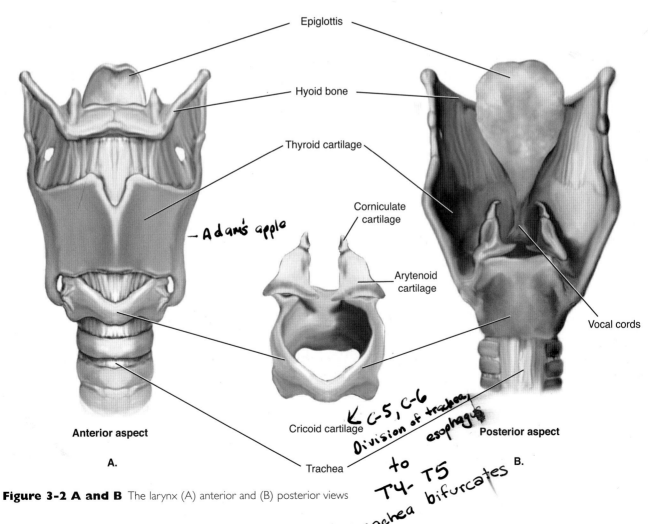

Figure 3-2 A and B The larynx (A) anterior and (B) posterior views

MUSCLES

Figure 3-3 details the construction of a **muscle**. Muscle cells are bundled together and then these bundles are grouped and surrounded by a covering called the **epimysium**. The bulky part of the muscle is called the **belly**. Each end tapers into a cordlike structure, a **tendon**, for attachment. One tendon, the **origin**, remains fixed and the other end, the **insertion**, is movable, analogous to the spring attached to a door frame and door. Generally the origin is proximal and the insertion distal. Some muscles have multiple or divided origins, with each division termed a **head**. Most muscles do not overlie the bone they move. **Skeletal** muscles, which are **striated** (having a striped appearance), are composed of thick and thin myofilaments. When a muscle is in a relaxed state a space exists between the thin **myofilaments**. With contraction the space closes and the muscle shortens. Figure 3-4 demonstrates this

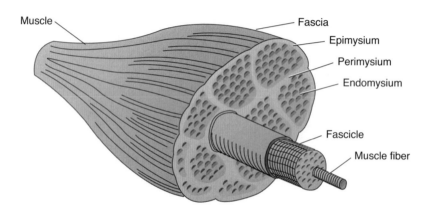

Figure 3-3 Oblique view and cross-section of muscle

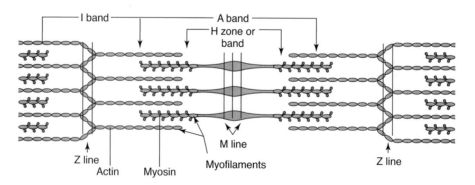

Figure 3-4 Construction of muscle—sliding filament theory

concept, the sliding filament theory of muscle contraction. Figure 3-5 shows two muscles working in opposition, allowing for extension and flexion of the forearm. Muscles acquire their name a number of ways: action, point of origin and insertion, shape, number of heads, size, location, and direction.

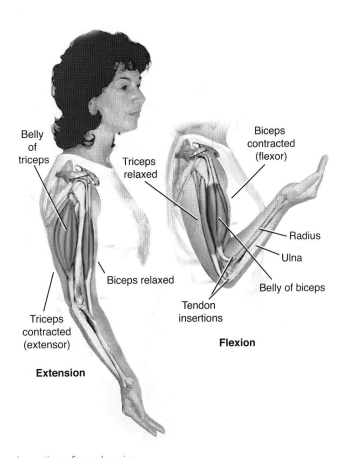

Belly of triceps

Triceps relaxed

Biceps contracted (flexor)

Biceps relaxed

Radius

Ulna

Belly of biceps

Tendon insertions

Triceps contracted (extensor)

Extension

Flexion

Figure 3-5 Opposing action of muscle pairs

Muscles of the Neck

Figure 3-6 shows some of the muscles seen in the neck. The **platysma** is the most anterior. What cannot be observed in this line drawing is that it is very thin. The **sternocleidomastoid**, or **SCM**, attaches to the mastoid superiorly and the sternum and medial aspect of the clavicle inferiorly. It moves anteriorly as axial CT cuts descend.

Seen on Figure 3-7 are the **sternohyoid/sternothyroid muscles**. For sectional anatomy purposes, they can be referred to collectively and are seen anterior to the hyoid bone, extending down in front of the thyroid cartilage with the point of origin being the sternum and medial aspects of the clavicle. Also on Figure 3-7 are the anterior, middle, and posterior **scalene muscles**, found lateral to the body

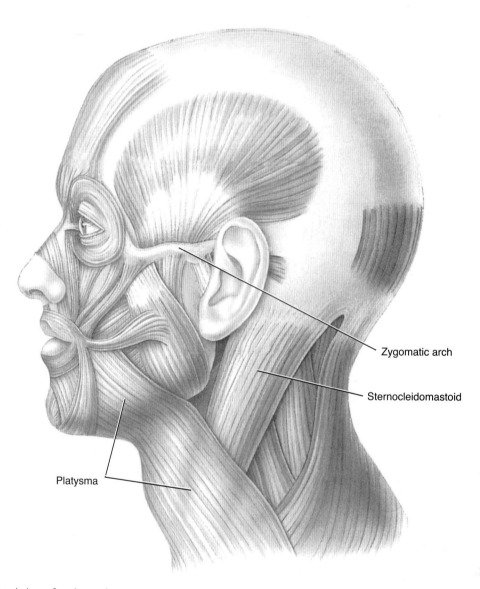

Zygomatic arch

Sternocleidomastoid

Platysma

Figure 3-6 Lateral view of neck muscles

of the vertebrae. At a higher level they also are referred to collectively but the anterior scalene can be separated from the middle and posterior scalene muscles at approximately the same level that the pharynx divides into the trachea and esophagus. Not shown are the **longus capitis** and

longus colli located in front of the bodies of the cervical vertebrae. They are identified as one until the level of the cricoid, at which time only the longus colli can be identified. Those muscles seen posterior to the vertebrae in the neck are the **erector spinae muscles**.

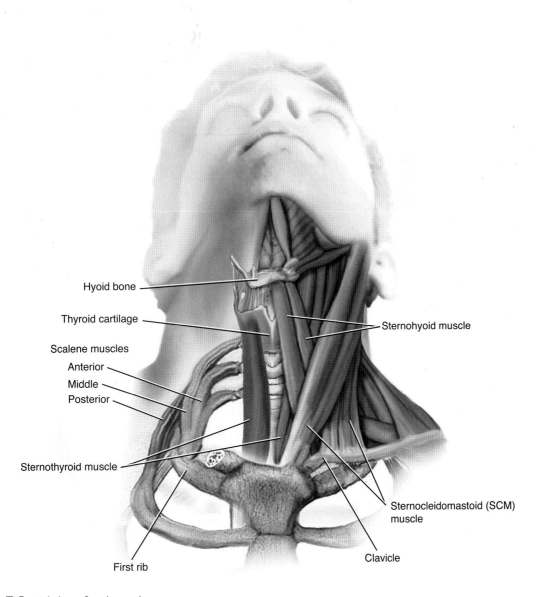

Figure 3-7 Frontal view of neck muscles

TRACHEA AND ESOPHAGUS

At the level of the cricoid cartilage the pharynx forms into the trachea anteriorly and the esophagus posteriorly. The trachea is protected anteriorly by C-shaped pieces of cartilage, **tracheal cartilage**, with the opening located posteriorly, allowing for protrusion of the esophagus in the tracheal space if larger pieces of food are being swallowed. The trachea extends down into the thoracic region, eventually splitting at approximately T4/T5 into the right and left primary bronchi, which enter the right and left lungs, respectively. As the trachea is an air-filled passageway, on axial CT cuts it appears hyperlucent with the posterior aspect being blunted. The esophagus, initially seen immediately behind the trachea, continues down through the thoracic region and diaphragm into the abdomen, where it joins the stomach. On axial CT cuts, the esophagus appears as an area of opacity, although occasionally a small bleb of air is seen within it.

THYROID GLAND   *Needs Iodine*

The **thyroid gland**, one of the endocrine glands, is found anterior to the lower part of the larynx. It has a right and left lobe connected in the middle by an isthmus. Some individuals have a smaller pyramidal lobe extending superiorly from the isthmus. Figure 3-8 places it in the neck region. In order to function properly the thyroid gland requires iodine, also found in iodinated contrast media, causing it to appear hyperopaque on CT axial cuts. It is initially seen on sectional images on the posterolateral and anterior aspect of the thyroid gland and extends below the level of the cricoid cartilage.

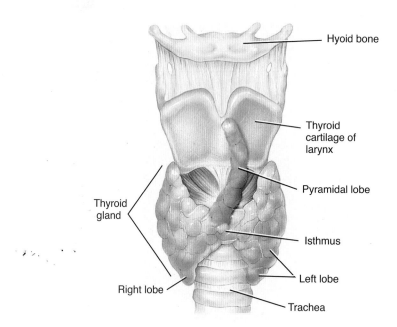

Figure 3-8 Frontal view of thyroid gland

SALIVARY GLANDS

There are three pairs of salivary glands, the **sublinguals**, **parotids**, and **submandibulars**. Figure 3-9 shows their anatomic location. The parotids are seen on sectional images as rounded masses posterior to the rami of the mandible and anterior to the SCM at a higher level in the neck. At the level of the hyoid bone the smaller submandibular glands are seen on either side of the hyoid bone, medial and posterior to the body of the mandible. The equally small sublingual glands are situated between the submandibular gland and mandible bilaterally.

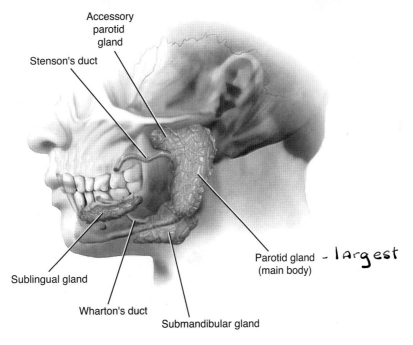

Accessory parotid gland

Stenson's duct

Parotid gland - largest
(main body)

Sublingual gland

Wharton's duct

Submandibular gland

Figure 3-9 Lateral view of salivary glands

BLOOD VESSELS

In the neck region, arteries and veins are demonstrated on sectional images with contrast medium administration. Contrast medium is used for locational purposes rather than to gain functional information. Doppler ultrasound is the preferred modality to demonstrate blood flow obstruction.

Arteries

In Chapter 1 the blood flow to the head was discussed. A quick review highlights the three major vessels arising off the arch of the aorta going from right to left: the right brachiocephalic, the left common carotid, and the left subclavian arteries. The brachiocephalic artery branches into the right common carotid and right subclavian arteries. At approximately C3/C4 the right and left common carotid arteries bifurcate into the external and internal carotid arteries bilaterally. Although the external carotid arteries were not of great interest when studying the brain they are visualized in the neck region. The carotid arteries are found medial to the SCM and medial to any veins. The internal and external carotid arteries are seen at or above the level of the hyoid bone, with the external carotid arteries being anterior to the internal carotid arteries. Below the level of the hyoid bone the anterior arteries are the common carotid arteries.

The right and left vertebral arteries arise from the right and left subclavian arteries and travel through the foramina of the transverse processes of the cervical vertebrae, entering the skull through the foramen magnum. Locating these foramina on CT axial cuts of the neck allows visualization of the vertebral arteries.

Veins

All blood returning from the brain, along with cerebrospinal fluid, drains first into the dural sinuses and then into the **internal jugular veins**. The internal jugular veins are medial to the SCM and lateral to the carotid arteries (common or external and internal). The internal jugular veins are usually the largest blood vessels in the neck, with the right generally being larger than the left. The **external jugular veins** drain those areas fed by the external carotid arteries and are a continuation of the **retromandibular veins** starting at the level of the parotid glands. They are lateral to the posterior aspect of the SCM. At a lower level the external jugular veins become more lateral, allowing them to drain into the **subclavian veins**. The size of the external jugular veins can vary but often they are inversely proportional in size to the other veins in the neck region. The **anterior jugular veins** are first seen on sectional images around the level of the hyoid bone anterior to the SCM and continue to be seen until they drain into the external jugular veins in the lower neck region. The size of the anterior jugular veins can vary but they are usually inversely proportional to the external jugular veins. Figure 3-10 demonstrates the drainage of the blood in the head into the internal and external jugular veins. Figure 3-11 is a schematic diagram of the venous blood flow of the head.

jugular veins anterior + lateral

internal jugular drains brain

external " " face, scalp — superficial

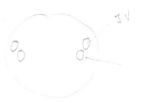

1st eca branch is the
Superior thyroidal artery.
cc &
int. c. has no branches

Know jugular veins
Know netter 70

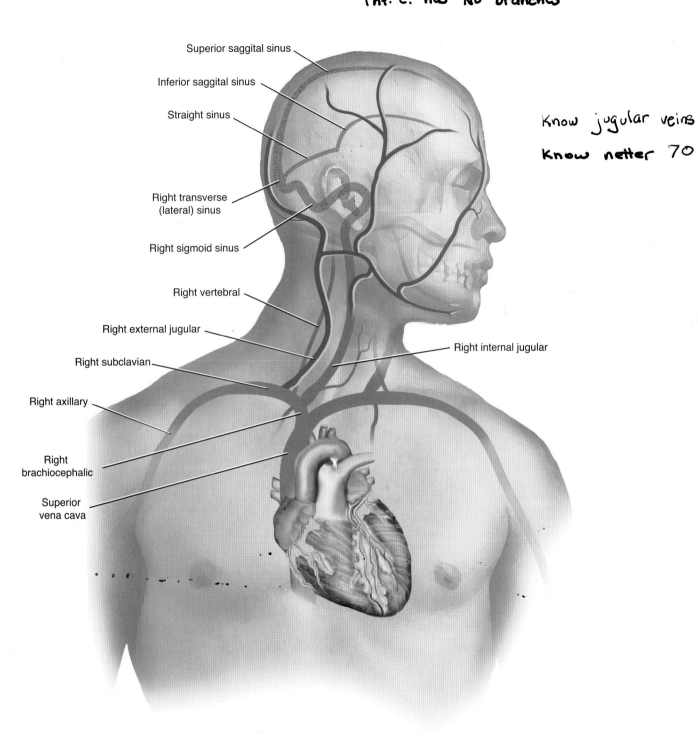

Superior saggital sinus

Inferior saggital sinus

Straight sinus

Right transverse
(lateral) sinus

Right sigmoid sinus

Right vertebral

Right external jugular

Right subclavian

Right axillary

Right
brachiocephalic

Superior
vena cava

Right internal jugular

Figure 3-10 Oblique view of venous blood flow of head

Scheme of Drainage

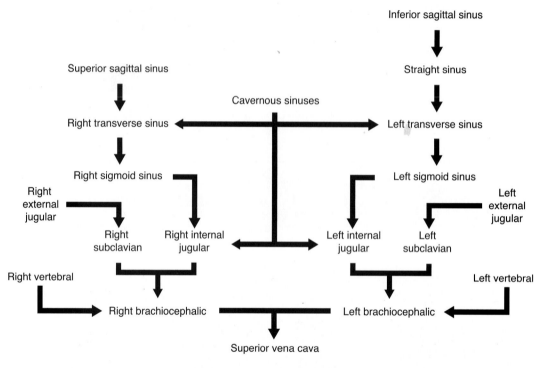

Figure 3-11 Schematic diagram of venous blood flow of head (Tortora, G. and Grabowski, S. R. [2000]. *Principles of Anatomy & Physiology* [9th ed.]. New York: John Wiley & Sons, Inc. This material is used by permission of John Wiley & Sons, Inc.)

CT IMAGES

Exam 1

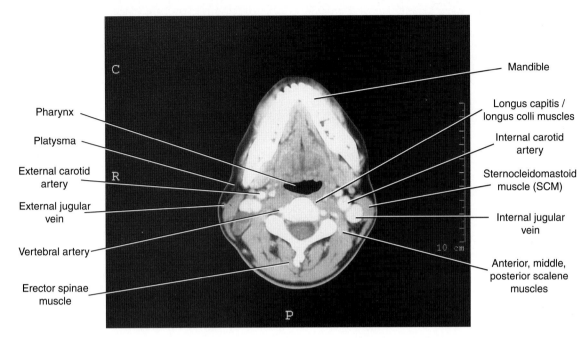

Mandible

Longus capitis / longus colli muscles

Internal carotid artery

Sternocleidomastoid muscle (SCM)

Internal jugular vein

Anterior, middle, posterior scalene muscles

Pharynx

Platysma

External carotid artery

External jugular vein

Vertebral artery

Erector spinae muscle

Figure 3-12 Not all films in this exam have been included. The first of the images, Figure 3-12, shows the sternocleidomastoid muscles posteriorly, but as the cuts descend, expect to see them more anteriorly. The internal and external carotid arteries, branches of the common carotid arteries, are evident on both sides of the neck. The external carotid arteries are anterior to the internal carotid arteries. The bifurcation of the common carotid arteries into the internal and external carotid arteries occurs at approximately the level of the hyoid bone. Of all the vessels in the neck, the internal jugular veins are usually the largest, although this particular case is atypical as the left internal jugular vein is larger than the right. The thin muscle seen along the anterior surface of the neck is the platysma.

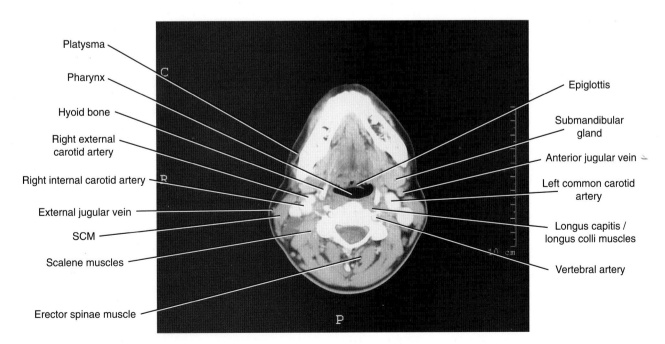

Platysma

Pharynx

Hyoid bone

Right external carotid artery

Right internal carotid artery

External jugular vein

SCM

Scalene muscles

Erector spinae muscle

Epiglottis

Submandibular gland

Anterior jugular vein

Left common carotid artery

Longus capitis / longus colli muscles

Vertebral artery

Figure 3-13 The hyoid bone is just starting to appear on Figure 3-13. On the left side the common carotid artery is seen but on the right the internal and external carotid arteries still are visible. The vertebral arteries are passing through the transverse foramina of the vertebra. Within the pharynx is the epiglottis, one of the nine pieces of cartilage making up the larynx.

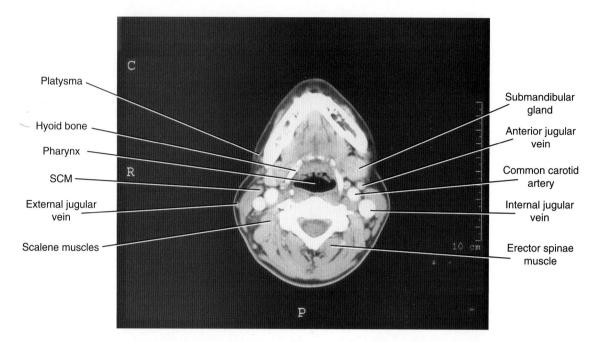

Figure 3-14 Figure 3-14 shows the submandibular glands on either side of the hyoid bone. The hyoid bone can be differentiated from the thyroid cartilage by its U shape and the absence of an opening anteriorly. The thyroid cartilage is more angulated and first appears with a gap anteriorly.

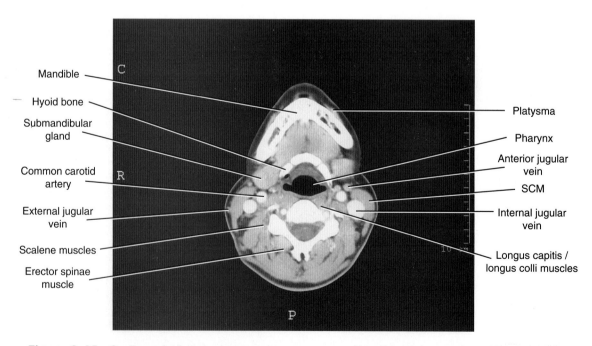

Figure 3-15 On Figure 3-15 the scalene muscles are seen on either side of the vertebra while the longus capitis/longus colli are found anterior to the vertebra.

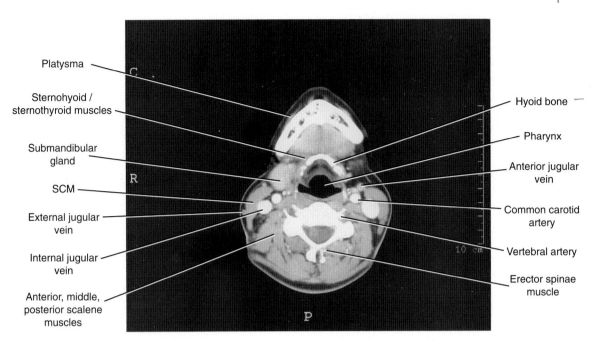

Figure 3-16 On the next cut, Figure 3-16, the sternohyoid/sternothyroid muscles are anterior to the hyoid bone. They continue down through the neck until the level of the sternum.

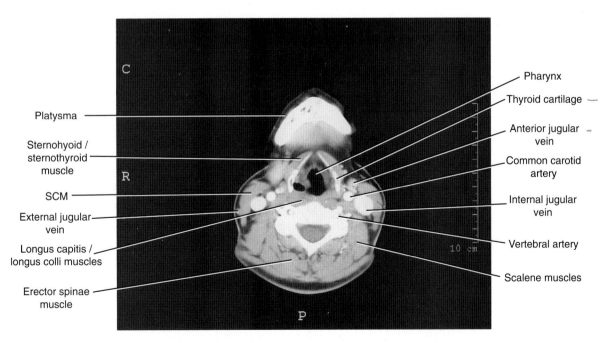

Figure 3-17 The hyoid bone has been replaced by the thyroid cartilage on Figure 3-17. Notice the anterior gap and its angular shape. Another indication that you are looking at thyroid cartilage is that only a small portion of the mandible remains. The SCM muscles are seen more anteriorly. The thin platysma, covering the length of the neck, is visible.

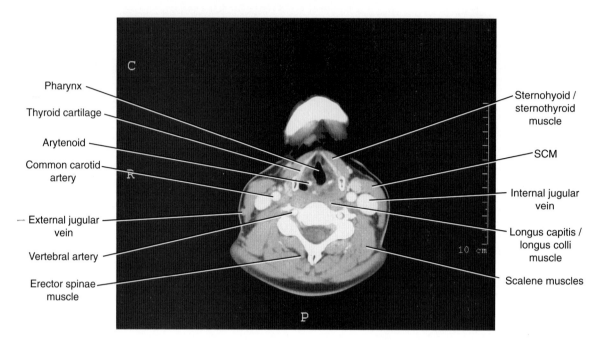

Pharynx

Thyroid cartilage

Arytenoid

Common carotid
artery

External jugular
vein

Vertebral artery

Erector spinae
muscle

Sternohyoid /
sternothyroid
muscle

SCM

Internal jugular
vein

Longus capitis /
longus colli
muscle

Scalene muscles

10 cm

Figure 3-18   Figure 3-18 shows the smaller arytenoids sitting atop the posterior aspect of the cricoid cartilage. Expect to see the cricoid cartilage soon.

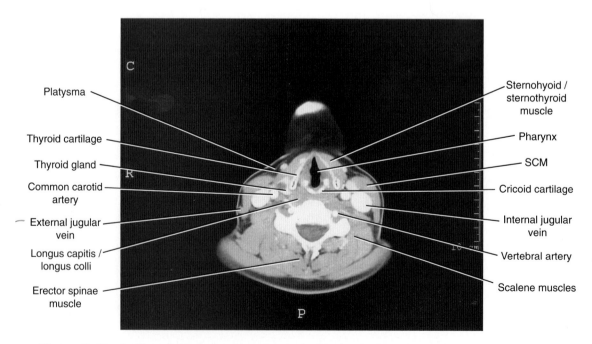

Platysma

Thyroid cartilage

Thyroid gland

Common carotid
artery

External jugular
vein

Longus capitis /
longus colli

Erector spinae
muscle

Sternohyoid /
sternothyroid
muscle

Pharynx

SCM

Cricoid cartilage

Internal jugular
vein

Vertebral artery

Scalene muscles

Figure 3-19   On Figure 3-19, the thyroid cartilage is closed anteriorly. The posterior portion of the cricoid cartilage has appeared behind the pharynx. The back of the cricoid cartilage is deeper than the front, explaining why only a portion of it is seen at this level. Look closely on the right side of the posterior aspect of the thyroid cartilage to detect the thyroid gland. It is quite opaque because of its high iodine content.

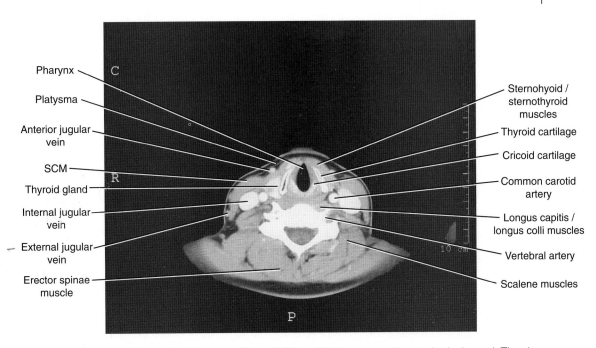

Figure 3-20 At the lower level shown on Figure 3-20, the SCM appears quite anterior in the neck. The pharynx is still oval in shape, an indication it has not divided into the trachea and esophagus.

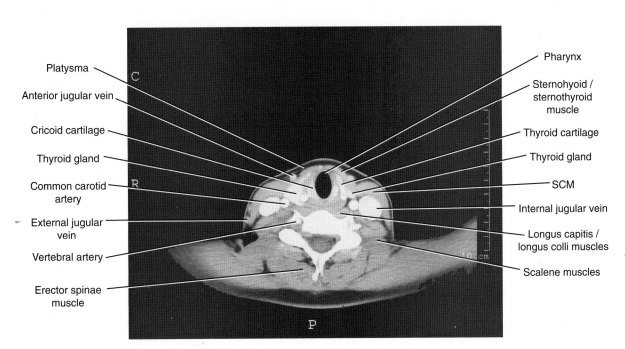

Figure 3-21 On Figure 3-21, the thyroid cartilage has all but disappeared while the cricoid cartilage almost encompasses the pharynx. The thyroid gland on the left is just starting to appear.

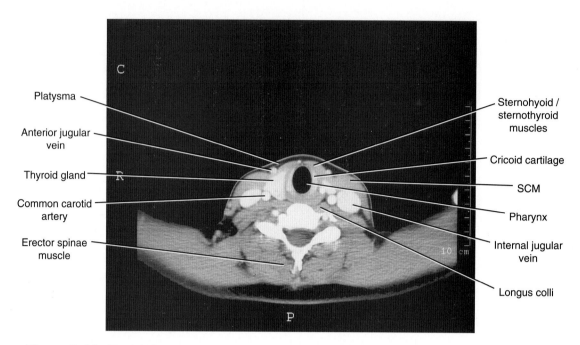

Figure 3-22   The fully formed cricoid cartilage now completely surrounds the pharynx on Figure 3-22. It is the only one of the nine pieces of the larynx to do so. At this level, only the longus colli remains anterior to the vertebra.

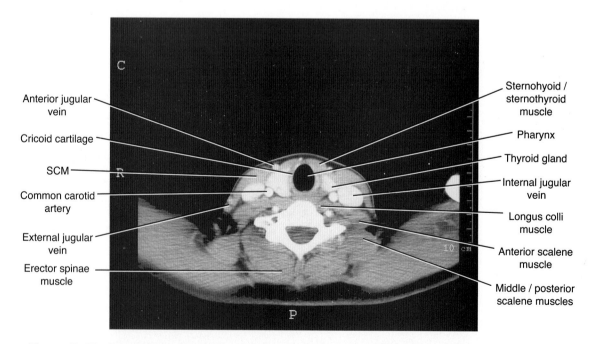

Figure 3-23   Figure 3-23 clearly demonstrates the thyroid gland, not to be confused with the thyroid cartilage of the larynx, on either side of the cricoid cartilage. The SCM is located very anteriorly in the neck. As the cricoid cartilage is the most inferior part of the larynx, expect to see the division of the pharynx into the trachea and esophagus next.

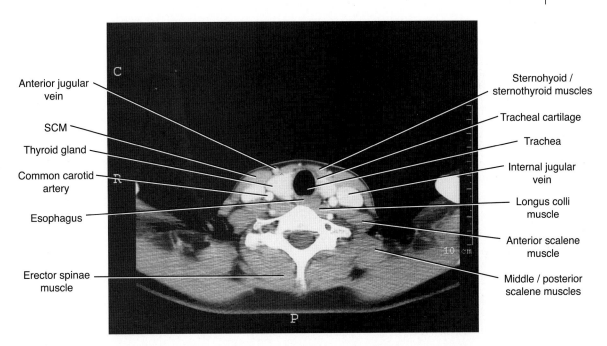

Anterior jugular vein

SCM

Thyroid gland

Common carotid artery

Esophagus

Erector spinae muscle

Sternohyoid / sternothyroid muscles

Tracheal cartilage

Trachea

Internal jugular vein

Longus colli muscle

Anterior scalene muscle

Middle / posterior scalene muscles

10 cm

Figure 3-24 On this last image of Exam 1, Figure 3-24, the air-filled structure in the neck has an indentation posteriorly. It is the trachea with the esophagus posterior to it. Anterior to the trachea is a tracheal cartilage. The numerous pieces of tracheal cartilage do not extend around the back of the trachea. The scalene muscles can now be sorted into anterior scalene muscles and the paired middle and posterior scalene muscles. Even at this low level, the sternohyoid/sternothyroid muscles are seen and remain visible until the level of the sternum.

Exam 2

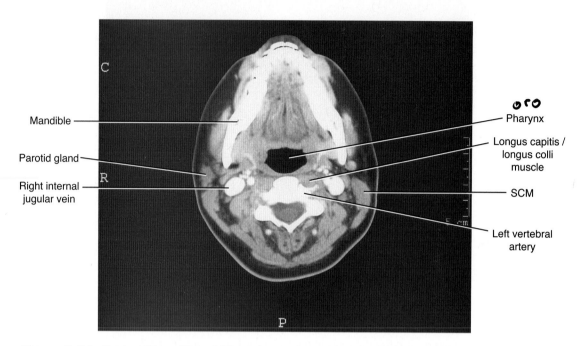

Figure 3-25   Barely visible on Figure 3-25 are the remnants of the parotid glands on the right side. The typical internal jugular veins are larger than any of the other vessels.

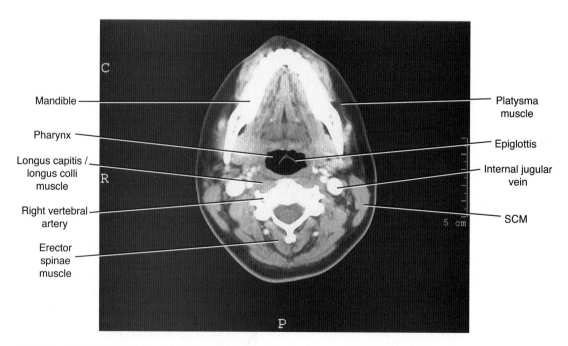

Figure 3-26   Figure 3-26, a cut at a fairly high level in the neck, places the sternocleidomastoid muscles posteriorly; however, as the cuts descend the SCM will appear more anteriorly in the neck.

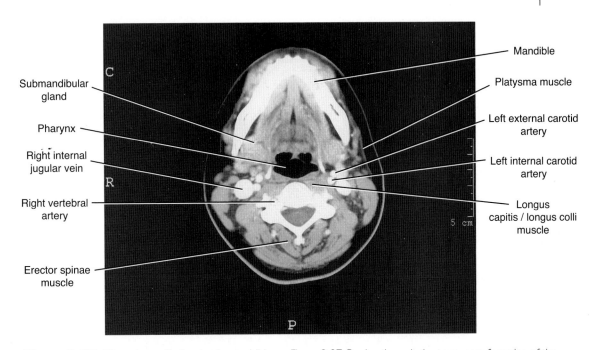

Submandibular gland

Pharynx

Right internal jugular vein

Right vertebral artery

Erector spinae muscle

Mandible

Platysma muscle

Left external carotid artery

Left internal carotid artery

Longus capitis / longus colli muscle

Figure 3-27 The submandibular glands are visible on Figure 3-27. Passing through the transverse foramina of the cervical vertebrae are the vertebral arteries.

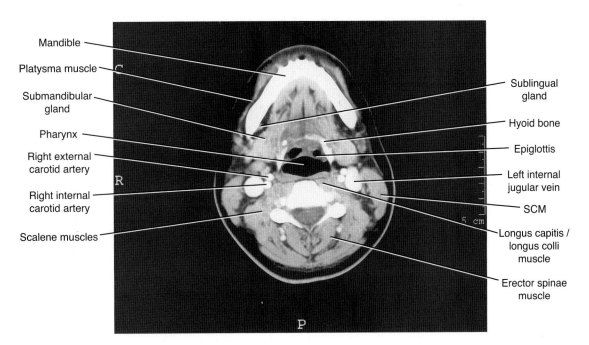

Mandible

Platysma muscle

Submandibular gland

Pharynx

Right external carotid artery

Right internal carotid artery

Scalene muscles

Sublingual gland

Hyoid bone

Epiglottis

Left internal jugular vein

SCM

Longus capitis / longus colli muscle

Erector spinae muscle

Figure 3-28 Figure 3-28 shows the upper edges of the hyoid bone. The apparent break in the pharynx is the epiglottis. The smaller sublingual glands are anterior to the submandibular glands.

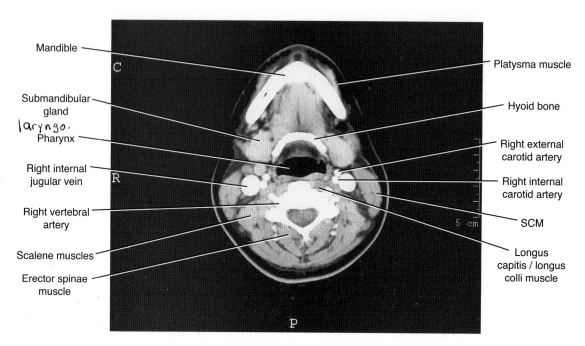

Mandible
Submandibular gland
laryngo.
Pharynx
Right internal jugular vein
Right vertebral artery
Scalene muscles
Erector spinae muscle

Platysma muscle
Hyoid bone
Right external carotid artery
Right internal carotid artery
SCM
Longus capitis / longus colli muscle

Figure 3-29 On Figure 3-29, the submandibular glands are quite prominent. Notice the platysma, the thin muscle covering the entire length of the anterior neck.

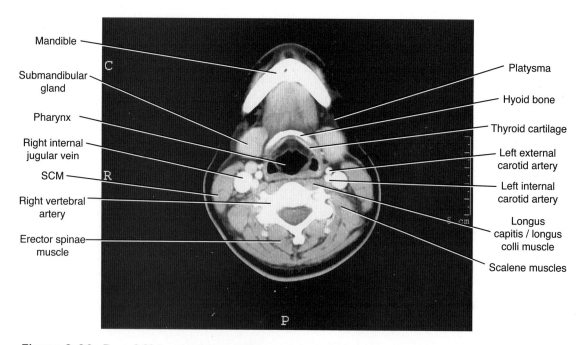

Mandible
Submandibular gland
Pharynx
Right internal jugular vein
SCM
Right vertebral artery
Erector spinae muscle

Platysma
Hyoid bone
Thyroid cartilage
Left external carotid artery
Left internal carotid artery
Longus capitis / longus colli muscle
Scalene muscles

Figure 3-30 Figure 3-30 is somewhat unusual because the hyoid bone is seen at the same level as the thyroid cartilage.

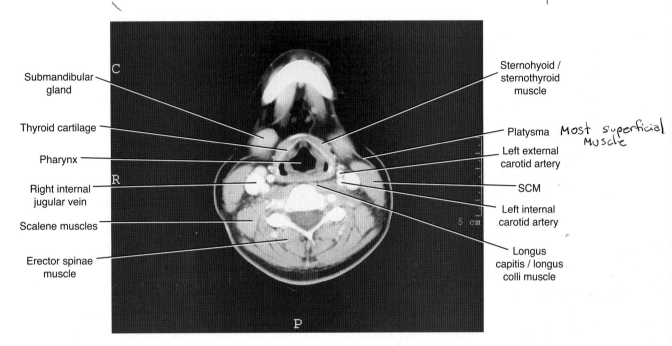

Submandibular gland

Thyroid cartilage

Pharynx

Right internal jugular vein

Scalene muscles

Erector spinae muscle

Sternohyoid / sternothyroid muscle

Platysma Most superficial Muscle

Left external carotid artery

SCM

Left internal carotid artery

Longus capitis / longus colli muscle

5 cm

Figure 3-31 The thyroid cartilage has assumed its full form anterior to the pharynx on Figure 3-31. Also appearing on this image is the sternohyoid/sternothyroid muscle.

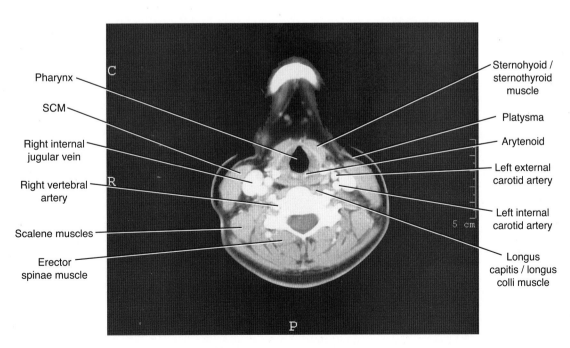

Pharynx

SCM

Right internal jugular vein

Right vertebral artery

Scalene muscles

Erector spinae muscle

Sternohyoid / sternothyroid muscle

Platysma

Arytenoid

Left external carotid artery

Left internal carotid artery

Longus capitis / longus colli muscle

5 cm

Figure 3-32 Figure 3-32 is an axial CT image taken below the level of the hyoid bone and yet the internal and external carotids are still visible, rather than the common carotids from which they arise. This is somewhat unusual.

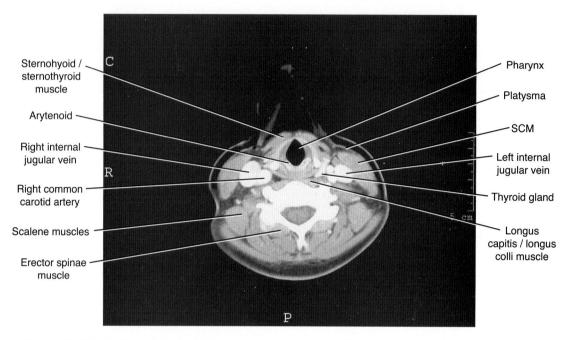

Sternohyoid / sternothyroid muscle

Arytenoid

Right internal jugular vein

Right common carotid artery

Scalene muscles

Erector spinae muscle

Pharynx

Platysma

SCM

Left internal jugular vein

Thyroid gland

Longus capitis / longus colli muscle

Figure 3-33   On Figure 3-33, the SCM has moved more anteriorly. The right internal jugular vein is larger than the left, which is quite common. The thyroid gland is now appearing on the left and the arytenoids sitting on top of the posterior cricoid cartilage are visible.

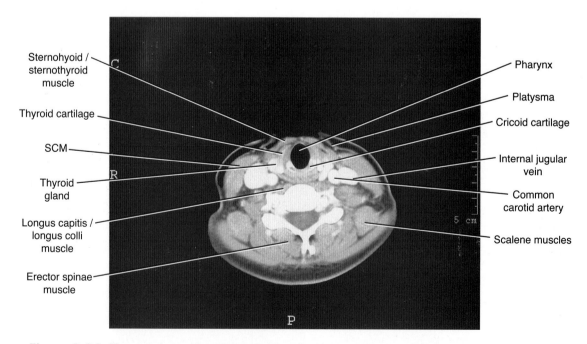

Sternohyoid / sternothyroid muscle

Thyroid cartilage

SCM

Thyroid gland

Longus capitis / longus colli muscle

Erector spinae muscle

Pharynx

Platysma

Cricoid cartilage

Internal jugular vein

Common carotid artery

Scalene muscles

Figure 3-34   The posterior portion of the cricoid cartilage is seen at the same level as the thyroid cartilage on Figure 3-34. This is expected as the posterior portion of the cricoid cartilage is deeper than the anterior portion.

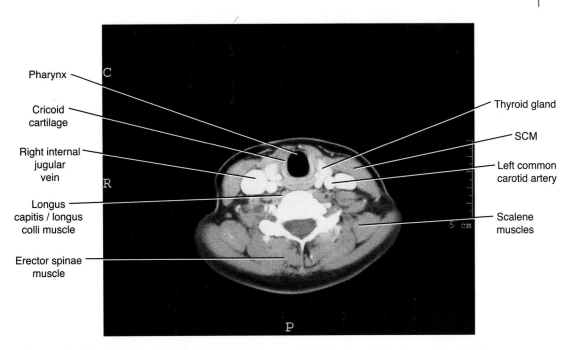

Figure 3-35 On Figure 3-35, the cricoid cartilage completely surrounds the pharynx. The SCM is very anterior and the thyroid gland is becoming more obvious.

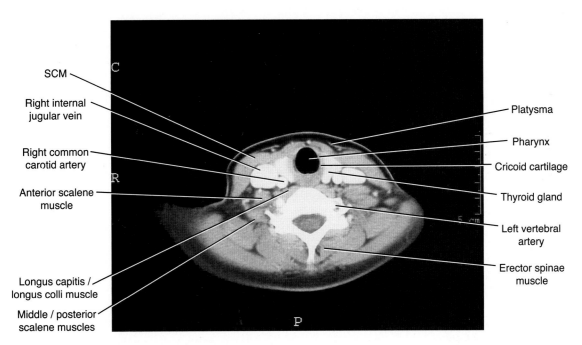

Figure 3-36 At this level, the scalene muscles can be sorted into anterior scalene muscles and the paired middle and posterior scalene muscles. Locate them on Figure 3-36.

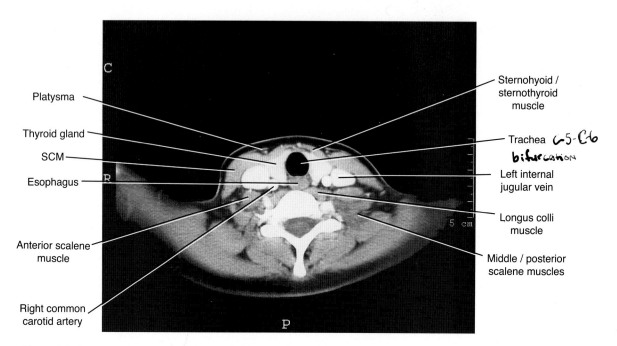

Platysma

Thyroid gland

SCM

Esophagus

Anterior scalene
muscle

Right common
carotid artery

Sternohyoid /
sternothyroid
muscle

Trachea C-5-C-6
bifurcation

Left internal
jugular vein

Longus colli
muscle

Middle / posterior
scalene muscles

5 cm

Figure 3-37 The last image included in this exam, Figure 3-37, demonstrates the division of the laryngeal pharynx into the trachea and the esophagus, with the esophagus more posterior. Not apparent, because of the opacity of the thyroid gland, is the tracheal cartilage sitting anterior to the trachea.

parathyroids are posterior to the thyroid

REVIEW QUESTIONS

1. The number of pieces of cartilage making up the larynx is
   a. 6.
   b. 7.
   c. 8.
   d. 9.
   e. 10.

2. The laryngeal cartilage associated with the bifurcation of the pharynx into the trachea and esophagus is the
   ___Cricoid_____ .

3. On axial CT images, which portion of the larynx is seen completely encircling the laryngeal pharynx?
   a. Epiglottis
   b. Arytenoid
   c. Thyroid
   d. Cricoid

4. The first laryngeal cartilage encountered on a series of axial CT images of the neck arranged in descending order is the
   a. hyoid bone.
   b. thyroid cartilage.
   c. epiglottis.
   d. cricoid cartilage.

5. Which of the following pieces of laryngeal cartilage is one of a pair?
   a. Cuneiform
   b. Thyroid cartilage
   c. Epiglottis
   d. Cricoid

6. The last laryngeal cartilage encountered on a series of axial CT images of the neck arranged in descending order is the
   a. epiglottis.
   b. arytenoid.
   c. thyroid cartilage.
   d. cricoid.
   e. hyoid.

7. Which of the following statements about muscles is true?
   I. Generally muscles overlie the bones they move.
   II. A "head" would be one of the divided origins of a muscle.
   III. Generally the origin of a muscle is distal.
   IV. The insertion of a muscle is fixed.
   a. I
   b. II
   c. III
   d. IV
   e. None of the statements is true.

8. Which muscle is seen most anteriorly on axial CT images of the neck?
   a. SCM (sternocleiodomastoid)
   b. Platysma
   c. Sternohyoid/sternothyroid
   d. Longus capitis/longus colli

9. On axial CT images of the neck the esophagus is posterior to the trachea.
   a. True
   b. False

10. Explain why the thyroid gland is so well visualized on CT sectional images of the neck.
    ___Iodine_____
    __Naturally____contains_____

11. What gland(s) is/are found lateral to the hyoid bone on axial CT images of the neck?
    a. Submandibular
    b. Parotid
    c. Sublingual
    d. Thyroid

12. Why is contrast medium administered when acquiring axial CT images of the neck?
    ___localization__of__vessels_____
    _____

13. In the region of the neck, arteries are lateral to the veins.
    a. True
    b. False

14. In the neck, the external carotid artery is anterior to the internal carotid artery.
    a. True
    b. False

15. Which of the following vessels in the neck is usually the largest?
    a. Internal carotid artery
    b. External carotid artery
    c. Internal jugular vein
    d. External jugular vein

Thorax

OUTLINE

BONY THORAX

The bony thorax includes the **sternum**, **ribs**, and **clavicles**, and serves to enclose and protect vital organs within the thorax, including the **lungs**, **heart**, and **great vessels**.

Sternum

The sternum is the bone found midline anteriorly in the thorax. It serves to protect the mediastinal organs and is a point of attachment for the ribs and clavicle, discussed next. It is composed of three sections. The uppermost section is the **manubrium**, articulating with the first 1½ pairs of ribs and the two clavicles, one on each side. The junction between the manubrium and clavicles is the **sternoclavicular** or **SC joint**. Along the superior border of the manubrium is a small indentation, the **jugular** or **suprasternal notch**. The body or **gladiolus** is the centrally located, largest portion of the sternum. It articulates with the manubrium at the **sternal angle** and the ribs bilaterally. The **xiphoid** or **ensiform process** is the most inferior portion of the sternum and has no ribs attached. Figure 4-1 is a line drawing of the sternum and its articulations.

Ribs

There are twelve pairs of ribs. The ribs are curved flat bones with a vertebral end and sternal end. The vertebral end has as landmarks a head, neck, and tubercle. Each of the twelve thoracic vertebrae has a pair of ribs attached, one on each side. The head of the rib articulates with the body of the vertebra and the tubercle articulates with the transverse process. Each rib turns at the angle anterior to

the tubercle to head in an anterior direction. The first seven pairs of ribs are considered true ribs, attaching indirectly with the lateral sternum via cartilage. The remaining five pairs of ribs are false ribs. Ribs 8, 9, and 10 each attach to the cartilage of the ribs above via cartilage. Ribs 11 and 12 are "floating ribs" with the sternal end unattached. Figure 4-1 is a line drawing including the ribs.

Clavicle

The bilateral clavicles are slender bones located in the anterior upper thorax. Each clavicle has a sternal end medially, articulating with the lateral margin of the manubrium of the sternum, and an acromial end laterally, articulating with the acromion of the scapula. The clavicles and their articulations with the manubrium are shown on Figure 4-1.

LUNGS

With appropriate windowing all structures in the thorax can be visualized on CT images, but not simultaneously. The contrast range and levels to visualize the lung tissue would not be adequate for the structures in the mediastinum and vice versa.

The bilateral lungs and the circulatory system are involved in providing the body with **oxygen** and the elimination of **carbon dioxide**. The lungs, as shown on Figure 4-2, rest on the dome-shaped muscle separating the thorax from the abdomen, the **diaphragm**. Compression by the liver makes the right lung shorter than the left lung. Fissures divide the right lung into three lobes, and the left

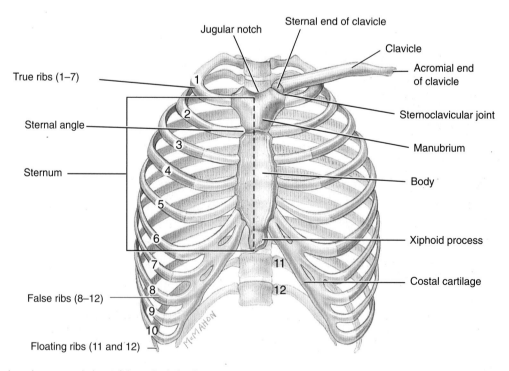

Figure 4-1 Anterior external view of thoracic skeletal structures

into only two, allowing space for the heart. There are further subdivisions of each lobe of the lung into segments, lobules, alveolar sacs, and finally **alveoli**. An alveolus is a tiny air sac where the incoming oxygen and outgoing carbon dioxide are temporarily stored. The superior, more pointed aspect of each lung is the **apex**, and the broader, dome-shaped, inferior portion is the base. Both lungs are enveloped by a vacuum-tight lining, the **pleura**, which folds inward, forming two layers. The inner layer in direct contact with the lung tissue is the **visceral** layer, and the outer layer in contact with the ribs is the **parietal** layer.

Located along the medial surface of each lung is a concave indentation, the **hilum**, with the left hilum slightly superior to the right. Entering and exiting the hilum are the airway structures, blood vessels, nerves, and lymphatic vessels, collectively referred to as the **root of the lung**. On the medial surface of the left lung is also found a larger concavity, the **cardiac notch**, accommodating the heart. The focus of this book is on the mediastinum, the region situated between the right and left lungs. Structures contained in the mediastinum include the heart, great vessels entering and exiting the heart, thymus, trachea, and esophagus.

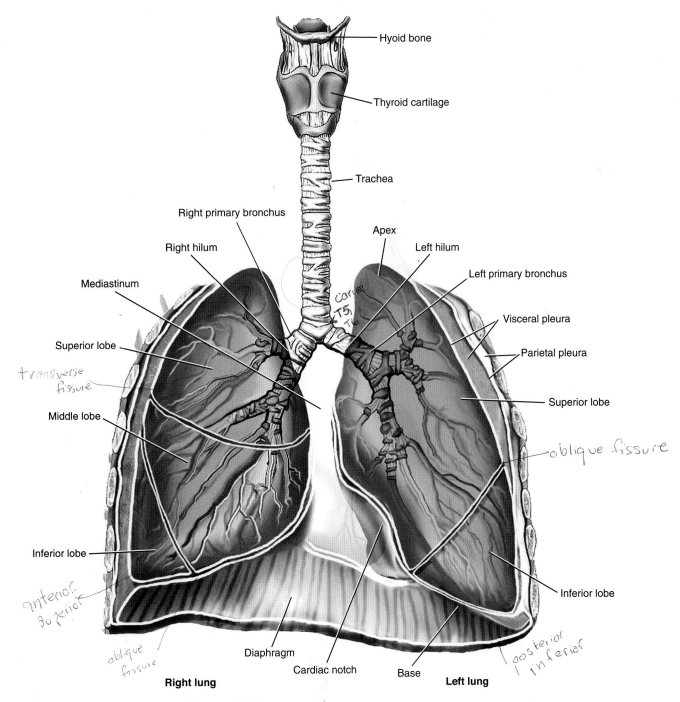

Figure 4-2 Anterior external view of right and left lungs

HEART

Put your right hand in a fist and you have the approximate shape and size of your heart. Place your fist so that the thumb is pointing toward your head at approximately a 45-degree angle to the right and heading in a posterior direction. This simulated upper surface of the heart is called the **base**. The inferior portion that projects anteriorly and to the left is called the apex, as labeled on Figure 4-3.

The heart is the organ responsible for circulating all the blood in the body. There are two major distributions, the **pulmonary** and **systemic circulation**. Pulmonary circulation involves all blood going from the heart to the lungs and the return route. Systemic circulation involves all blood going from the heart to the entire body and the return route.

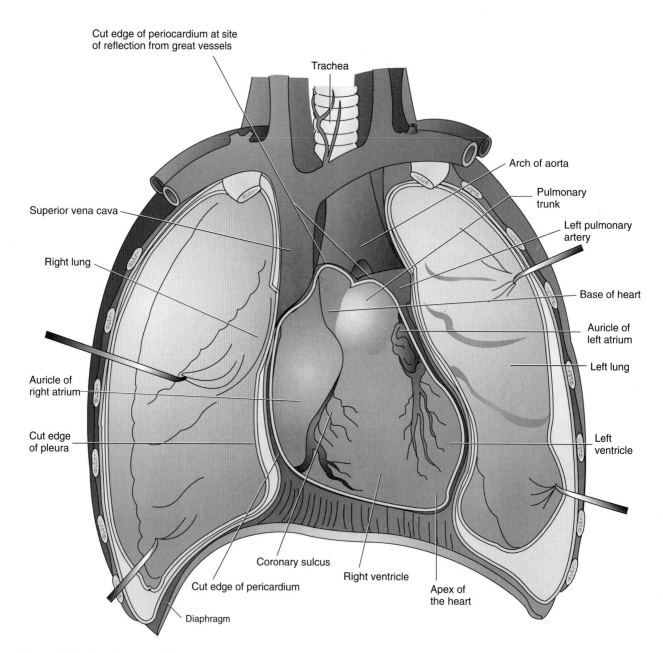

Figure 4-3 Anterior external view of the heart situated in the mediastinum

Linings

The heart is encased in a sac or lining, with the opening of the sac adhering to the great vessels entering and exiting the heart. This lining, the **pericardium**, drawn on Figure 4-4, is composed of two layers: the outermost layer or **fibrous pericardium** and the innermost layer or **serous pericardium**. The serous pericardium itself has two layers, the external parietal layer and the internal visceral layer. The visceral layer, or the **epicardium**, is in direct contact with the actual heart muscle itself, the **myocardium**. The **endocardium** lines the inside of the heart.

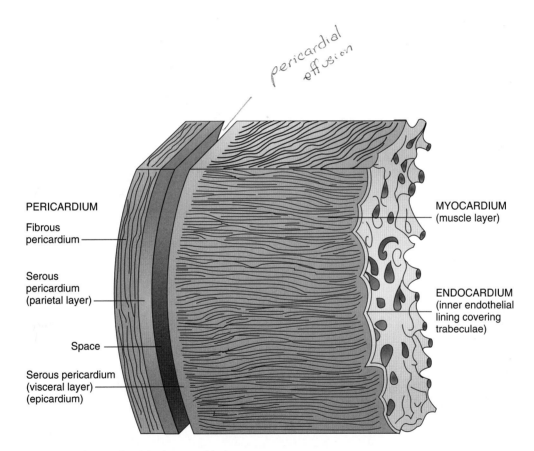

Figure 4-4 Cross-section of the walls of the heart and its layers

Chambers

The heart, as shown on Figure 4-5, is subdivided into four chambers, the two upper **atria**, and two lower **ventricles**. Septa separate the right chambers from the left chambers and act as a barrier, preventing blood exchange. The **interatrial septum** is between the right and left atria, and the **interventricular septum** is between the right and left ventricles. In the fetus an opening exists in the interatrial septum, the **foramen ovale**. The atria receive incoming blood while the ventricles pump blood. Consequently the heart muscle is typically thicker in the lower chambers because it works harder. In particular, the left ventricle must provide the most exertion and thus has the thickest walls.

Of the four chambers, the right ventricle is the most anterior, and the left atrium is the most posterior chamber. A rough configuration of all four chambers as seen on axial images is drawn on Figure 4-6. Because the heart sits obliquely in the mediastinum, transverse cuts at some levels demonstrate both upper and lower chambers.

Valves

Associated with the heart are numerous **valves** that, if functioning properly, prevent backflow of blood. The **tricuspid valve** is located between the right atrium and right ventricle and the **bicuspid** or **mitral valve** is found between the left atrium and left ventricle. Both can generically be termed **atrioventricular valves** and are seen on

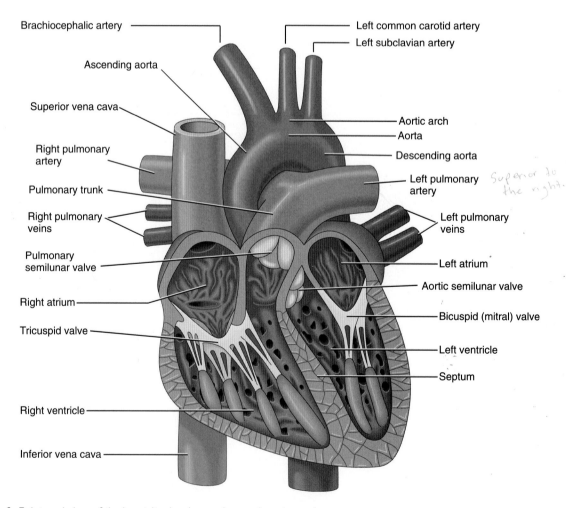

Figure 4-5 Internal view of the heart, its chambers, valves, and great vessels

Figure 4-5. The **semilunar** valves, situated where vessels enter and exit the heart, are discussed with the associated vessels.

Great Vessels

Numerous vessels enter and exit the heart, and are those previously referred to as the great vessels. Figure 4-5 assists in identifying them.

Entering

There are three significant vessels entering the right atrium of the heart, all carrying deoxygenated blood. The one bringing in blood from the heart itself is the **coronary sinus**. The valve situated at its point of entry is the **thebesian valve**. The **superior vena cava (SVC)** returns all blood from above the level of the heart to the right atrium and the **inferior vena cava (IVC)** brings in blood from below the level of the heart. The blood then passes from the right atrium through the tricuspid valve into the right ventricle.

Those vessels entering the left atrium include the two right and two left **pulmonary veins**. These veins return freshly oxygenated blood from the lungs. From the left atrium the blood flows through the bicuspid or mitral valve into the left ventricle.

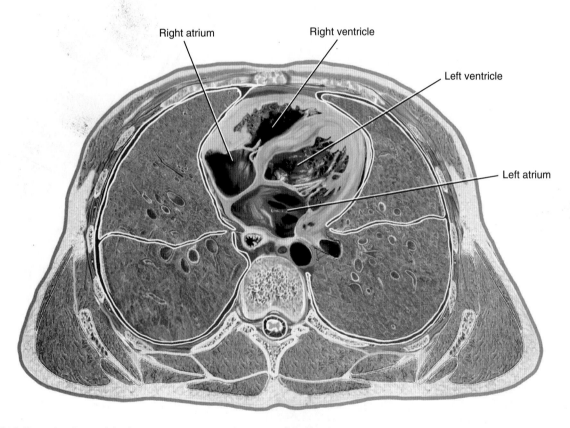

Figure 4-6 Four chambers of the heart as seen on a transverse sectional image

Exiting

The great vessel exiting the superior aspect of the right ventricle is the **pulmonary trunk**, with the blood first passing through the **pulmonary semilunar valve**. The pulmonary trunk bifurcates into the right and left **pulmonary arteries**, transporting deoxygenated blood to the right and left lungs. The pulmonary arteries are the only arteries in the adult human body carrying deoxygenated blood. In the lungs the arteries branch into smaller and smaller branches, ending as **capillaries**. These capillaries surround the alveoli in the lungs (see Figure 4-7). Diffusion occurs with carbon dioxide transferred from the cap-

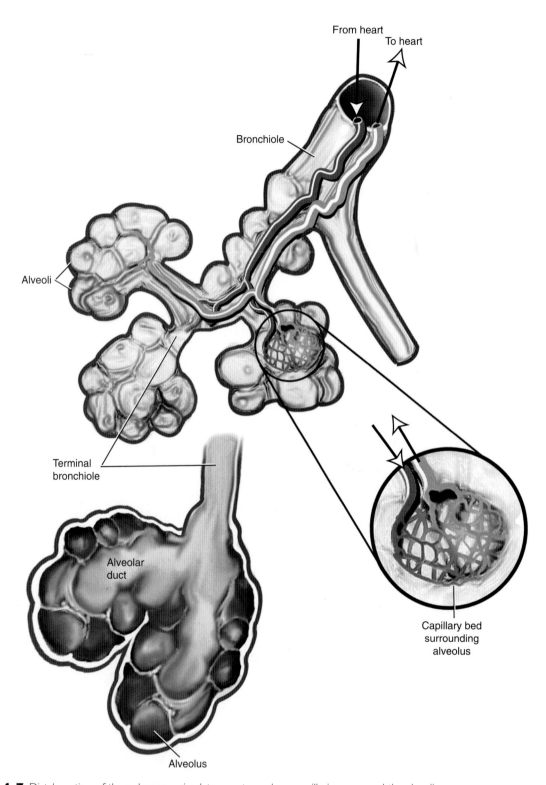

Figure 4-7 Distal portion of the pulmonary circulatory system where capillaries surround the alveoli

illaries into the alveoli and oxygen entering the capillaries from the alveoli. The capillaries then merge into venules and finally into the pulmonary veins, returning the freshly oxygenated blood to the left atrium. This circuit, beginning with the pulmonary trunk and ending with the pulmonary veins, is pulmonary circulation, and is the source of freshly oxygenated blood for the entire body.

The great vessel exiting the superior aspect of the left ventricle via the **aortic semilunar valve** is the **aorta**. The aorta is the largest vessel in the body. The **coronary arteries**, immediate branches off the originating aorta, provide the heart itself with freshly oxygenated blood. The aorta continues in a superior direction, this portion being termed the **ascending aorta**. The ascending aorta is found central to the four chambers of the heart, a notable point when studying axial sectional images. The aorta distributes oxygenated blood to the entire body and ultimately makes its return route to the heart by way of the superior and inferior vena cava, a circuit known as the systemic circulation. The demand on the left ventricle to apply enough force for this far-reaching distribution accounts for the thickness of the myocardium of this chamber.

Blood Flow of the Heart

A review of the blood flow of the heart finds deoxygenated blood entering the right atrium via the superior vena cava, inferior vena cava, and coronary sinus. From the right atrium the blood enters the right ventricle through the tricuspid valve and then exits the right ventricle through the pulmonary semilunar valve into the pulmonary trunk. The pulmonary trunk divides into the right and left pulmonary arteries and the deoxygenated blood is delivered to the right and left lungs, where the carbon dioxide is given off and oxygen picked up. The oxygen-rich blood starts the return route to the heart by way of the right and left pulmonary veins. Once there it enters the left atrium and then passes through the bicuspid or mitral valve into the left ventricle. Finally, the freshly oxygenated blood exits through the aortic semilunar valve into the ascending aorta where the systemic circulation commences. Review this pathway on Figure 4-8.

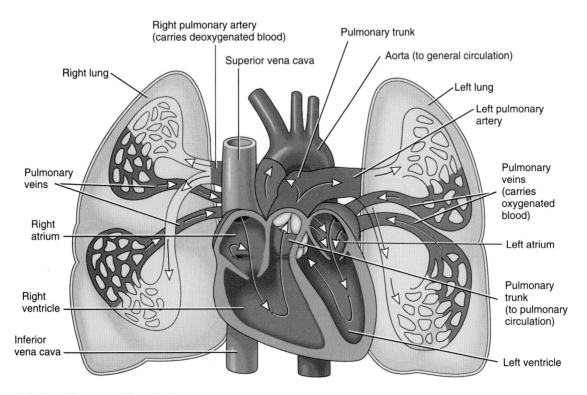

Figure 4-8 Blood flow to and from the heart

BLOOD VESSELS

Vessels involved in forming the IVC and SVC, along with the other great vessels and many of their branches are visible on sectional images.

Superior Vena Cava

The bilateral external jugular veins of the head drain into the right and left subclavian veins, which carries deoxygenated blood from the arms. The subclavian veins then join with the internal jugular veins of the head to form the right and left **brachiocephalic** or innominate **veins**. In the upper thorax the left brachiocephalic vein sweeps over to the right to meet the right brachiocephalic vein, forming the superior vena cava. The sweep is apparent on axial images above the level of the heart. The newly formed superior vena cava is found on the right, and appears smaller than the aorta. As the superior vena cava drains into the superior aspect of the right atrium, axial images at the level of, or below the right atrium do not demonstrate the SVC.

Inferior Vena Cava

The inferior vena cava, draining most of the blood from below the level of the heart into the right atrium, originates in the lower pelvic cavity at approximately L5 with the merger of the right and left **common iliac veins**. The IVC enters the inferior aspect of the right atrium so is often not seen on axial images of the chest arranged in descending order until almost below the level of the heart. Figure 4-9 shows the formation of the superior vena cava and inferior vena cava.

Pulmonary Trunk

Also seen above the level of the heart is the bifurcation of the pulmonary trunk into the right and left pulmonary arteries. The three vessels take on the appearance of an inverted Y with the right pulmonary artery seen posterior to the superior vena cava and ascending aorta as drawn on Figure 4-5. The left pulmonary artery is slightly superior to the right.

Pulmonary Veins

The right and left pulmonary veins, also labeled on Figure 4-5, are a continuation of the pulmonary circuit leaving the right and left lungs. Vessels seen entering the left atrium on axial sectional images are either the right or left pulmonary veins. Compared to other structures composing the root of the lung, the pulmonary veins exit the lungs at a slightly lower level.

Aorta

The aorta, as stated, provides the entire body with oxygenated blood. Once the aorta leaves the left ventricle three main sections are identified: the ascending aorta, the arch of the aorta, and the **descending aorta**.

Ascending Aorta

The ascending aorta, the segment with the greatest diameter, has an immediate branch at the root, the aortic sinus. The aortic sinus gives rise to the right and left coronary arteries. At approximately the level of the sternal angle the ascending aorta sweeps to the left and in a posterior direction. This sweep is the arch of the aorta.

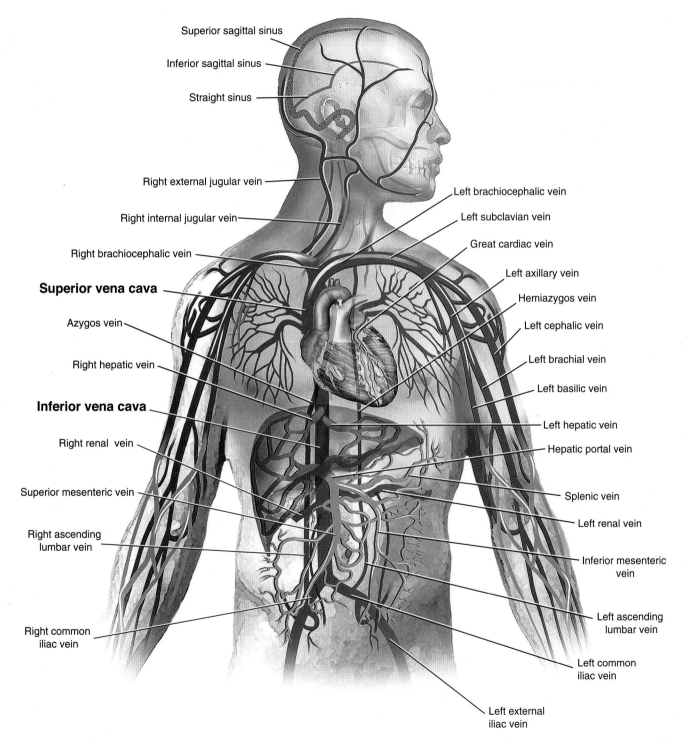

Figure 4-9 Formation of the SVC and IVC

Arch of the Aorta

In previous chapters we encountered the branches off the arch of the aorta. They included the right brachiocephalic artery, the left common carotid artery, and the left subclavian artery, in that order. At a higher level the three branches of the arch of the aorta are centered between the right and left brachiocephalic veins. The configuration is shown on Figure 4-10. Before it becomes the right subclavian artery, the brachiocephalic artery has a branch heading in a superior direction, the right common carotid artery. Thus, if four vessels are seen on axial cuts in addition to the right and left brachiocephalic veins, they can be identified as the right subclavian artery, right common carotid artery, left common carotid artery, and left subclavian artery. Reviewing Chapter 1 will remind you that the right and left common carotid arteries ultimately supply the anterior and middle portions of the brain with blood.

The bilateral vertebral arteries, branches heading in a superior direction off the right and left subclavian arteries, ultimately supply the posterior aspect of the brain with blood. On descending axial CT images of the mediastinum, the branches off the arch are seen first along with the brachiocephalic veins. Then the arch of the aorta appears at approximately the same level that the left brachiocephalic vein is seen running transversely to join the right brachiocephalic vein, prior to forming the SVC. The arch of the aorta then begins its downward descent to become the descending aorta.

Descending Aorta

Having turned 180 degrees from the originating ascending aorta, the descending aorta is now seen more on the left and much more posteriorly. It can be found just slightly to the left of and anterior to the spine. The cir-

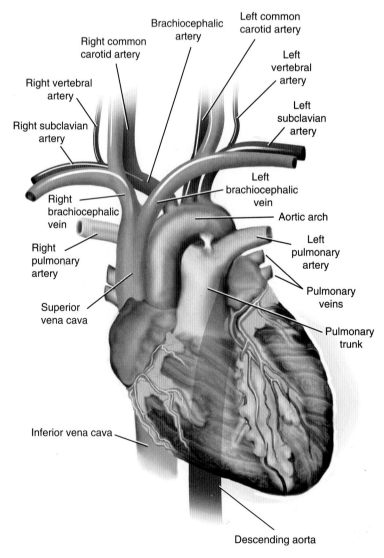

Figure 4-10 Anterior external view of the vessels arising from the arch of the aorta

cumference of the descending aorta is smaller than the ascending aorta. The descending aorta acquires names determined by the region through which it is passing: the **thoracic** and the **abdominal descending aorta**. Eventually the descending aorta will bifurcate in the pelvic region to become the right and left **common iliac arteries**.

Azygos/Hemiazygos Veins

In a preceding section the statement was made that the inferior vena cava drained *most* of the blood from below the level of the heart. Some blood drains through an alternate route. Refer to Figure 4-9 and you will see that there are small branches off the right and left common iliac veins, the right and left **ascending lumbar veins**, which continue as the **azygos vein** on the right and the **hemiazygos vein** on the left. Eventually the hemiazygos vein joins the azygos vein at approximately T7–T9. The azygos vein is often seen on axial CT images in the region of the thorax as a small vessel anterior and to the right of the vertebrae. Just below the level of the arch of the aorta the azygos vein abruptly swings forward (the **arch of the azygos**) to empty into the superior vena cava.

THYMUS

The **thymus**, pictured on Figure 4-11, is part of the endocrine system, producing a number of hormones, all of which are involved in the maturation of T cells. T cells are a type of white blood cell essential to the immune system. The thymus is quite large in infants but after puberty tends to atrophy in size. It is found immediately behind the manubrium, the superior portion of the sternum. Because it tends to decrease in size with age, it is more apparent on axial sectional images of younger patients.

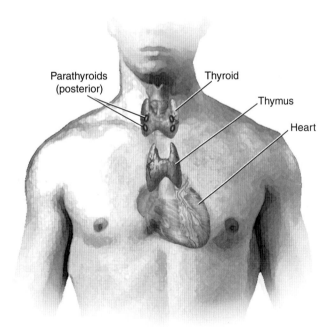

Figure 4-11 The location of the thymus in the chest

TRACHEA

Referring back to Chapter 3, recall that the trachea, along with the esophagus, originated from the pharynx at the inferior aspect of the larynx. The trachea is located anterior to the esophagus, posterior to the superior vena cava and ascending aorta, and anterior to the vertebrae. It eventually bifurcates into the right and left primary **bronchi** at approximately T4/T5, or the same level as the sternal angle. The **carina**, the ridge at the point of this bifurcation, is posterior to the right pulmonary artery. The right and left primary bronchi enter into the hilum of the right and left lungs, respectively. The right primary bronchus is wider and more vertical than the left, making the right lung more susceptible to aspiration of foreign bodies. The primary bronchi are seen as linear areas of lucency running transversely on axial CT images at approximately the same level as the split of the pulmonary trunk into the right and left pulmonary arteries. This is not a coincidence but

explained by the fact that both are involved in forming the root of the lung. Like an inverted tree, each primary bronchus gives rise to secondary bronchi, one for each lobe of the lung. The branching process continues until the smallest airways reach the alveoli. The root of each of the lungs is found above the level of the heart but below the level of the arch of the aorta, so other structures seen on axial images at this level include the superior vena cava, and ascending and descending aorta. Refer to Figure 4-12.

ESOPHAGUS

Also shown on Figure 4-12 is the other division arising from the distal pharynx, the esophagus, which is posterior to the trachea but may be seen either slightly to the left or right. Occasionally on axial images, it contains a bleb of air. Otherwise, it is identified as a small area of opacity between the vertebral bodies and trachea.

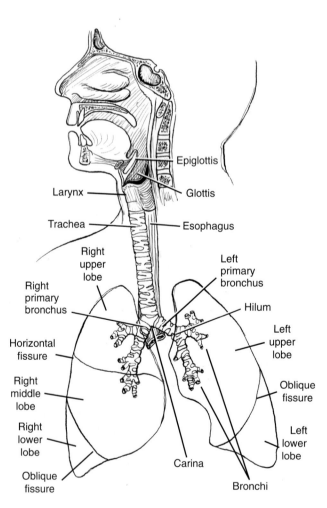

Figure 4-12 Slightly oblique view of the trachea, bronchi, and esophagus

CHAPTER 4 | Thorax **137**

A quick review of the order of appearance of structures in the mediastinum on axial images presented in descending order is listed below:

1. The right and left brachiocephalic veins flank the three vessels arising from the arch of the aorta: the right brachiocephalic artery, left common carotid artery, and left subclavian artery. These last three vessels assume the shape of the arch with the right brachiocephalic artery located on the right.

2. The arch of the aorta sweeps from the right to the left and in a posterior direction. Anterior to the arch of the aorta, the left brachiocephalic vein passes transversely to the right to join with the right brachiocephalic vein.

3. Next appear the ascending and descending aorta, and superior vena cava.

4. Following this the pulmonary trunk is seen with its two branches, the right and left pulmonary arteries, along with the split of the trachea at the carina into the right and left bronchi.

5. The superior chambers of the heart, the right and left atria, then appear.

6. All four chambers of the heart with the ascending aorta central to the chambers become evident. The descending aorta, anterior and slightly to the left of the vertebral column, can be identified. The superior vena cava disappears once the right atrium presents itself.

7. The ascending aorta is no longer apparent. The atria, the first chambers of the heart to appear, are the first to disappear. The inferior vena cava appears.

8. The right hemidiaphragm and liver appear.

CT IMAGES

Exam 1

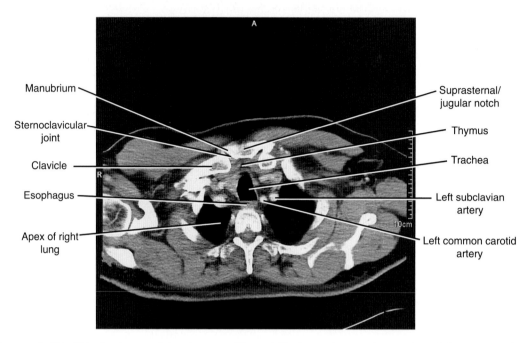

Figure 4-13   This first image of the thorax on Figure 4-13 shows the superior portion of the sternum, the manubrium, and its articulation with the clavicles, the sternoclavicular (SC) joints. The thymus is located posterior to the manubrium. The trachea is anterior to the esophagus. The upper portion of the lungs, the apex, is identified. The arteries supplying the head and upper extremities are evident.

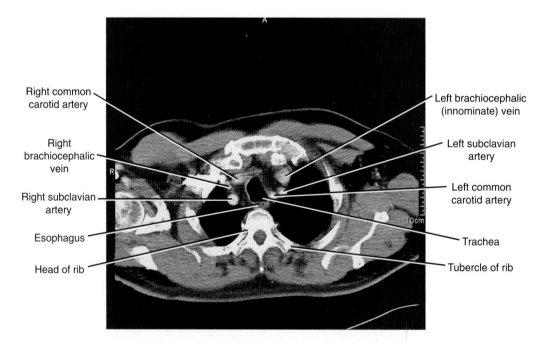

Figure 4-14   On Figure 4-14, the brachiocephalic or innominate veins become more obvious. These veins drain the upper extremities; draining into them is the deoxygenated blood from the head.

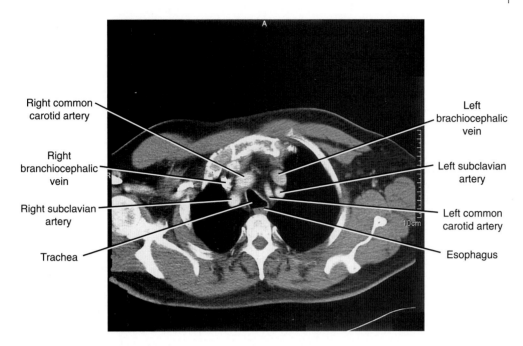

Right common carotid artery

Right branchiocephalic vein

Right subclavian artery

Trachea

Left brachiocephalic vein

Left subclavian artery

Left common carotid artery

Esophagus

Figure 4-15 Branches of the right brachiocephalic artery, the right subclavian and right common carotid arteries, are labeled on Figure 4-15.

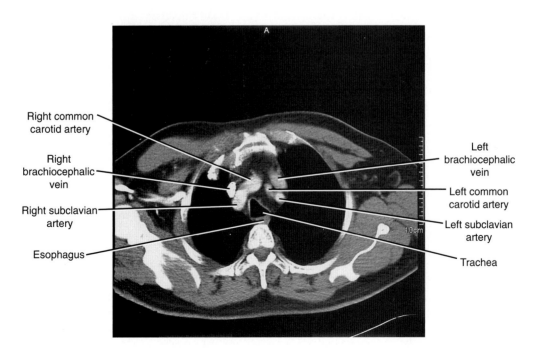

Right common carotid artery

Right brachiocephalic vein

Right subclavian artery

Esophagus

Left brachiocephalic vein

Left common carotid artery

Left subclavian artery

Trachea

Figure 4-16 On Figure 4-16, the two branches of the right brachiocephalic artery, the right subclavian and right common carotid arteries, are becoming indistinct. The left brachiocephalic vein is starting to arch across to the right where it will meet with the right brachiocephalic vein to form the superior vena cava (SVC).

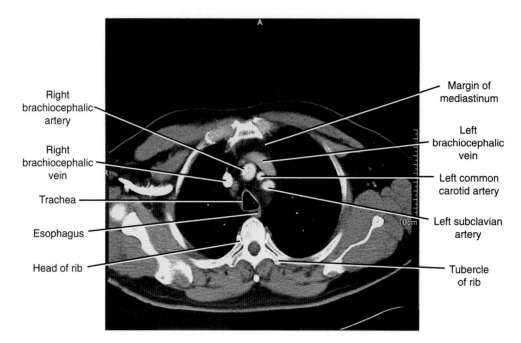

Figure 4-17   The left brachiocephalic vein continues to swing to the right on Figure 4-17. The three major branches off the arch of the aorta are distinctly seen in the order they appear: the right brachiocephalic, left common carotid, and left subclavian arteries.

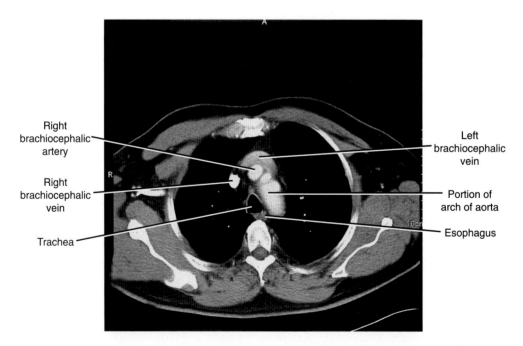

Figure 4-18   The merger of the right and left brachiocephalic veins is almost complete on Figure 4-18. The only branch off the arch of the aorta clearly identifiable is the right brachiocephalic artery as the arch of the aorta is starting to appear.

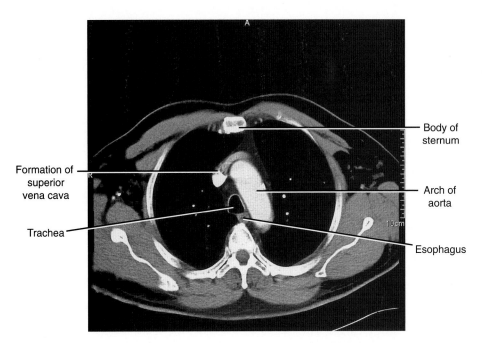

Figure 4-19 The formation of the SVC is nearing completion on Figure 4-19. The arch of the aorta, sweeping from the right to the left and in a posterior direction, is clearly visible. The esophagus is still seen posterior to the trachea but seems slightly off center to the trachea, which is not uncommon.

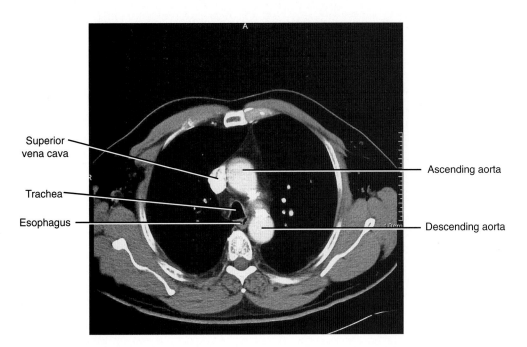

Figure 4-20 On Figure 4-20, the SVC is fully formed. Starting to appear is the ascending aorta, the start of the arch of the aorta, along with the descending aorta, seen slightly anterior and to the left of the vertebra.

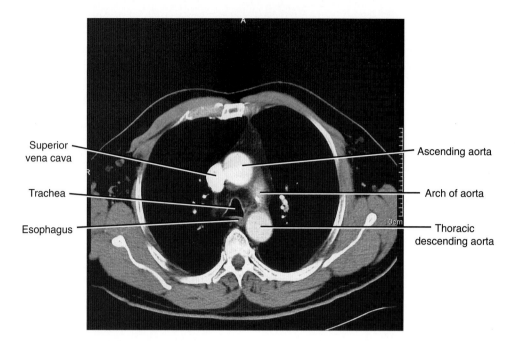

Figure 4-21   The superior vena cava is seen to the right of the ascending aorta on Figure 4-21. Notice the thoracic descending aorta. It will continue to be seen through the thorax until it penetrates the diaphragm, where it will then be termed the abdominal descending aorta. The remnants of the arch of the aorta are barely visible.

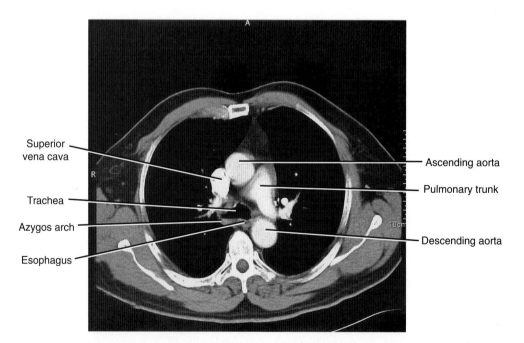

Figure 4-22   On Figure 4-22, the vessel arising from the right ventricle, the pulmonary trunk, appears. It branches into the right and left pulmonary arteries and is the beginning of the pulmonary circulation. Notice the trachea starting to stretch out. It will soon be bifurcating. The azygos vein is seen sweeping anteriorly via the azygos arch where it empties into the superior vena cava.

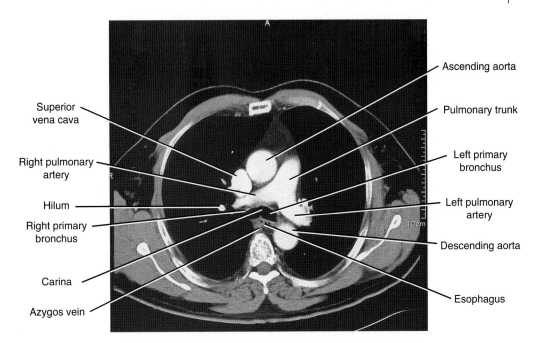

Figure 4-23 The pulmonary trunk, along with the right and left pulmonary arteries, is clearly seen on Figure 4-23. Also evident are the right and left primary bronchi, a result of the bifurcation of the trachea. The point where the division occurs is the carina. Both the pulmonary arteries and primary bronchi are seen on the same plane as they enter the lung at the same point, the hilum. The collection of structures entering and exiting the lungs is called the root of the lung. The azygos vein is seen anterior to the vertebra.

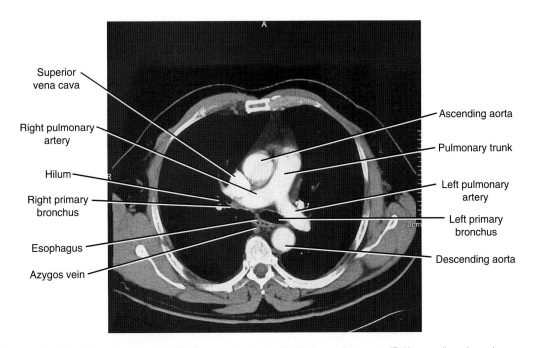

Figure 4-24 Still apparent are the SVC, ascending aorta (AA), descending aorta (DA), as well as the pulmonary trunk and its branches, the right and left pulmonary arteries on Figure 4-24. The right and left primary bronchi are labeled. The esophagus, containing a bleb of air, is labeled, and will continue to be seen through the length of the thorax. It will eventually penetrate the diaphragm, terminating in the stomach.

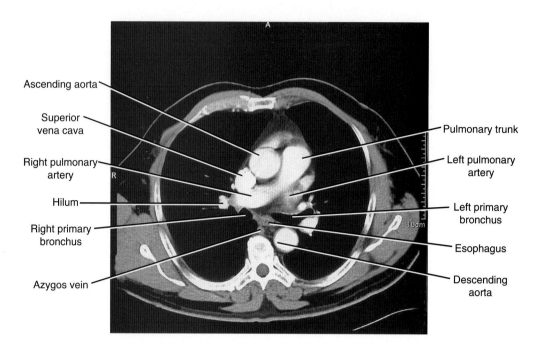

Ascending aorta
Superior vena cava
Right pulmonary artery
Hilum
Right primary bronchus
Azygos vein

Pulmonary trunk
Left pulmonary artery
Left primary bronchus
Esophagus
Descending aorta

Figure 4-25   On Figure 4-25, the pulmonary arteries are entering the lungs at the hila. Once in the lungs they will eventually branch into smaller and smaller vessels, ultimately surrounding the alveoli where diffusion of blood gases will occur.

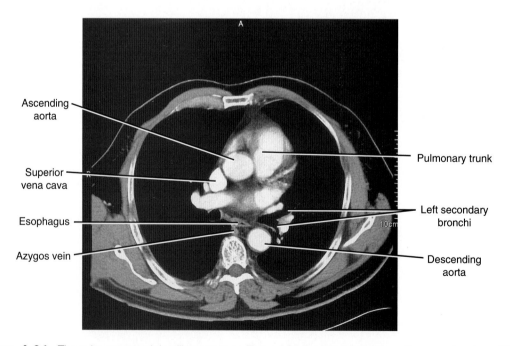

Ascending aorta
Superior vena cava
Esophagus
Azygos vein

Pulmonary trunk
Left secondary bronchi
Descending aorta

Figure 4-26   The pulmonary trunk is still apparent on Figure 4-26. Seen at this level are the secondary bronchi on the left. There is one secondary bronchi associated with each lobe of the lungs.

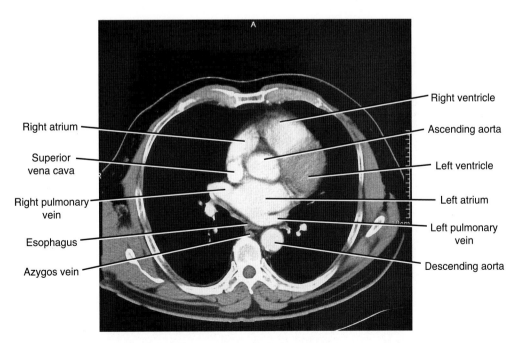

Right atrium
Ascending aorta
Superior
vena cava
Right pulmonary
vein
Esophagus
Azygos vein

Left atrium
Left pulmonary
vein
Descending aorta

Figure 4-27 On Figure 4-27, the superior chambers of the heart, the right and left atria, are taking shape.

Right atrium
Superior
vena cava
Right pulmonary
vein
Esophagus
Azygos vein

Right ventricle
Ascending aorta
Left ventricle
Left atrium
Left pulmonary
vein
Descending aorta

Figure 4-28 The right and left pulmonary veins drain into the left atrium on Figure 4-28. The superior vena cava drains into the superior aspect of the right atrium. Both are apparent on this image. Also starting to appear are the right and left ventricles. As the heart sits obliquely in the mediastinum, it is possible at times to see both the upper and lower chambers of the heart.

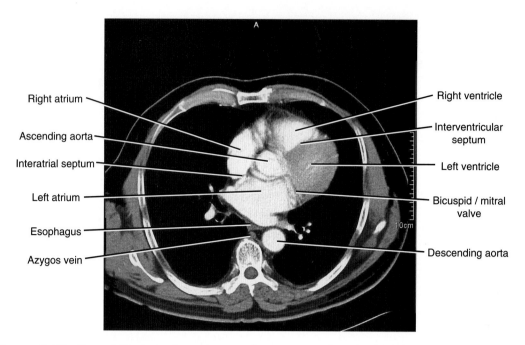

Figure 4-29 Figure 4-29 clearly shows the ascending aorta central to the four chambers of the heart. The interatrial septum and interventricular septum separate the right and left atria and ventricles, respectively. The right ventricle is seen most anteriorly and the left atrium most posteriorly. The valve between the left atrium and left ventricle, the bicuspid or mitral valve, appears to be closed.

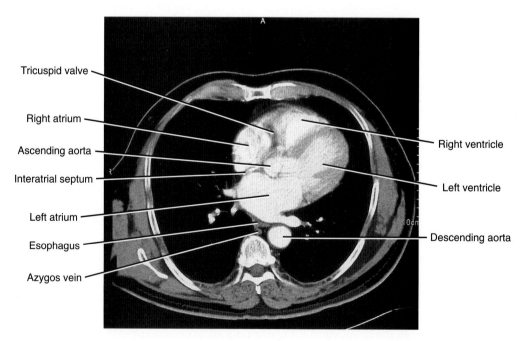

Figure 4-30 The ascending aorta appears to be diminishing in size on Figure 4-30. The septum separating the atria is distinct. In this image, the tricuspid valve found between the right atrium and right ventricle appears to be closed.

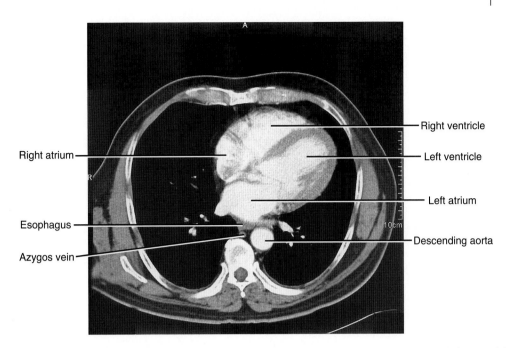

Right ventricle

Left ventricle

Right atrium

Left atrium

Esophagus

Descending aorta

Azygos vein

Figure 4-31 On Figure 4-31, the right atrium appears to be disappearing; this is not unusual as it is one of the two superior chambers of the heart.

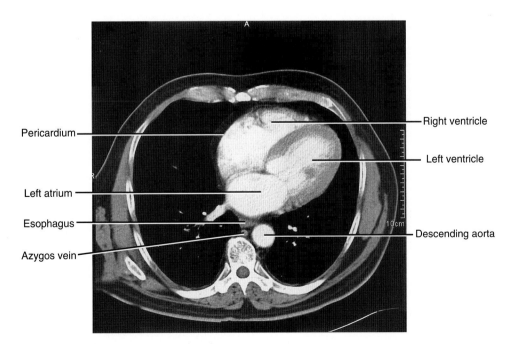

Right ventricle

Pericardium

Left ventricle

Left atrium

Esophagus

Descending aorta

Azygos vein

Figure 4-32 On Figure 4-32, only three chambers of the heart remain, the right and left ventricles and the left atrium. The pericardium, surrounding the heart, can be identified.

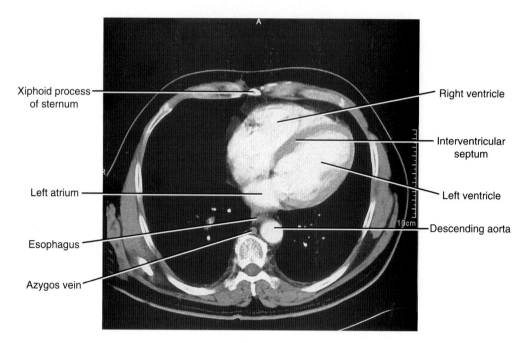

Figure 4-33 The left atrium is also starting to disappear on Figure 4-33; again, this is not unusual as the atria are the superior chambers of the heart.

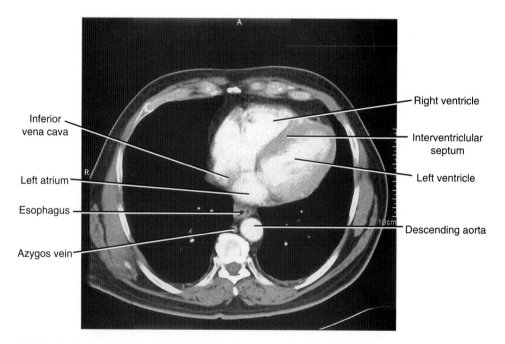

Figure 4-34 Starting to appear on Figure 4-34 is the inferior vena cava, which drains almost all the deoxygenated blood from below the level of the heart. It empties into the inferior aspect of the right atrium.

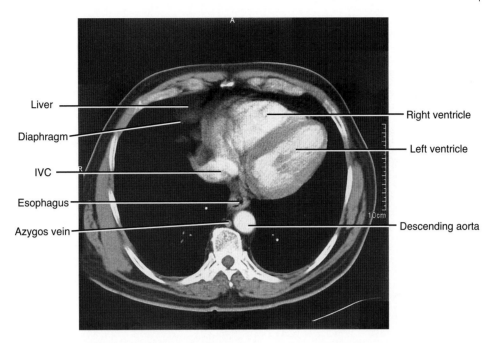

Liver
Diaphragm
IVC
Esophagus
Azygos vein

Right ventricle
Left ventricle
Descending aorta

Figure 4-35 On Figure 4-35, the only chambers of the heart still visible are the two ventricles. The IVC is seen, along with the superior aspect of the liver on the right side, which is an indication that this slice is at the level of a portion of the diaphragm. The diaphragm is a dome-shaped muscle so abdominal organs will appear gradually as we slice down. The liver is the largest organ in the body and, as a result, pushes up the right hemidiaphragm. This explains why the right lung is shorter than the left, despite having three lobes as compared to the left lung, which has only two.

Exam 2

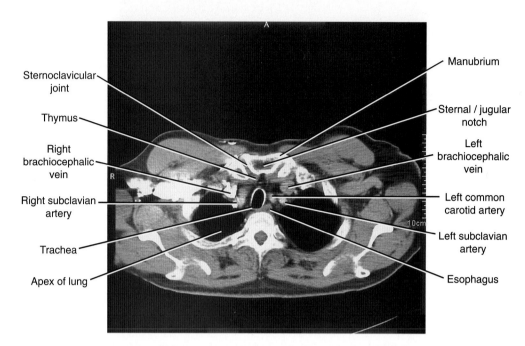

Figure 4-36   The first image of the second study selected (Figure 4-36) shows the upper portion of the sternum, the manubrium, behind which lies the thymus. The right subclavian artery, a continuation of the right brachiocephalic artery, is demonstrated. Both brachiocephalic veins, right and left, flank the arteries off the arch of the aorta.

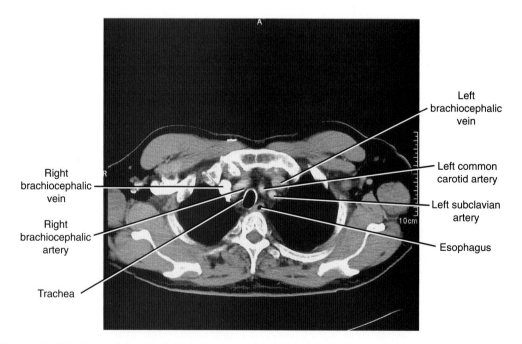

Figure 4-37   Some of the vessels arising from the arch of the aorta are identified on Figure 4-37: the right brachiocephalic, left common carotid, and left subclavian arteries. The esophagus is seen posterior and slightly to the left of the trachea.

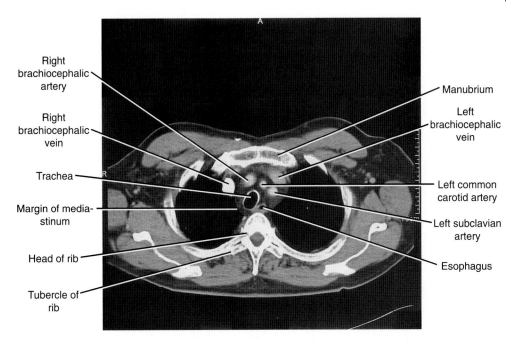

Right
brachiocephalic
artery

Right
brachiocephalic
vein

Trachea

Margin of media-
stinum

Head of rib

Tubercle of
rib

Manubrium

Left
brachiocephalic
vein

Left common
carotid artery

Left subclavian
artery

Esophagus

Figure 4-38 On Figure 4-38, the left brachiocephalic vein is starting to sweep across to join with the right brachiocephalic vein. They will eventually merge to form the superior vena cava. The three vessels arising from the arch of the aorta are easily identifiable: the right brachiocephalic, left common carotid, and left subclavian arteries. Notice the edge of the mediastinum.

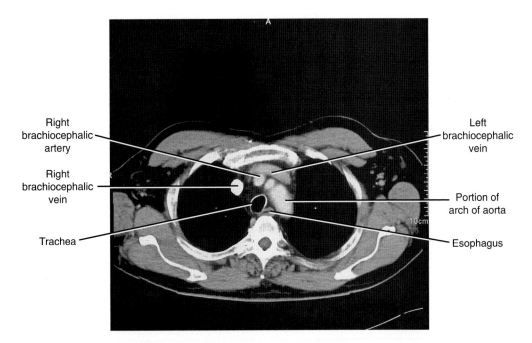

Right
brachiocephalic
artery

Right
brachiocephalic
vein

Trachea

Left
brachiocephalic
vein

Portion of
arch of aorta

Esophagus

Figure 4-39 The left brachiocephalic vein continues to run transversely toward the right brachiocephalic vein on Figure 4-39. Although the right brachiocephalic artery is still identifiable, the other vessels arising from the arch of the aorta are less distinct because the arch is taking shape.

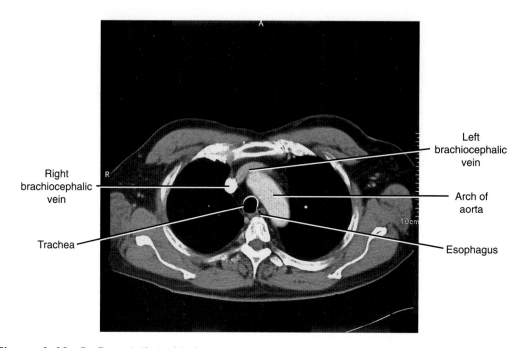

Figure 4-40   On Figure 4-40, the fully formed arch of the aorta is now apparent, while the left brachiocephalic vein moves closer to the right.

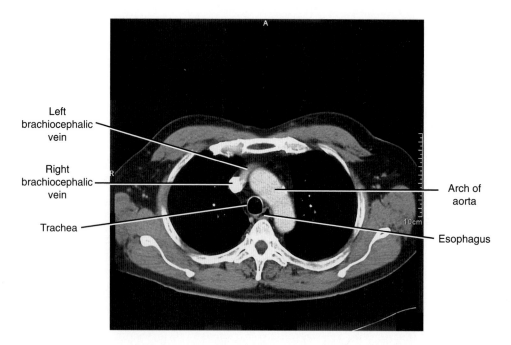

Figure 4-41   The formation of the superior vena cava is almost complete on Figure 4-41. The esophagus is just anterior to the vertebra and posterior to the trachea. The center of the arch of the aorta is seen clearly.

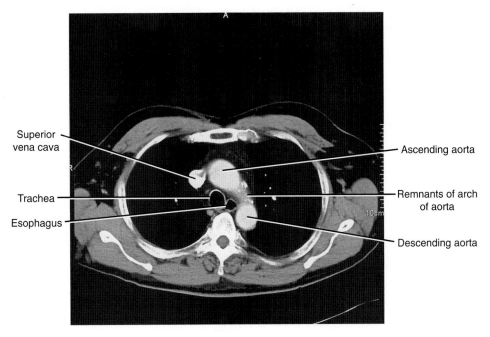

Figure 4-42 As we approach the lower arch of the aorta, the ascending and descending aorta start to take shape on Figure 4-42. The esophagus is seen containing a sizeable amount of air.

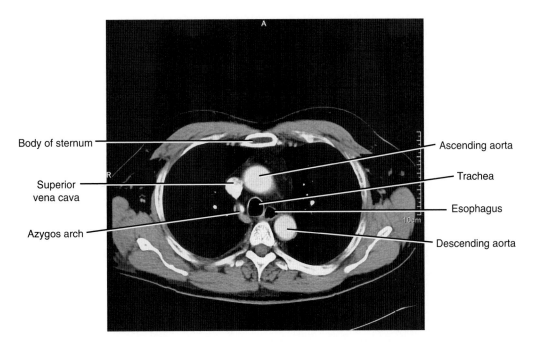

Figure 4-43 On Figure 4-43, the azygos arch empties the azygos vein into the superior vena cava. Three of the great vessels can be identified: the superior vena cava, and the ascending and descending aorta.

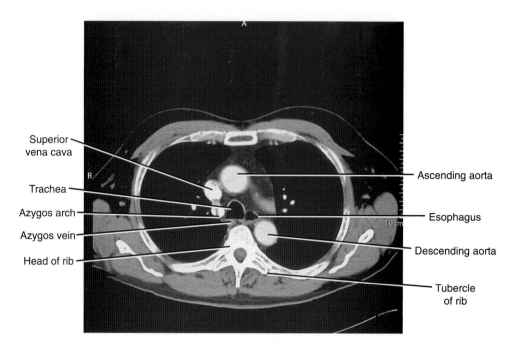

Figure 4-44   The azygos vein is seen along with the azygos arch on Figure 4-44. The esophagus still contains air.

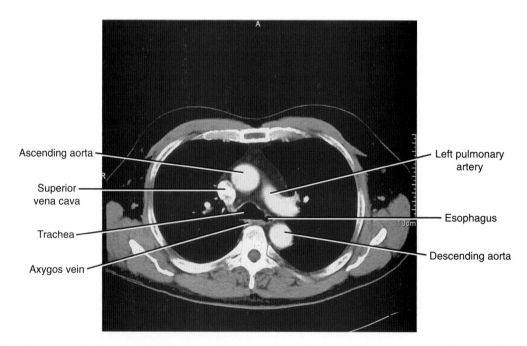

Figure 4-45   On Figure 4-45, the trachea appears to be stretching out in preparation for its bifurcation. The left pulmonary artery is seen anterior to the descending aorta.

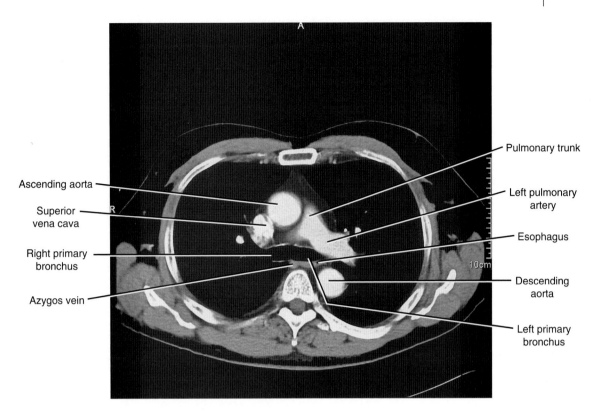

Ascending aorta

Superior
vena cava

Right primary
bronchus

Azygos vein

Pulmonary trunk

Left pulmonary
artery

Esophagus

Descending
aorta

Left primary
bronchus

Figure 4-46 Starting to make its appearance is the pulmonary trunk on Figure 4-46. The trachea has almost completed its bifurcation into the right and left primary bronchi. The azygos vein is seen anterior to the vertebra. The superior vena cava, ascending aorta, and descending aorta are all identified.

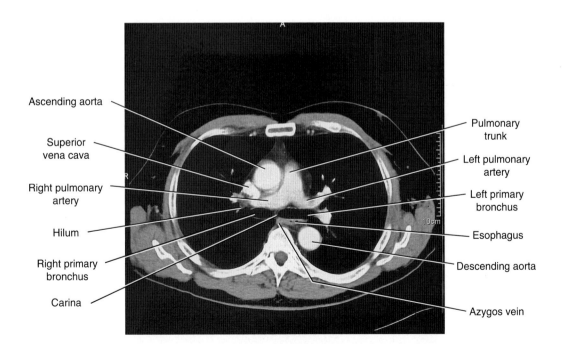

Ascending aorta

Superior
vena cava

Right pulmonary
artery

Hilum

Right primary
bronchus

Carina

Pulmonary
trunk

Left pulmonary
artery

Left primary
bronchus

Esophagus

Descending aorta

Azygos vein

Figure 4-47 The image on Figure 4-47 is definitely at the level of the hilum as both primary bronchi along with the right and left pulmonary arteries are seen. The esophagus is apparent, as is the azygos vein and the carina of the trachea.

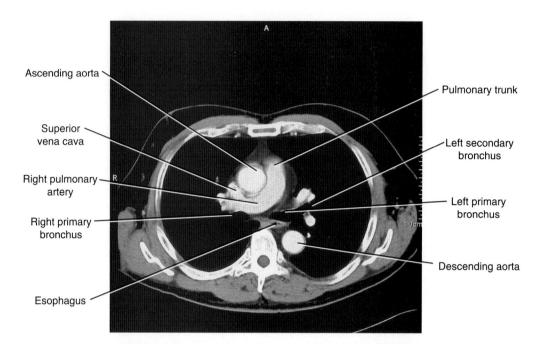

Figure 4-48 The secondary bronchi on the left are discernable on Figure 4-48. There is one secondary bronchus for each lobe of the lung. The pulmonary trunk and right pulmonary artery are still present.

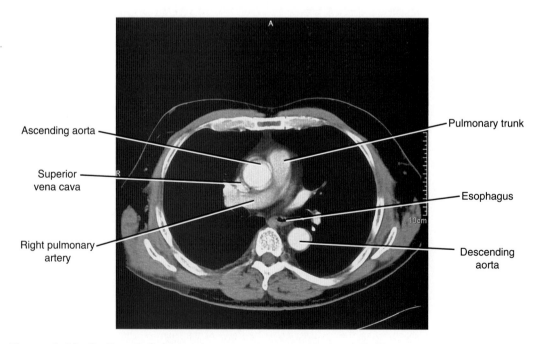

Figure 4-49 On Figure 4-49, the superior vena cava appears to be narrowing. The ascending and descending aorta are in typical locations within the mediastinum.

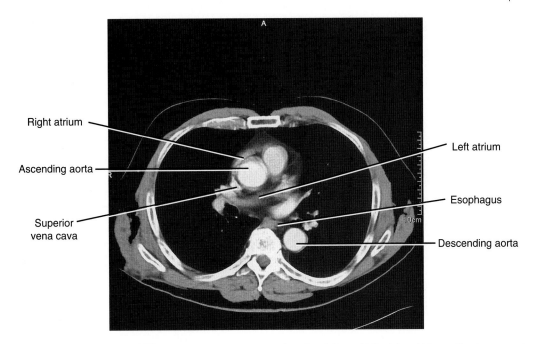

Figure 4-50 On Figure 4-50, new structures are appearing, the right and left atria, which are the two superior heart chambers.

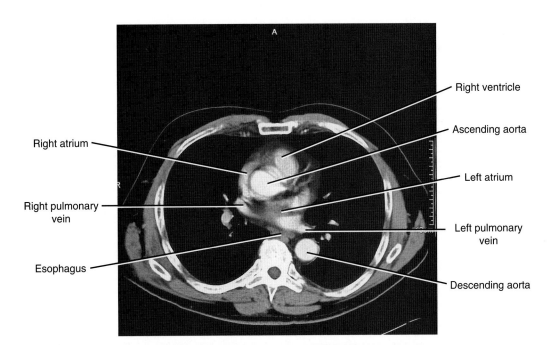

Figure 4-51 The superior vena cava, which drains into the superior aspect of the right atrium, has disappeared with the appearance of the right atrium on Figure 4-51. Draining into the left atrium are the right and left pulmonary veins. The ascending aorta is seen central to the chambers of the heart.

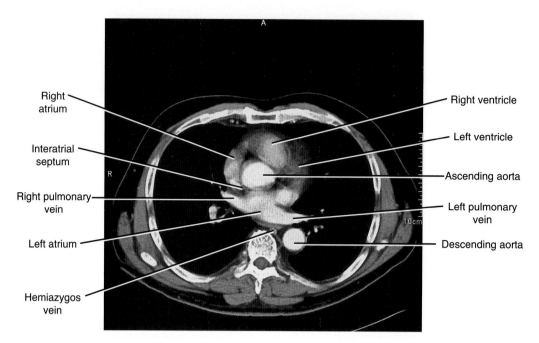

Right
atrium

Interatrial
septum

Right pulmonary
vein

Left atrium

Hemiazygos
vein

Right ventricle

Left ventricle

Ascending aorta

Left pulmonary
vein

Descending aorta

Figure 4-52   The four chambers of the heart are present on Figure 4-52. Because the heart sits obliquely in the mediastinum, upper and lower chambers can be identified on some slices. Notice the hemiazygos vein anterior to the left of the vertebra. The interatrial septum separates the two atria.

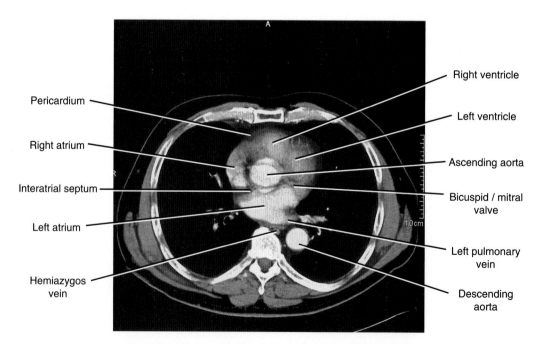

Pericardium

Right atrium

Interatrial septum

Left atrium

Hemiazygos
vein

Right ventricle

Left ventricle

Ascending aorta

Bicuspid / mitral
valve

Left pulmonary
vein

Descending
aorta

Figure 4-53   The pericardium is shown encasing the heart on Figure 4-53. The interatrial septum divides the two upper chambers of the heart. The bicuspid or mitral valve, located between the left atrium and ventricle, appears to be closed.

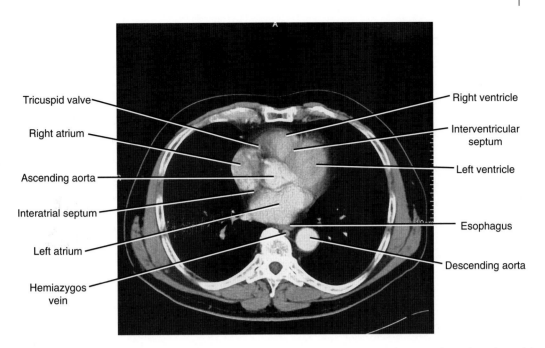

Figure 4-54 On Figure 4-54, the interatrial and interventricular septa are seen between the atria and ventricles, respectively. On this image, the tricuspid valve, connecting the right atrium and ventricle, is seen closed. We continue to see the esophagus and hemiazygos vein, along with the descending aorta.

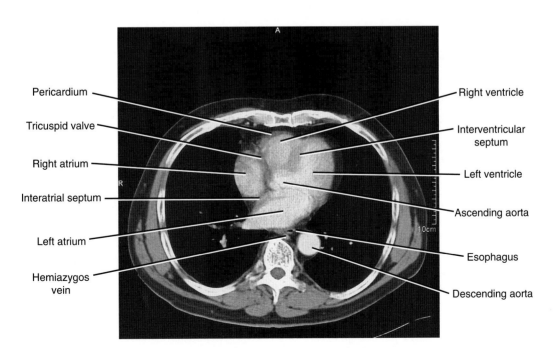

Figure 4-55 On Figure 4-55, again notice the pericardium surrounding the heart. The tricuspid valve still appears closed. Little of the ascending aorta, which arises from the superior aspect of the left ventricle, is seen. The two septa between the atria and ventricles are labeled.

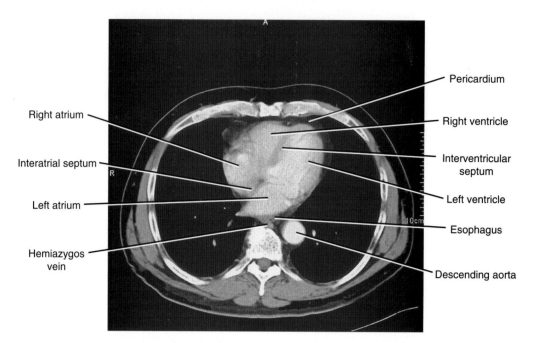

Figure 4-56   The left atrium is diminished in size on Figure 4-56. One of the first chambers to appear, it will be one of the first to disappear. Again we see the interatrial and interventricular septa.

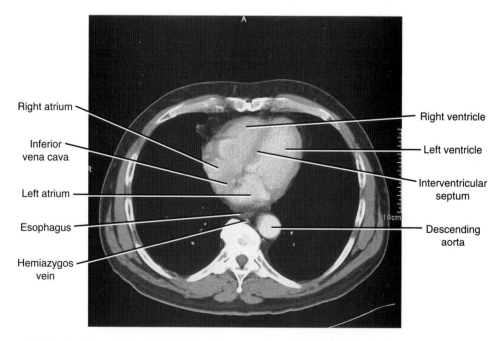

Figure 4-57   On Figure 4-57, a faint shadow of a new structure is starting to appear, the inferior vena cava. Still seen are the esophagus, hemiazygos vein, and descending aorta. They will continue to be seen into the level of the abdomen.

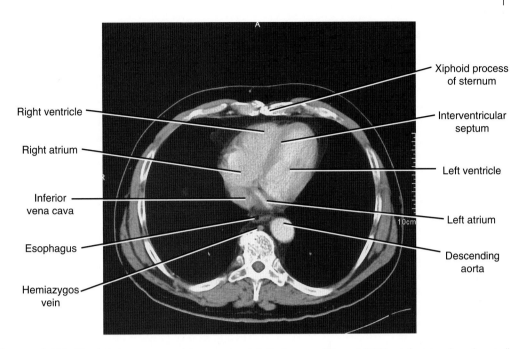

Right ventricle

Right atrium

Inferior
vena cava

Esophagus

Hemiazygos
vein

Xiphoid process
of sternum

Interventricular
septum

Left ventricle

Left atrium

Descending
aorta

Figure 4-58 The inferior vena cava takes a more definite form on Figure 4-58. The left atrium has almost disappeared. The esophagus, containing a bleb of air, is identified.

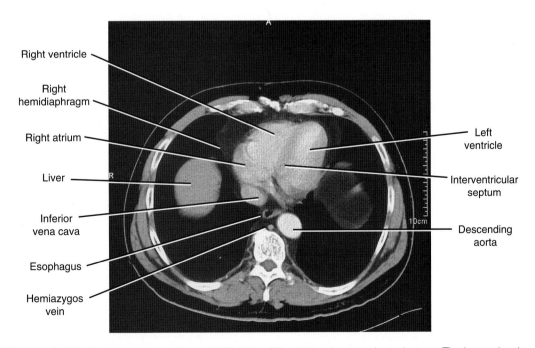

Right ventricle

Right
hemidiaphragm

Right atrium

Liver

Inferior
vena cava

Esophagus

Hemiazygos
vein

Left
ventricle

Interventricular
septum

Descending
aorta

Figure 4-59 On this last image (Figure 4-59), little of the right atrium remains to be seen. The lower chambers of the heart, the ventricles, separated by the interventricular septum, are still present. The largest organ in the body, the liver, is seen on the right, which is an indication that this cut is at the level of a portion of the diaphragm. Because the liver pushes up the right lung, the right lung is shorter than the left.

REVIEW QUESTIONS

1. All but one of the following statements is true. Identify the incorrect statement.
   - I. The right lung is shorter than the left. T
   - II. The left lung has two lobes. T
   - III. The layer of the pleura in direct contact with the lungs is the visceral layer. T
   - IV. The left hemidiaphragm is usually higher than the right.
   - a. I
   - b. II
   - c. III
   - d. IV

2. The portion of the sternum first seen on CT axial images arranged in descending order is the
   - a. ensiform process.
   - b. body.
   - c. manubrium.
   - d. xiphoid process.

3. The most superior aspect of the heart is the apex.
   - a. True
   - b. False

4. In which direction does the apex of the heart project?
   - a. Anterior and to the left
   - b. Anterior and to the right
   - c. Posterior and to the left
   - d. Posterior and to the right

5. Identify the outermost lining of the heart.
   - a. Endocardium
   - b. Epicardium
   - c. Visceral layer of serous pericardium
   - d. Parietal layer of serous pericardium
   - e. Fibrous pericardium

6. The innermost lining of the chambers of the heart is the
   - a. endocardium.
   - b. parietal layer of serous pericardium.
   - c. visceral layer of serous pericardium.
   - d. epicardium.
   - e. fibrous pericardium.

Match the following:

____ 7. Thickest myocardium   a. Right atrium

____ 8. Most anterior chamber   b. Left atrium

____ 9. Most posterior chamber   c. Right ventricle

                                   d. Left ventricle

10. The atria are the pumping chambers of the heart.
    - a. True
    - b. False

11. Which valve is seen on sectional images separating the left atrium from the left ventricle?
    - a. Pulmonic semilunar
    - b. Tricuspid valve
    - c. Aortic semilunar valve
    - d. Mitral valve
    - e. Thebesian valve

Match the following vessels with the appropriate heart chamber:

____ 12. Pulmonary trunk   a. Right atrium

____ 13. Pulmonary veins   b. Right ventricle

____ 14. SVC and IVC   c. Left atrium

____ 15. Aorta   d. Left ventricle

16. On axial CT images the inferior vena cava (IVC) is central to the four chambers of the heart.
    - a. True
    - b. False

17. Which vessels merge together to form the superior vena cava (SVC)?
    - a. Right and left internal jugular veins
    - b. Right and left subclavian veins
    - c. Right and left brachiocephalic veins
    - d. Right and left external jugular veins

18. Describe in which direction the aortic arch sweeps.

    _____

    _____

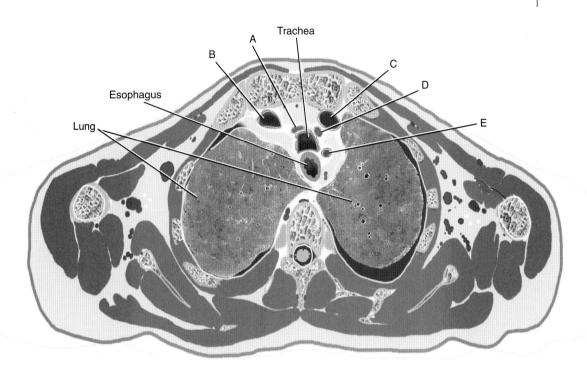

Trachea
A
B
Esophagus
C
D
Lung
E

Match the following great vessels with their location on the line drawing:

____ 19. Right brachiocephalic vein

____ 20. Right brachiocephalic artery

____ 21. Left common carotid artery

____ 22. Left subclavian artery

____ 23. Left brachiocephalic vein

24. Where is the descending aorta located in the mediastinum?
    a. Anterior and to the left
    b. Posterior and to the left
    c. Anterior and to the right
    d. Posterior and to the right

25. The azygos and hemiazygos veins are a continuation of the
    a. right and left ascending lumbar veins.
    b. right and left common iliac veins.
    d. right and left internal iliac veins.
    e. right and left external iliac veins.

26. Into which vessel does the azygos vein empty?
    a. Right internal jugular vein
    b. Superior vena cava
    c. Right external jugular vein
    d. It empties directly into the right atrium.

27. The thymus is located posterior to the body of the sternum and typically appears larger in children on sectional images.
    a. True
    b. False

28. The carina is
    a. the location of the bifurcation of the pharynx into the trachea and the esophagus.
    b. the location of the bifurcation of the trachea into the right and left primary bronchi.
    c. located at T4/T5.
    d. a and c.
    e. b and c.

29. On axial CT images one expects to find the right and left pulmonary arteries branching off the pulmonary trunk at approximately the same level as the bifurcation of the trachea.
    a. True
    b. False

30. The esophagus is posterior to the trachea on sectional images.
    a. True
    b. False

Chapter 5

Abdomen

CONTRAST MEDIUM

Most abdominal and pelvic CT scans employ IV administration of iodinated contrast medium, either ionic or nonionic. Additionally, oral contrast media, either water-soluble or barium dilutions, may be used. Certain types of pathology may contraindicate the use of contrast medium.

ABDOMINAL CAVITY

The diaphragm is a dome-shaped muscle separating the thoracic cavity from the abdominal cavity. It attaches posteriorly to the lumbar vertebrae by way of the **crus** of the diaphragm. The points of attachment are seen on transaxial CT sectional images as thin curvilinear opacities anterior to the bodies of the lumbar vertebrae. Along the anterior surface of the abdominal wall the muscular insertions of the diaphragm on the rib cage if seen, appear as V-shaped structures. Three openings are present in the diaphragm. Listed anteriorly to posteriorly they are the **caval hiatus** for the inferior vena cava, the **esophageal hiatus** for the esophagus, and the **aortic hiatus** for the aorta. Figure 5-1 is a line drawing of the diaphragm.

No such structure divides the inferior portion of the abdominal cavity from the pelvic cavity. The definition of the boundary between the two can vary from textbook to textbook. This book will choose an imaginary transverse line at the level of the iliac crests, L4/L5. A superficial indication of this landmark on CT images is an indentation on the anterior abdomen, midline, where the umbilicus exists. Those organs found in the abdominal cavity include the blood vessels, liver, gallbladder, pancreas, spleen, esophagus, stomach, intestines, kidneys, and adrenals.

BLOOD VESSELS

Aorta

The section of the aorta after passing through the diaphragm is the abdominal descending aorta. Located in the posterior abdomen, it is just slightly anterior to and to the left of the vertebral column. Before bifurcating at approximately L4 into the right and left common iliac arteries there are numerous arteries that branch off, as shown on Figure 5-2.

Celiac Axis

The first branch off the abdominal aorta, the **celiac axis**, **artery**, or **trunk**, arises from the anterior aorta almost immediately after the descending aorta passes through the diaphragm. The celiac axis trifurcates into three separate vessels: the **splenic**, **left gastric**, and **common hepatic arteries**.

Splenic Artery

The splenic artery is directed transversely to the left and passes along the superior surface of the pancreas; it provides the spleen with freshly oxygenated blood.

Left Gastric Artery

The left gastric artery, the smallest of the three branches, heads upward and slightly to the left, going into the lesser curvature of the stomach.

Common Hepatic Artery

The common hepatic artery passes to the right and runs along the inferior surface of the pancreas; one of the

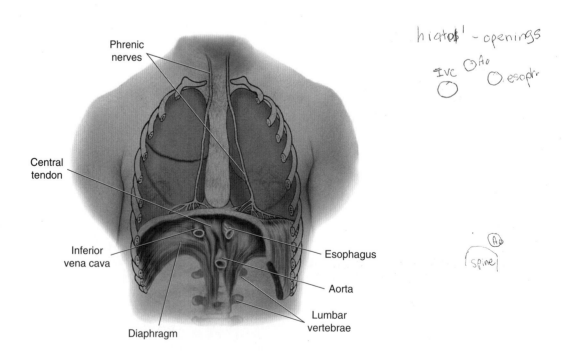

Figure 5-1 Diaphragm separating the thoracic region from the abdominopelvic region

two major blood sources to the liver, it supplies oxygenated blood.

Superior Mesenteric Artery

The second vessel to arise off the descending abdominal aorta (also anteriorly) is the **superior mesenteric artery (SMA)**. The SMA supplies most of the small intes-

tine, the ascending colon, and about one-half of the transverse colon (all of which are covered in a subsequent section in this chapter) with oxygenated blood. After branching off the aorta about 1 cm below the celiac axis, it is found coursing down for quite a distance anterior and slightly to the right of the aorta and to the left of the superior mesenteric vein.

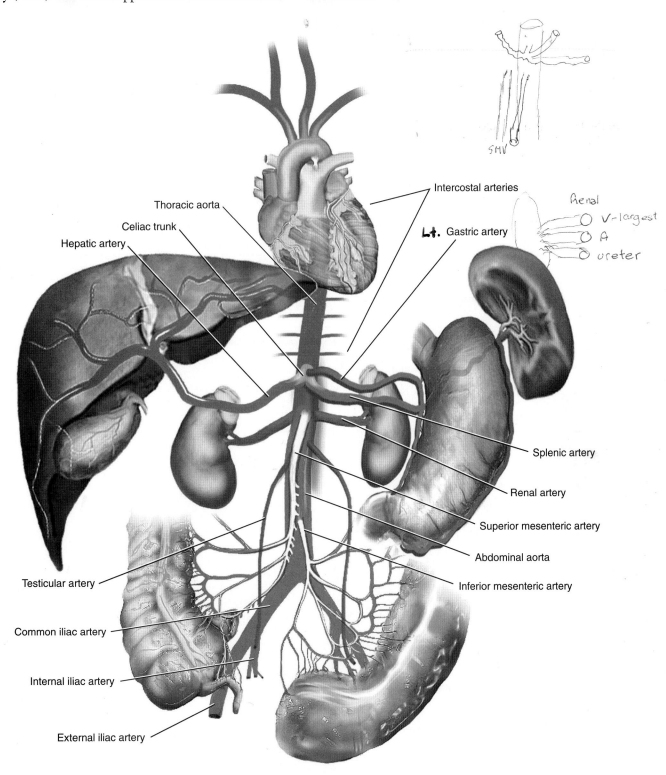

Figure 5-2 Abdominal descending aorta with its branches

Renal Arteries

The bilateral **renal arteries** extend laterally off the abdominal aorta at approximately L1–L2. Generally, the left renal artery appears first as it supplies the left kidney and the liver pushes down the right kidney. The right renal artery, seen posterior to the IVC, is longer as it must travel from the descending aorta, located to the left of the vertebral column, over to the right kidney. It is not uncommon for an individual to have more than one renal artery on at least one side, more frequently the left.

Inferior Mesenteric Artery

The **inferior mesenteric artery**, or **IMA**, is not often seen on axial CT images; it is the last vessel to branch off the abdominal descending aorta before its bifurcation into the right and left common iliac arteries at L4, the level of the crests. The IMA supplies the left half of the transverse colon, descending colon, sigmoid, and most of the rectum, all of which are discussed later in this chapter. Figure 5-3 is a schematic diagram of all the major branches off the abdominal aorta.

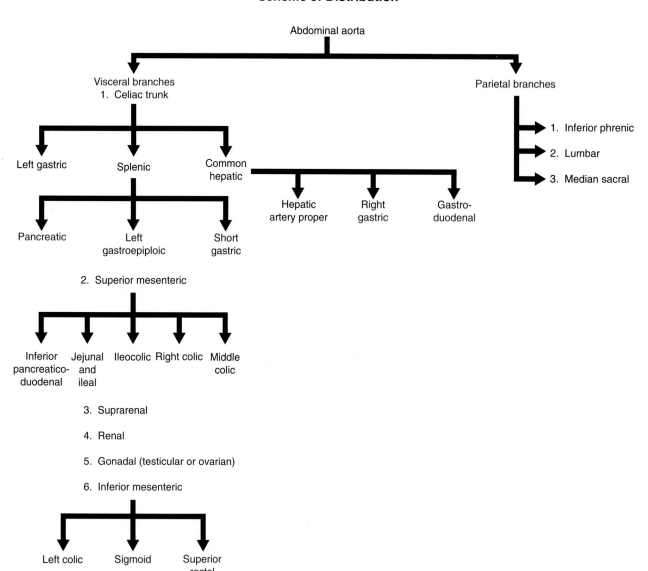

Scheme of Distribution

Abdominal aorta

Visceral branches
1. Celiac trunk

Left gastric   Splenic   Common hepatic

Pancreatic   Left gastroepiploic   Short gastric

Hepatic artery proper   Right gastric   Gastro-duodenal

2. Superior mesenteric

Inferior pancreatico-duodenal   Jejunal and ileal   Ileocolic   Right colic   Middle colic

3. Suprarenal

4. Renal

5. Gonadal (testicular or ovarian)

6. Inferior mesenteric

Left colic   Sigmoid   Superior rectal

Parietal branches
1. Inferior phrenic
2. Lumbar
3. Median sacral

Figure 5-3 Schematic diagram of the abdominal descending aorta (Tortora, G. and Grabowski, S. R. [2000]. *Principles of Anatomy & Physiology* [9th ed.]. New York: John Wiley & Sons, Inc. This material is used by permission of John Wiley & Sons, Inc.)

Inferior Vena Cava

In the abdominal region, the veins tend to be larger than the arteries. The inferior vena cava begins at L5 slightly to the right of the aorta with the merger of the right and left common iliac veins. At higher levels in the abdomen the IVC is anterior to the aorta. The formation of the IVC is seen on Figure 5-4.

Renal Veins

The bilateral **renal veins** empty into the inferior vena cava. Because the inferior vena cava is on the right the left renal vein is longer. Typically, the right renal vein is at a lower level than the left. If visualized on axial CT images the left renal vein is seen crossing in front of the aorta. The renal arteries can be differentiated from the renal veins by noting which vessel (aorta or inferior vena cava) the vessel in question is entering or exiting. Generally, the renal veins are larger than the renal arteries. Because the IVC is anterior to the descending aorta in this region, the renal veins will be anterior to the renal arteries.

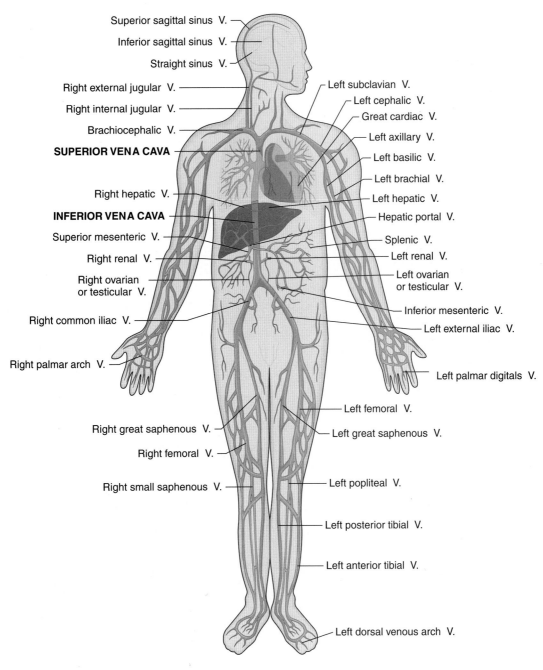

Figure 5-4 Inferior vena cava

Portal Circulation

The liver has two major sources of blood. One is the common hepatic artery, which was previously discussed. The other is the **portal vein**.

Portal Vein

The portal vein is formed by the union of the **splenic vein**, carrying the venous blood from the spleen, and the **superior mesenteric vein (SMV)**. Prior to the union, the splenic vein runs along the posterior aspect of the pancreas. The superior mesenteric vein begins in the lower quadrant and is seen to the right of and slightly anterior to the superior mesenteric artery. As a rule, the SMV is larger than the SMA. The SMV and splenic vein join in the vicinity of the head of the pancreas. Occasionally the **inferior mesenteric vein (IMV)** is identifiable on axial sectional images posterior to the SMA to the left of the aorta. If the location of the SMV and SMA are reversed, the fact that the veins are larger than the arteries should help in identifying them. Both the IMV and the **left gastric vein** (not seen on CT axial images) drain into the splenic vein prior to its merger with the SMV. Although the blood in the portal vein is no longer oxygenated, it is rich in nutrients, acquired primarily through the SMV, and pigmentation from the breakdown products of the spleen. The major contributors to the portal vein are demonstrated on Figure 5-5.

Hepatic Veins

The blood leaves the superior liver by way of three veins, the right, middle, and left **hepatic veins**, going directly into the inferior vena cava, also visualized on Figure 5-5. The middle hepatic vein drains the medial segment of the left lobe and the anterior portion of the right lobe, while the right and left hepatic veins drain the remaining portions of the right and left lobes, respectively.

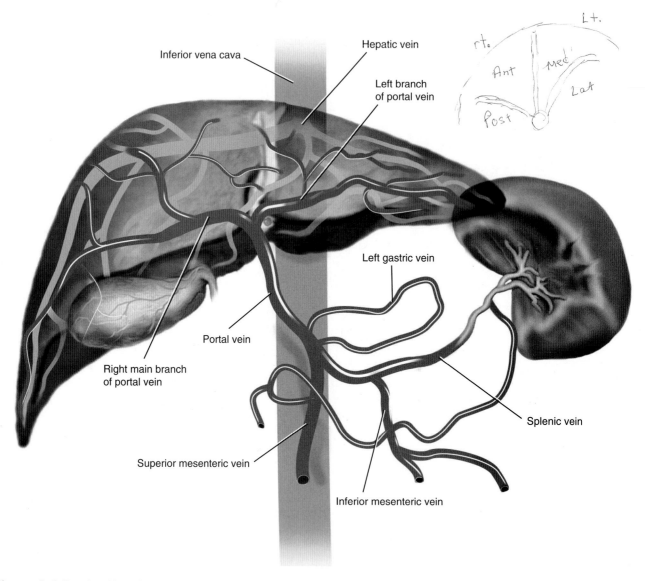

Figure 5-5 Portal and hepatic veins

ACCESSORY DIGESTIVE ORGANS

A number of accessory organs are involved in the digestive process. They are the liver, gallbladder, pancreas, and spleen.

Liver

Figure 5-6 is a drawing of the largest organ in the body, the **liver**, primarily located in the right upper quadrant of the abdominal cavity, but extending into the left quadrant. It is composed of two major lobes, a right and left, as well as two smaller lobes, the **caudate** and ~~quadrate lobes. Textbooks may vary in classifying the two smaller lobes, but in theory, they are considered part of the right lobe.~~ The **falciform ligament** both separates the upper anterior larger right lobe from the left lobe and attaches the liver to the diaphragm and anterior abdominal wall. The **longitudinal fissure** is a groove beginning at the **umbilical notch** on the anterior inferior surface of

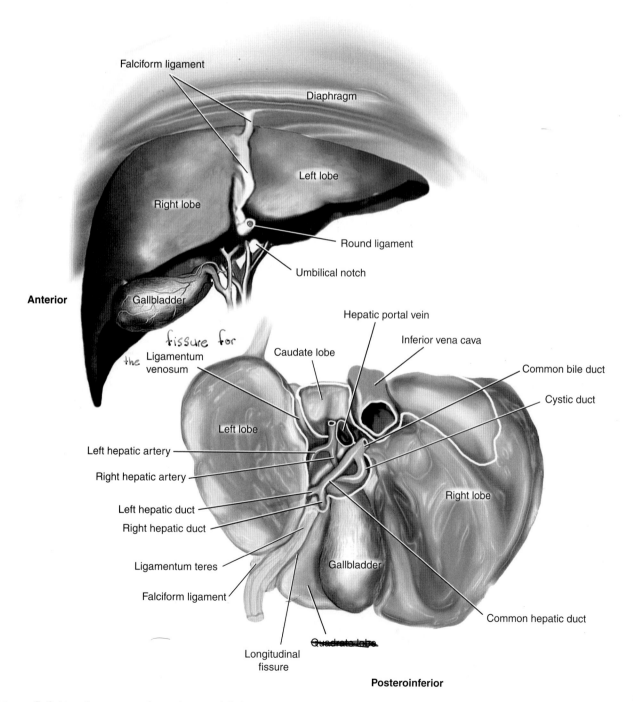

Figure 5-6 Liver from an anterior and posteroinferior perspective

the liver between the right and left lobes. It continues in a superior direction along the posterior aspect of the liver and serves to separate the right and left lobes. The caudate lobe is located superiorly in the liver, anterior to the inferior vena cava. It is separated from the left lobe by the **ligamentum venosum**, the remnant of the obliterated fetal **ductus venosus**. The quadrate lobe, situated medially and inferiorly within the right lobe, is anterior to the gallbladder. The **ligamentum teres**, or **round ligament**, a remnant of the umbilical vein found in the fetus, begins at the umbilicus and rises to join the free edge of the falciform ligament at its base. It is found between the quadrate and left lobe of the liver. The opening for structures to enter and exit the liver is the **porta hepatis**. The **hepatic ducts**, draining the bile manufactured by the liver, exit here and then join together, forming the **common hepatic duct**.

Gallbladder

The **gallbladder** is an organ located on the inferior surface of the liver, more or less anteriorly, where the right and left lobes separate (see Figure 5-6). Although the gallbladder is seen on CT images, CT is not the best modality to demonstrate pathology. If **choleliths**, or gallstones, are present, they tend to gravitate to the posterior gallbladder when the patient is supine. The bile stored in the gallbladder drains out through the **cystic duct** to merge with the common hepatic duct forming the **common bile duct** (refer to Figure 5-7).

Pancreas

The **pancreas**, a mixed gland as it is both an endocrine and exocrine gland, has a unique mottled appearance on CT axial images. It is posterior to the stomach. Shaped something like a fish, it has a tail, body, and head. Although the body runs transversely, the tail is usually seen at a higher level. Refer back to the discussion about the splenic artery and recall that it runs along the superior surface of the pancreas. The splenic vein runs posterior to the body of the pancreas before merging with the superior mesenteric vein to become the portal vein in the vicinity of the head of the pancreas. The indentation near the head of the pancreas is the **neck**. The **pancreatic duct** travels through the pancreas to drain the digestive enzymes from the exocrine portion of the pancreas. When barium is administered orally prior to a CT of the abdomen, the head of the pancreas is seen lying within the duodenum. This relationship is shown on Figure 5-7.

Spleen

The **spleen**, as shown on Figure 5-8, is located in the left upper quadrant, adjacent to the posterior rib cage and posterior to the greater curvature of the stomach. It is at the level of the esophagastric junction and is supplied with oxygenated blood via the splenic artery, a branch of the celiac axis. The blood drains from the spleen by way of the splenic vein, which proceeds to run along the posterior

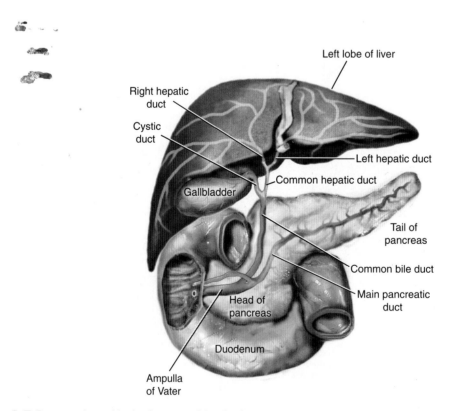

Right hepatic duct

Cystic duct

Gallbladder

Left lobe of liver

Left hepatic duct

Common hepatic duct

Tail of pancreas

Common bile duct

Main pancreatic duct

Head of pancreas

Duodenum

Ampulla of Vater

Figure 5-7 Pancreas situated in the first part of the duodenum

border of the pancreas and join with the superior mesenteric vein to form the portal vein. The splenic artery and vein enter and exit the spleen at the hilum, where the tail of the pancreas can also be found. The spleen has many functions including filtering and destroying old red blood cells, acting as a reservoir for blood, and producing lymphocytes and monocytes after birth. The byproduct of the red blood cell destruction contains the pigment that reaches the liver through the portal vein and gives bile its coloration.

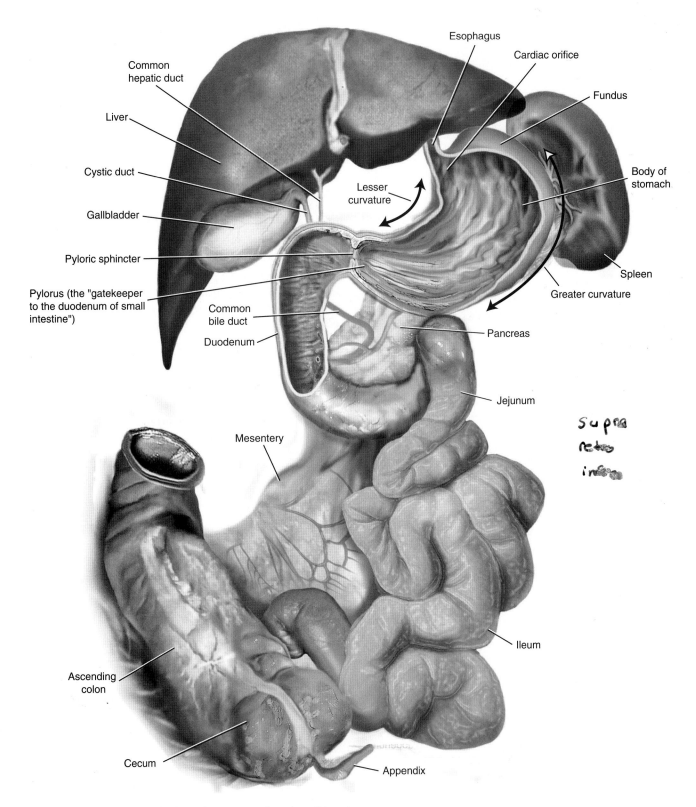

Figure 5-8 The spleen, distal esophagus, stomach, and small intestine

DIGESTIVE ORGANS

The location of any existing air fluid levels within the abdominal cavity will be dependent upon the position of the patient. If a patient is supine, the levels appear anteriorly and vice versa.

Esophagus

The esophagus emerges through the esophageal hiatus, one of the three openings in the diaphragm, into the abdomen, eventually emptying into the stomach through the **cardiac orifice**, at the **esophagogastric junction**. Figure 5-8 allows you to identify these landmarks as well as those mentioned in the following discussion on the stomach and small intestine.

Stomach

The **stomach** is seen on CT axial images about the level of the spleen. The esophagus empties into it below the level of the **fundus** along the medial border. The **greater curvature of the stomach** is on the lateral border and the **lesser curvature** is on the medial border. The partially digested food contents pass into the **pyloric antrum** and empty into the **duodenum**, the first part of the **small intestine**, through the **pyloric sphincter**.

Intestines

The intestines are divided according to diameter into two sections, the small and large intestines. It is within the small intestine that most digestion occurs and from there that the body absorbs most nutrients and liquid. The remaining liquid absorbed by the body comes from the waste products passing through the large intestine.

Small Intestine

There are three sections to the **small intestine**, totaling approximately 20 feet. The duodenum originates at the pylorus at the level of L1 when the stomach is empty. If contrast medium is administered, the initial C-shaped portion of the duodenum is seen curving around the head of the pancreas. The most distal portion of the duodenum is at the level of L4. Both the bile from the liver and gallbladder, passing through the dilated distal portion of the common bile duct, the **ampulla of Vater**, and the pancreatic enzymes, passing through the pancreatic duct, empty into the duodenum. In some individuals the pancreatic duct empties into the common bile duct prior to its entry into the duodenum. When oral contrast medium is administered, its purpose is to fill the intestines, thereby allowing for delineation of other organs, rather than to visualize pathology within the small and **large intestines**. The remaining portions of the small intestine include the **jejunum** in the umbilical region, and **ileum** in the hypogastric and pelvic region. The jejunum begins at the level of L2.

Large Intestine

The ileum empties into the cecum, part of the large intestine, through the **ileocecal valve**. The length of the large intestine is approximately 5 feet. The labeled areas of the large intestine, as seen on Figure 5-9, include the **cecum** with its appendage the **appendix** or **vermiform appendix**, the segments of the colon, the **ascending**, **transverse**, **descending**, and **sigmoid**, and the **rectum**. The **hepatic** and **splenic flexures** are bends on the right and left of the transverse colon, respectively, with the splenic flexure higher than the hepatic flexure. The rectum empties externally through the **anus**.

Most of the large intestine is located within the abdominal cavity, as defined by this textbook, but the cecum, vermiform appendix, sigmoid colon, and rectum are found in the pelvic cavity and are discussed more extensively in Chapter 6.

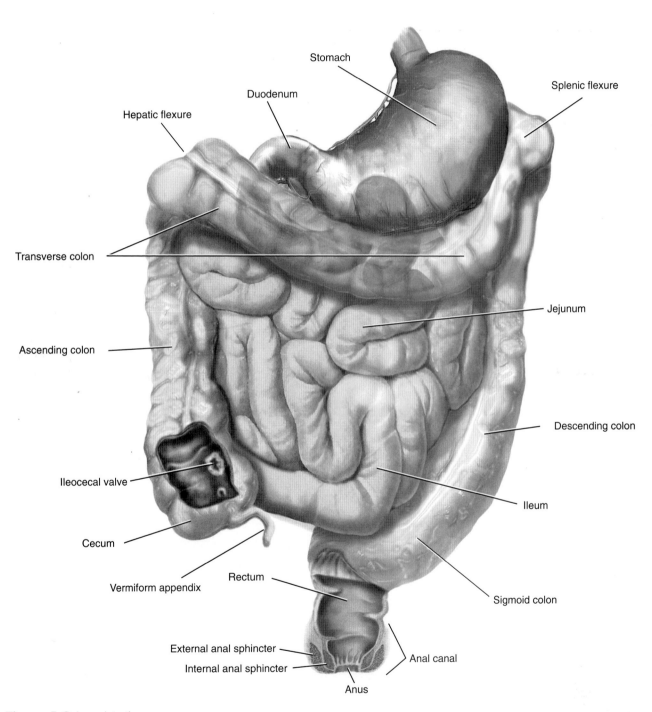

Figure 5-9 Large intestine

KIDNEYS

A number of structures are involved in the urinary system. They include the bilateral **kidneys** and **ureters**, and a single bladder and urethra, demonstrated on Figure 5-10. Those located within the abdominal region are the kidneys and the upper portion of the ureters. The right and left kidneys are located on either side of the vertebral column with the right kidney most often at a slightly lower level because the liver pushes it down. Shaped like a kidney bean, the outermost section is the cortex and the more central region is the medulla. Along the medial border is an indentation, the hilum, through which blood vessels, nerves, lymphatic vessels, and the ureters enter or exit. At the hilum of the kidneys from anterior to posterior are the renal vein, renal artery, and ureter. After urine is manufactured through a filtration process within the kidney, it drains into minor and then major **calyces** and finally into the collecting area for urine, the **renal pelvis**, adjacent to

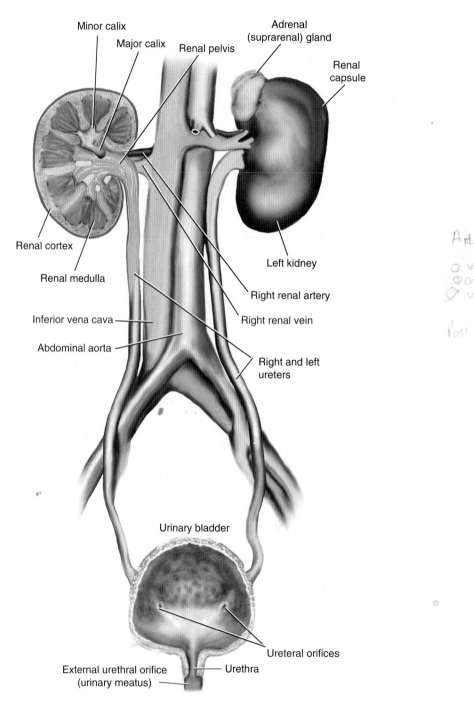

Figure 5-10 Organs of the urinary system

the hilum. The urine drains out through the ureter, which descends in an anterior and medial direction, eventually emptying into the bladder. Because of peristalsis the ureters may not be visible on all sectional images, even with administration of contrast medium. Contrast medium obscures kidney stones.

ADRENAL GLANDS

The **adrenal glands** or **suprarenals** are endocrine glands found superiorly on the kidneys, separated by perirenal fat, generally around the level of the crus of the diaphragm. The left adrenal is included on Figure 5-10. As seen on CT axial images, the adrenals can vary considerably in shape, with the right adrenal resembling an inverted V or slash mark caused by compression by the liver, and the left an inverted Y. As the right kidney is often lower, the left adrenal gland usually appears before the right. CT is often done to identify tumors of the adrenals. If calcifications are present, this may be an indication of cancer; therefore, if the adrenals are of interest on CT scans, no contrast medium is administered.

PERITONEUM

The **peritoneum**, which has two layers, a parietal and visceral layer, is a **serous membrane** lining the abdominal cavity. The visceral layer covers those organs within the peritoneal cavity, including the liver, gallbladder, spleen, stomach, and most of the intestines. It surrounds many abdominal viscera but other organs are found in the region behind the peritoneum, the **retroperitoneal space**.

Retroperitoneal Space

Unlike those organs within the peritoneal cavity, the location of organs in the retroperitoneal space does not vary much from one individual to another. The retroperitoneal space can be divided into three sections, identified on Figure 5-11: the anterior **pararenal** space, posterior pararenal space, and **perirenal** space. Within the anterior pararenal space are portions of the ascending and descending colon, the pancreas, and most of the duodenum. The posterior pararenal space contains mostly fat and some vessels while the perirenal space contains the kidneys, ureters, perirenal fat, adrenal glands, aorta, and IVC.

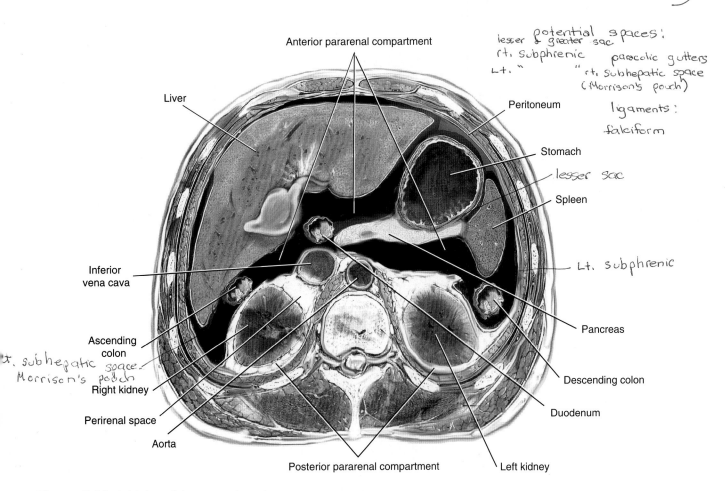

Figure 5-11 Axial view of the retroperitoneal space

MUSCLES

In learning the muscles of the abdomen, it is probably easier to divide them into groups: those that are constant in both the abdomen and pelvic area and those seen only in the abdominal region.

The first of the constant muscles are the bilateral **psoas muscles**, seen on either side of the vertebral body. They originate at approximately T12 and end at the level of the femur, although at the lower level they have merged with the bilateral **iliacus muscles** to form the **iliopsoas muscles** (refer to Figure 5-12). The second group of constant muscles are the erector spinae muscles seen posteri-orly on either side of the spinous processes. The last of the constant muscles are the **rectus abdominis**. They are found on the anterior abdominal wall originating at the pubic bone and inserting at the fifth, sixth, and seventh rib cartilage. The **linea alba**, created by the convergence of the three lateral muscles anteriorly, is a tendinous membrane separating the right and left rectus abdominis muscles midline. In studying Figure 5-13, note that the rectus abdominis muscle becomes foreshortened as CT axial imaging descends.

Those muscles that are seen only in the abdominal region are the **external** and **internal oblique muscles**,

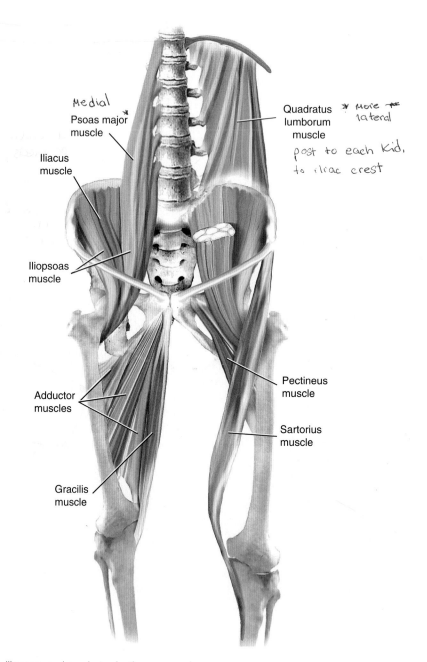

Figure 5-12 Iliacus, psoas, iliopsoas, and quadratus lumborum muscles

the **transversus abdominis**, and the **quadratus lumborum**. The external oblique, internal oblique, and transversus abdominis are seen along the lateral abdominal walls from the level of the lower ribs until approximately the level of the crest. They extend medially in the order they have been listed. They are included on Figure 5-13. The quadratus lumborum is also seen bilaterally in the region of the kidney, adjacent to the transverse processes of the vertebrae. Figure 5-12 demonstrates that it extends only from T12 to the level of the crest.

Cancer in pelvic organs may metastasize to adjacent muscles, often before spreading to the skeleton.

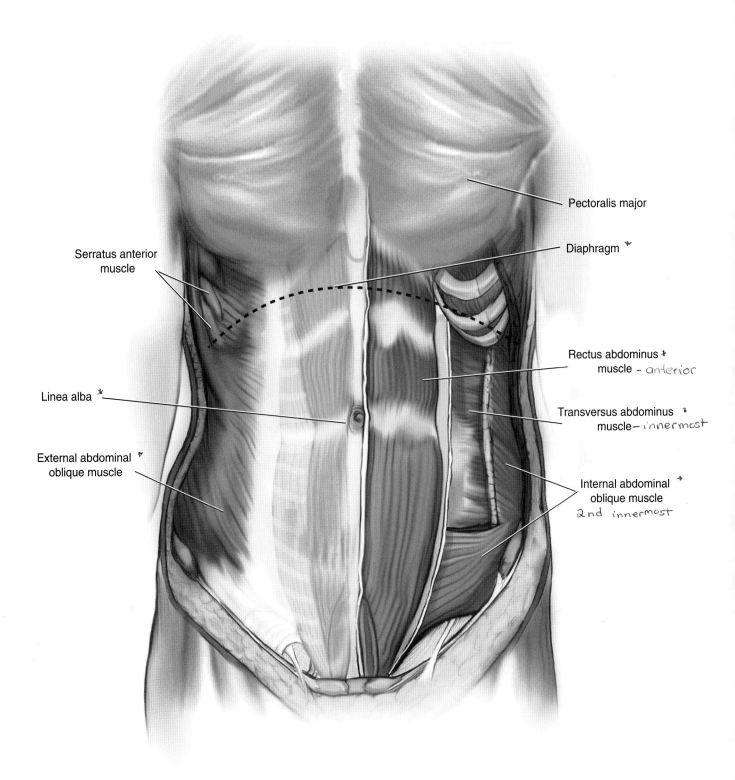

Pectoralis major

Diaphragm ✱

Serratus anterior muscle

Rectus abdominus ✱
muscle - anterior

Linea alba ✱

Transversus abdominus ✱
muscle — innermost

External abdominal ✱
oblique muscle

Internal abdominal ✱
oblique muscle
2nd innermost

Figure 5-13 Abdominopelvic muscles

CT IMAGES

Exam 1

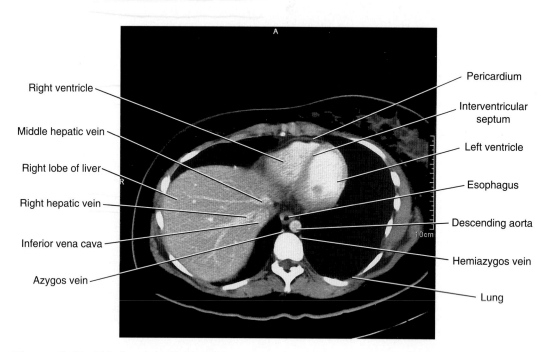

Figure 5-14   This first abdominal image (see Figure 5-14) demonstrates the first organ to appear within the abdomen below the level of the diaphragm, the liver. Within the liver are the right and middle hepatic veins, which drain into the inferior vena cava. The right and left ventricles of the heart are still evident, along with the interventricular septum and pericardium. The azygos and hemiazygos veins are anterior to the body of the vertebra.

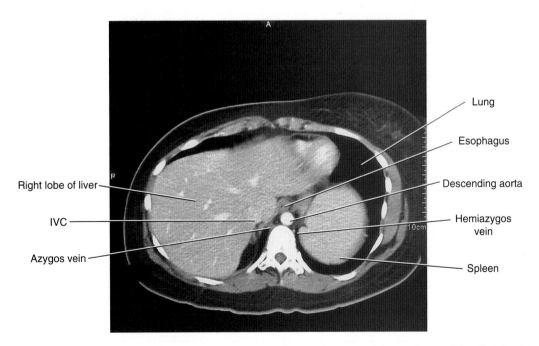

Right ventricle

Middle hepatic vein

Right lobe of liver

Right hepatic vein

IVC

Azygos vein

Interventricular septum

Left ventricle

Descending aorta

Hemiazygos vein

Spleen

Lung

Figure 5-15 For this patient, the spleen is the second abdominal organ to appear (see Figure 5-15). Less lung tissue is apparent. The inferior vena cava appears to be imbedded in the medial aspect of the liver. The two ventricles of the heart are discernable.

Right lobe of liver

IVC

Azygos vein

Lung

Esophagus

Descending aorta

Hemiazygos vein

Spleen

Figure 5-16 On Figure 5-16, the liver continues to spread across the upper abdomen. Eventually it will fill the right upper quadrant and a portion of the left upper quadrant. At this level, it is difficult to isolate the various lobes of the liver (right, left, caudate, and quadrate). The esophagus is seen anterior to the descending aorta.

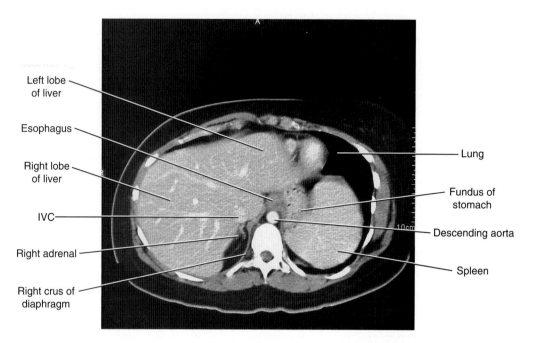

Figure 5-17   The esophagus is located medial to the fundus of the stomach on Figure 5-17. On the right the crus of the diaphragm runs anterior to the body of the vertebrae, serving to anchor the diaphragm. The right adrenal gland is seen, an indication that the right kidney will probably be the first kidney to appear. More commonly, the left kidney appears at a higher level because the liver tends to push down the right kidney.

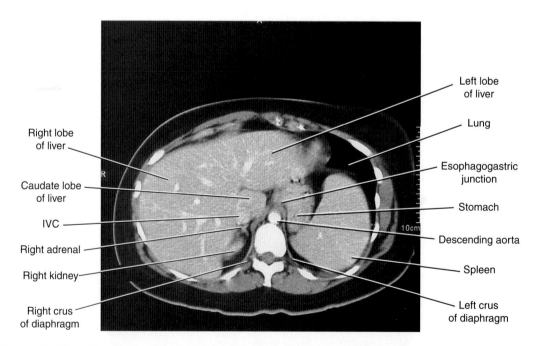

Figure 5-18   A faint shadow of the right kidney is seen on Figure 5-18, while the right adrenal gland is still visible. Anterior to the inferior vena cava is the caudate lobe of the liver. Although no apparent line of demarcation is visible, the right and left lobes of the liver can be identified by location. The esophagogastric junction is seen along with the crus of the diaphragm on the right and left.

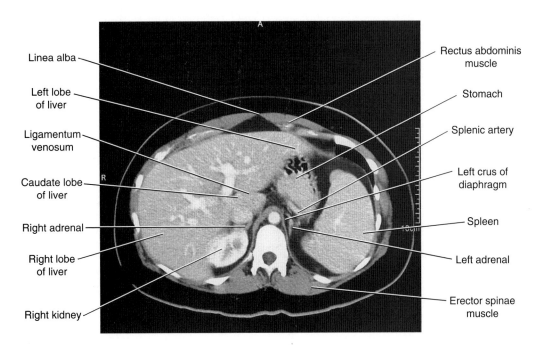

Ligamentum venosum

Caudate lobe of liver

Right lobe of liver

IVC

Right adrenal

Right kidney

Right crus of diaphragm

Left lobe of liver

Greater curvature of stomach

Stomach

Lesser curvature of stomach

Descending aorta

Left crus of diaphragm

Spleen

Figure 5-19 The greater and lesser curvatures of the stomach are identified on Figure 5-19 laterally and medially, respectively. The ligamentum venosum (a remnant of the obliterated ductus venosus) separates the caudate lobe of the liver from the left lobe. The descending aorta and inferior vena cava continue to be evident as the descending aorta does not bifurcate until L4 and the inferior vena cava is formed at L5.

Linea alba

Left lobe of liver

Ligamentum venosum

Caudate lobe of liver

Right adrenal

Right lobe of liver

Right kidney

Rectus abdominis muscle

Stomach

Splenic artery

Left crus of diaphragm

Spleen

Left adrenal

Erector spinae muscle

Figure 5-20 On Figure 5-20, this patient appears to be supine as air is seen in the anterior stomach (air rises). The splenic artery is evident. The splenic artery is a branch of the celiac axis and runs along the superior aspect of the pancreas. The left adrenal is seen. Abdominal muscles that can be identified are the rectus abdominis, separated by the linea alba, and the erector spinae.

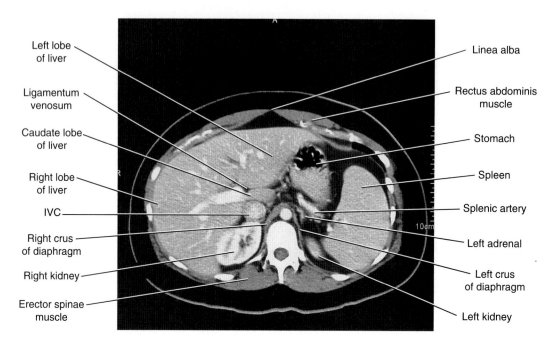

Left lobe of liver

Ligamentum venosum

Caudate lobe of liver

Right lobe of liver

IVC

Right crus of diaphragm

Right kidney

Erector spinae muscle

Linea alba

Rectus abdominis muscle

Stomach

Spleen

Splenic artery

Left adrenal

Left crus of diaphragm

Left kidney

Figure 5-21   On Figure 5-21, the caudate lobe of the liver is still apparent anterior to the inferior vena cava, along with the ligamentum venosum, which is found between the caudate lobe and left lobe of the liver. The left kidney is barely visible. We continue to see the crus of the diaphragm.

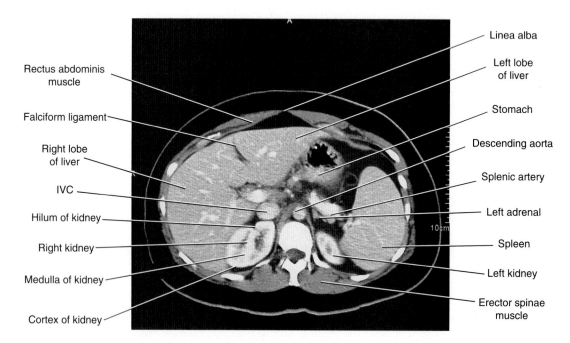

Rectus abdominis muscle

Falciform ligament

Right lobe of liver

IVC

Hilum of kidney

Right kidney

Medulla of kidney

Cortex of kidney

Linea alba

Left lobe of liver

Stomach

Descending aorta

Splenic artery

Left adrenal

Spleen

Left kidney

Erector spinae muscle

Figure 5-22   This next image (Figure 5-22) shows the falciform ligament on the anterior border of the liver. Besides dividing the right and left lobes of the liver, the falciform ligament also anchors the liver to the anterior abdominal wall and the diaphragm. The splenic artery is still apparent. The cortex, medulla, and hilum of the right kidney are labeled along with the left adrenal gland and kidney.

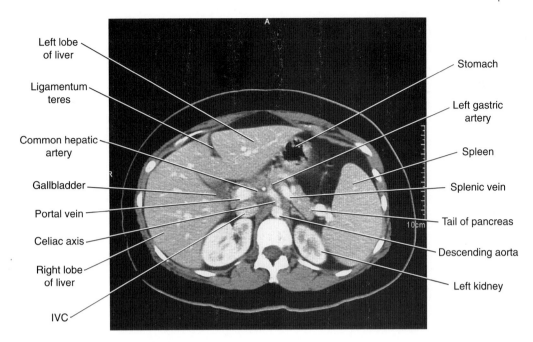

Figure 5-23 On Figure 5-23, the celiac axis (trunk, artery), the first branch off the descending aorta, is identified, along with two of the three associated vessels, the common hepatic artery and left gastric artery. The gallbladder is visible for the first time. The uppermost portion of the pancreas, the tail, is seen with a small segment of the splenic vein found posterior to the pancreas. Anterior to the inferior vena cava is the portal vein, one of the two vessels entering the liver. The ligamentum teres (the remnant of the umbilical vein) is to the right of the left lobe.

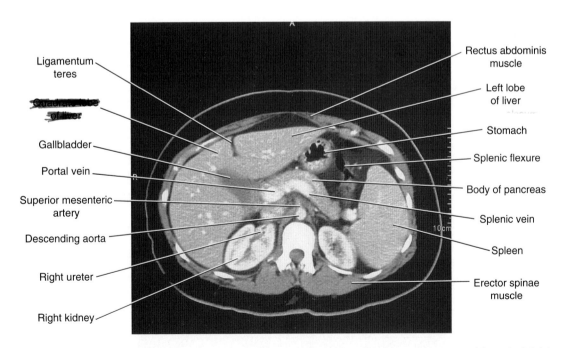

Figure 5-24 The quadrate lobe of the liver is found anterior to the gallbladder and is separated from the left lobe of the liver by the ligamentum teres on Figure 5-24. The stomach continues to be seen. The body of the pancreas is now evident behind which lies the splenic vein merging with the superior mesenteric vein to form the portal vein. The splenic flexure of the large intestines is found medial to the spleen. Typically the splenic flexure is higher than the hepatic flexure. Notice the superior mesenteric artery arising from the anterior border of the descending aorta. Also note the right ureter exiting the right kidney.

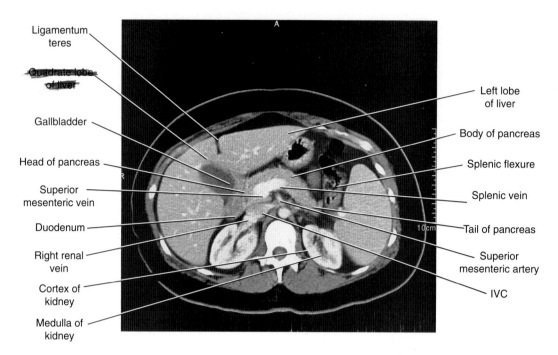

Figure 5-25 Again we see the gallbladder, quadrate lobe of the liver, ligamentum teres, and left lobe of the liver on Figure 5-25. The entire pancreas (tail, body, and head) is seen along with the actual merging of the superior mesenteric vein and splenic vein. More of the splenic flexure can be identified. The first part of the duodenum is located wrapping around the head of the pancreas. The superior mesenteric artery is still apparent. The right renal vein can be seen draining the venous blood from the right kidney into the inferior vena cava. The cortex and medulla can be located in the left kidney.

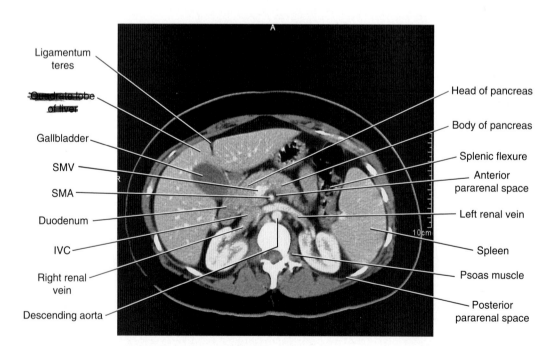

Figure 5-26 Figure 5-26 shows both the right and left renal veins with the left running anterior to the descending aorta. The posterior and anterior pararenal spaces are labeled. The posterior pararenal space contains mostly fat while the anterior pararenal space contains a number of organs, including the pancreas and ascending and descending colon. This image also demonstrates the superior mesenteric vein and superior mesenteric artery. The superior mesenteric vein is always larger than the superior mesenteric artery. A new muscle, the psoas, has appeared lateral to the body of the vertebra and will continue to be evident throughout the remaining abdomen and into the pelvis.

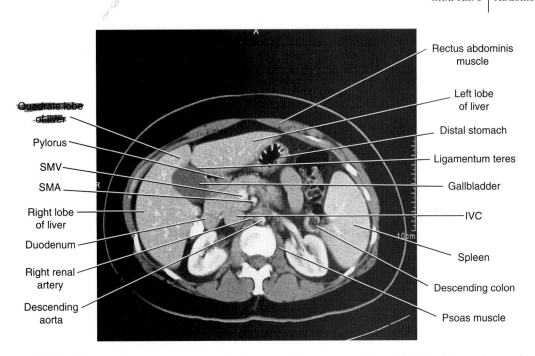

Quadrate lobe of liver

Pylorus

SMV

SMA

Right lobe of liver

Duodenum

Right renal artery

Descending aorta

Rectus abdominis muscle

Left lobe of liver

Distal stomach

Ligamentum teres

Gallbladder

IVC

Spleen

Descending colon

Psoas muscle

Figure 5-27 The superior mesenteric vein and artery are still apparent on Figure 5-27. The right renal artery is seen leaving the descending aorta. The distal stomach and pylorus are apparent on this image. Three of the lobes of the liver (right, left, and quadrate) are still visible, as well as the gallbladder and ligamentum teres. The rectus abdominis is seen on the anterior abdominal wall.

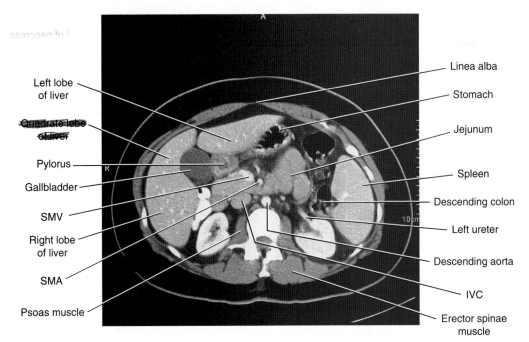

Left lobe of liver

Quadrate lobe of liver

Pylorus

Gallbladder

SMV

Right lobe of liver

SMA

Psoas muscle

Linea alba

Stomach

Jejunum

Spleen

Descending colon

Left ureter

Descending aorta

IVC

Erector spinae muscle

Figure 5-28 On Figure 5-28, the liver and gallbladder are diminishing in size, as is the spleen. The stomach and pylorus are again identified. Still apparent are the superior mesenteric vein and artery. The erector spinae and psoas muscles are labeled.

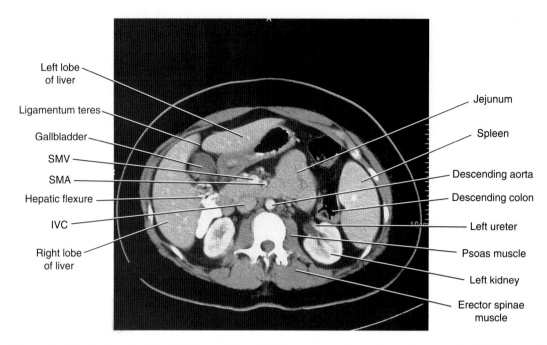

Figure 5-29   On the left side of this image (Figure 5-29) we see the descending colon, most of which is located retroperitoneally. The superior mesenteric vein and artery remain evident. A structure appears adjacent to the anterior left kidney, the left ureter. The upper part of the hepatic flexure is first identified. Typically, the hepatic flexure is at a lower level than the splenic flexure.

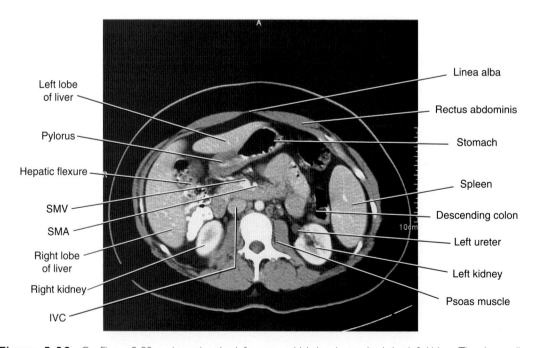

Figure 5-30   On Figure 5-30, again notice the left ureter, which has just exited the left kidney. The descending colon continues coursing downward. More of the hepatic flexure is apparent. Note the presence of the rectus abdominis muscle, separated by the linea alba.

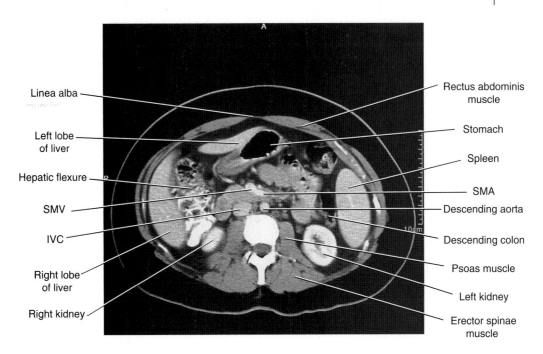

Linea alba

Left lobe
of liver

Hepatic flexure

SMV

IVC

Right lobe
of liver

Right kidney

Rectus abdominis
muscle

Stomach

Spleen

SMA

Descending aorta

Descending colon

Psoas muscle

Left kidney

Erector spinae
muscle

Figure 5-31 On Figure 5-31, we see the inferior right and left lobes of the liver. The right kidney is quickly disappearing. The descending colon is seen as is the hepatic flexure. Although the superior mesenteric vein is clearly identifiable, the superior mesenteric artery appears to be splitting into feeder vessels. Muscles at this level include the rectus abdominis, psoas, and erector spinae.

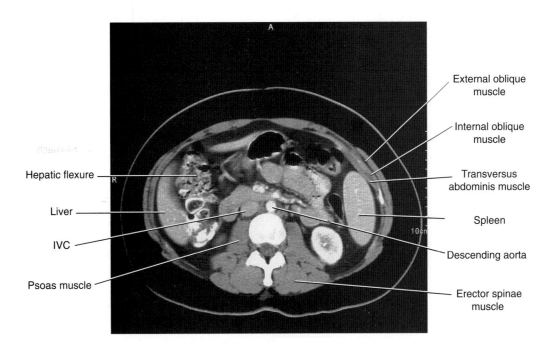

Hepatic flexure

Liver

IVC

Psoas muscle

External oblique
muscle

Internal oblique
muscle

Transversus
abdominis muscle

Spleen

Descending aorta

Erector spinae
muscle

Figure 5-32 This image (Figure 5-32) allows you to identify the three lateral muscles: the external and internal oblique, and transversus abdominis. Notice their placement with respect to each other. Little of the liver remains. The inferior vena cava and descending aorta continue to be seen.

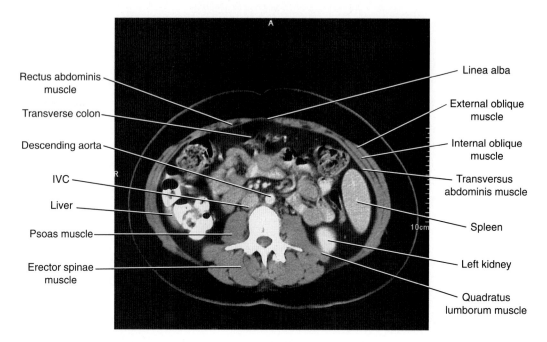

Figure 5-33 Be aware that the interslice gap between Figures 5-33 through 5-35 is greater than that for previous images. On Figure 5-33, almost all the liver has disappeared. Only the inferior part of the spleen is apparent. The transverse colon is seen for the first time on this set of images extending across the anterior abdomen from the hepatic flexure to the splenic flexure. Again notice the following muscles: external and internal oblique, transversus abdominis, psoas, and erector spinae. A new muscle has appeared in the vicinity of the transverse processes of the vertebra, the quadratus lumborum. Only a small amount of the left kidney remains.

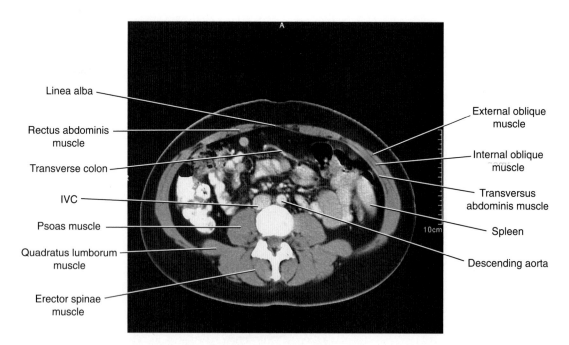

Figure 5-34 This image (Figure 5-34) is useful for identifying many of the muscles. Those that will continue to be seen into the pelvic region are the psoas and rectus abdominis. The inferior vena cava and descending aorta have not changed positions, or divided. The spleen has all but disappeared.

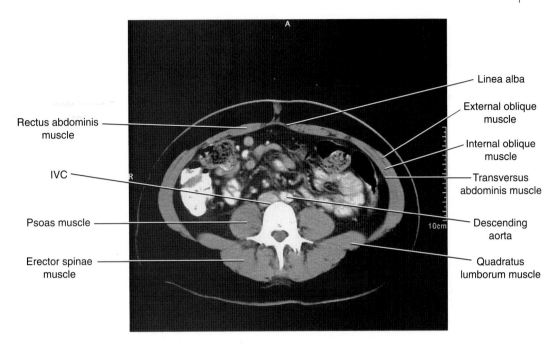

Rectus abdominis muscle

IVC

Psoas muscle

Erector spinae muscle

Linea alba

External oblique muscle

Internal oblique muscle

Transversus abdominis muscle

Descending aorta

Quadratus lumborum muscle

10cm

Figure 5-35 On Figure 5-35, you can discern the cleavage of the descending aorta. Arising from this bifurcation will be the right and left common iliac arteries. As a reminder, the descending aorta bifurcates at approximately L4 and the inferior vena cava forms from the right and left common iliac veins at L5. Take a moment to study the muscles.

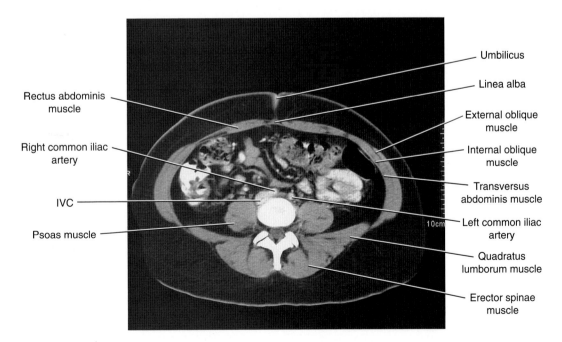

Rectus abdominis muscle

Right common iliac artery

IVC

Psoas muscle

Umbilicus

Linea alba

External oblique muscle

Internal oblique muscle

Transversus abdominis muscle

Left common iliac artery

Quadratus lumborum muscle

Erector spinae muscle

10cm

Figure 5-36 Figure 5-36 demonstrates the right and left common iliac arteries, vessels that arose from the bifurcation of the distal descending aorta. Notice the umbilicus along the anterior abdominal wall.

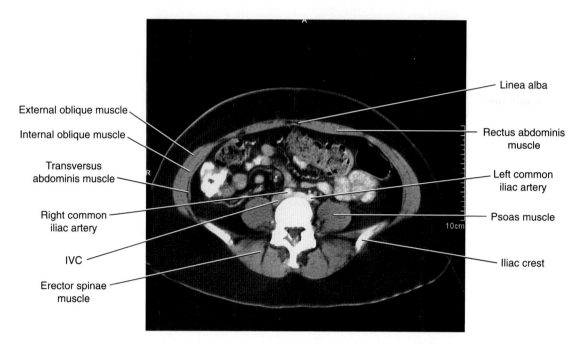

External oblique muscle

Internal oblique muscle

Transversus abdominis muscle

Right common iliac artery

IVC

Erector spinae muscle

Linea alba

Rectus abdominis muscle

Left common iliac artery

Psoas muscle

Iliac crest

10cm

Figure 5-37 The interslice gap between Figures 5-36 and 5-37 reverts to that seen with the earlier images of this exam. Figure 5-37 demonstrates the upper portion of the ilium, the iliac crest, which is a marker used by this author as a point of demarcation between the abdomen and pelvis. Compared to the previous image, a wider space separates the right and left common iliac arteries.

This particular study included examination of both the abdomen and pelvis. The first set of CT images in Chapter 6 on the pelvis will continue this exam into the pelvic region.

Exam 2

For the following study the interslice gap is larger for Figures 5-38 through 5-44 and 5-51 through 5-60. For those slices in the middle, Figures 5-45 through 5-50, smaller interslice gaps are chosen to more clearly demonstrate anatomy.

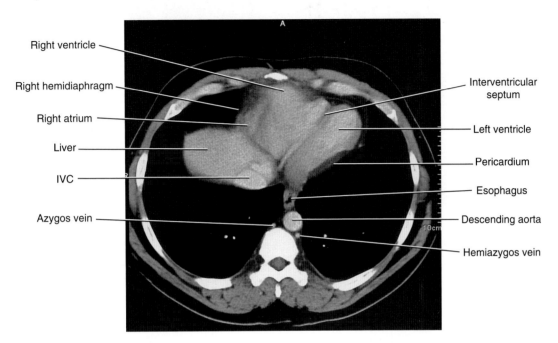

Figure 5-38 The first image of Exam 2, seen on Figure 5-38, demonstrates the transition from the thorax to the abdomen. Visualized are the right and left ventricles of the heart separated by the interventricular septum. A small amount of the right atrium is evident. The superior portion of the liver is just starting to appear. Notice the azygos and hemiazygos veins.

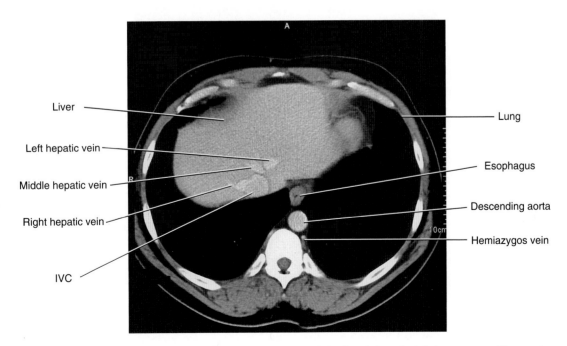

Figure 5-39 On Figure 5-39, notice that the hepatic veins drain directly into the inferior vena cava. The esophagus is identified anterior to the descending aorta.

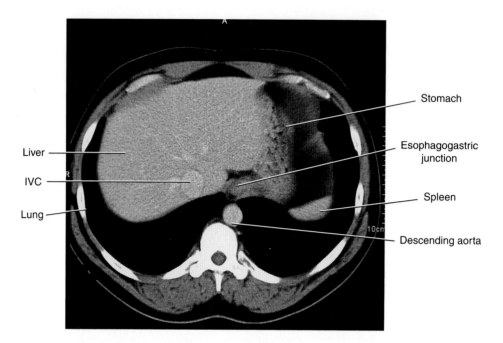

Figure 5-40 On Figure 5-40, a good portion of the stomach is seen in the left anterior upper abdomen, along with the esophagogastric junction. This is an indication that this image is just below the fundus of the stomach. Posterior to the stomach is the spleen. Individual patient differences determine whether the stomach or spleen is seen more superiorly.

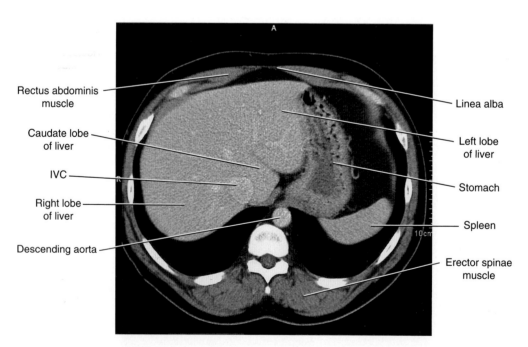

Figure 5-41 The next image (Figure 5-41) permits identification of some of the lobes of the liver: right, left, and caudate. The caudate lobe of the liver is found anterior to the IVC. Also labeled are the rectus abdominis muscles, separated by the linea alba, and the erector spinae muscles, seen posteriorly.

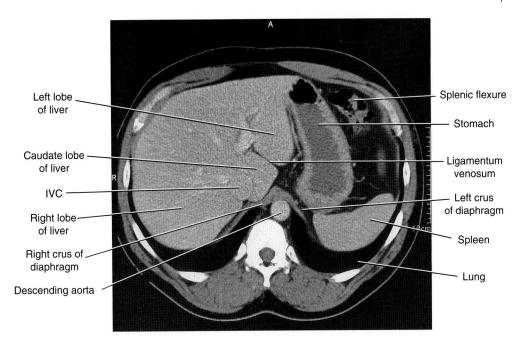

Figure 5-42 On Figure 5-42, the air seen in the anterior stomach indicates that the patient is supine. On the right and left, the crus of the diaphragm, anchoring the diaphragm posteriorly, is visible. The ligamentum venosum, a remnant of the fetal ductus venosus, separates the caudate lobe of the liver from the left lobe. Appearing in this image is the superior aspect of the splenic flexure on the left, which is typically higher than the hepatic flexure.

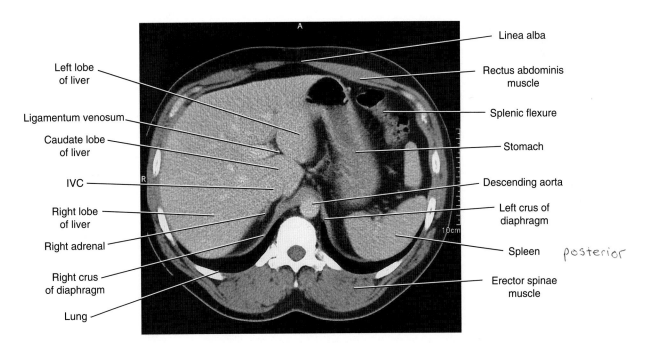

Figure 5-43 Structures that can be identified on Figure 5-43 are the stomach, spleen, right, left, and caudate lobes of the liver, IVC, and descending aorta. Notice the right adrenal behind the IVC. A small amount of lung tissue is still apparent. Coupled with the fact that the crus of the diaphragm is still evident, one can assume that this image is not below the level of the diaphragm.

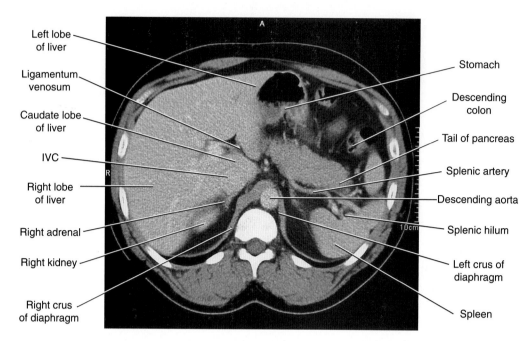

Left lobe of liver
Ligamentum venosum
Caudate lobe of liver
IVC
Right lobe of liver
Right adrenal
Right kidney
Right crus of diaphragm

Stomach
Descending colon
Tail of pancreas
Splenic artery
Descending aorta
Splenic hilum
Left crus of diaphragm
Spleen

Figure 5-44   A number of new organs have appeared on Figure 5-44. They include the tail of the pancreas, found to the left and at a higher level than the remaining sections of the pancreas. A small portion of the right kidney is now seen. This is somewhat atypical as normally the liver pushes the right kidney down to a level slightly lower than the left. A vessel is seen posterior to the pancreas, originating at the hilum of the spleen. The splenic artery typically runs along the superior aspect of the pancreas but on this series it appears posterior to the pancreas. Note the descending colon.

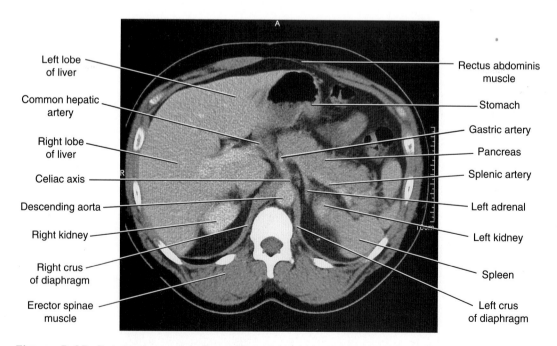

Left lobe of liver
Common hepatic artery
Right lobe of liver
Celiac axis
Descending aorta
Right kidney
Right crus of diaphragm
Erector spinae muscle

Rectus abdominis muscle
Stomach
Gastric artery
Pancreas
Splenic artery
Left adrenal
Left kidney
Spleen
Left crus of diaphragm

Figure 5-45   Probably the most significant difference between this image (Figure 5-45) and the previous one is the appearance of the celiac axis. The celiac axis is the first vessel to arise from the abdominal descending aorta and has three branches, the splenic artery, gastric artery, and common hepatic artery. All are identified on this image. The left adrenal gland and left kidney are seen for the first time.

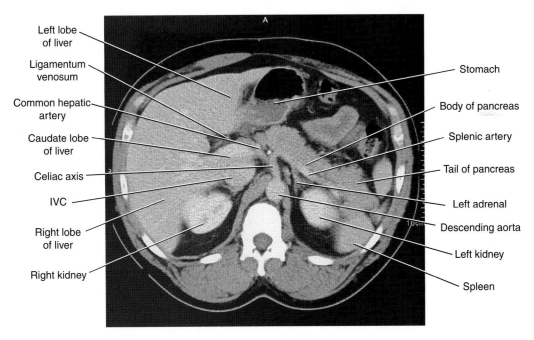

Left lobe
of liver

Ligamentum
venosum

Common hepatic
artery

Caudate lobe
of liver

Celiac axis

IVC

Right lobe
of liver

Right kidney

Stomach

Body of pancreas

Splenic artery

Tail of pancreas

Left adrenal

Descending aorta

Left kidney

Spleen

Figure 5-46 More of the pancreas appears on this image (Figure 5-46). Both kidneys are now seen, and the left adrenal particularly obvious. We continue to see the celiac axis, common hepatic artery, and splenic artery. Again, identify the right, left, and caudate lobes of the liver and the ligamentum venosum, which separates the caudate and left lobes.

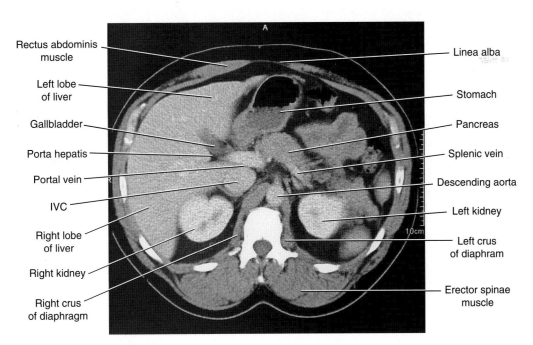

Rectus abdominis
muscle

Left lobe
of liver

Gallbladder

Porta hepatis

Portal vein

IVC

Right lobe
of liver

Right kidney

Right crus
of diaphragm

Linea alba

Stomach

Pancreas

Splenic vein

Descending aorta

Left kidney

Left crus
of diaphram

Erector spinae
muscle

Figure 5-47 A new organ has appeared on Figure 5-47, the gallbladder, an indication that this image is located more inferiorly in the liver. Also seen is the portal vein entering the porta hepatis of the liver. A small portion of the splenic vein is posterior to the pancreas. Locate the erector spinae and rectus abdominis muscles.

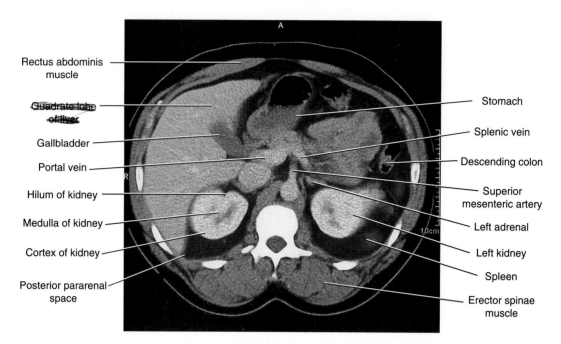

Rectus abdominis muscle

Quadrate lobe of liver

Gallbladder

Portal vein

Hilum of kidney

Medulla of kidney

Cortex of kidney

Posterior pararenal space

Stomach

Splenic vein

Descending colon

Superior mesenteric artery

Left adrenal

Left kidney

Spleen

Erector spinae muscle

Figure 5-48   On Figure 5-48, anterior to the gallbladder is the fourth lobe of the liver, the quadrate lobe. Identify the portal vein. The second vessel to arise off the abdominal descending aorta is the superior mesenteric artery (SMA). The SMA supplies the small intestines, cecum, ascending colon, and about one-half of the transverse colon with freshly oxygenated blood. The regions of the right kidney, the cortex and medulla, can be seen, as well as the hilum. Behind the kidney is the posterior pararenal space, in which is found mostly fat.

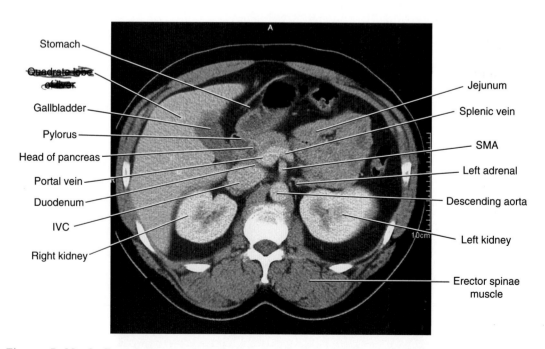

Stomach

Quadrate lobe of liver

Gallbladder

Pylorus

Head of pancreas

Portal vein

Duodenum

IVC

Right kidney

Jejunum

Splenic vein

SMA

Left adrenal

Descending aorta

Left kidney

Erector spinae muscle

Figure 5-49   On Figure 5-49, we can see the pylorus and distal stomach. The pylorus drains the stomach contents into the duodenum, which wraps around the head of the pancreas. This image shows the formation of the portal vein by the merger of the splenic vein and SMV, behind the head of the pancreas. A cross-section of the SMA is now apparent. The SMA will continue to descend for a while. Notice the quadrate lobe of the liver anterior to the gallbladder.

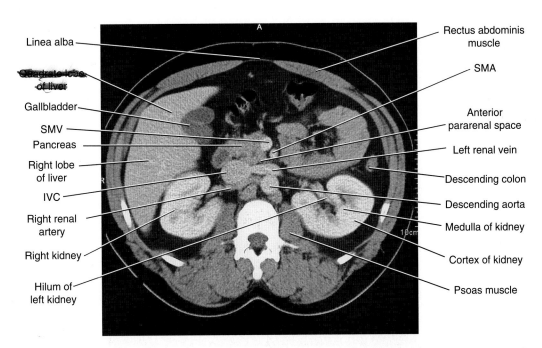

Figure 5-50 On Figure 5-50, the SMV and SMA are identified. The SMV is larger in circumference than the SMA and typically found to the right of the SMA. The left renal vein can be identified passing from the left kidney to the IVC. New muscles, the psoas, have appeared on either side of the body of the vertebra. We will observe the psoas muscles into the pelvic region, where they eventually will merge with the iliacus muscles to form the iliopsoas muscles.

Figure 5-51 The right renal artery connects the descending aorta with the right kidney on Figure 5-51. Identify the cortex, medulla, and hilum of the left kidney. The left renal vein is still apparent. Included in the anterior pararenal space are the pancreas and the descending colon. Still evident are the centrally located SMV and SMA. Both the right and quadrate lobes of the liver, along with the gallbladder, are visible, as is the descending aorta. The psoas muscles are increasing in size.

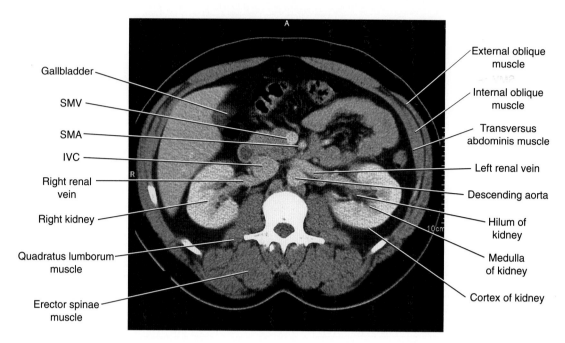

Figure 5-52 Newly labeled on Figure 5-52 are the three lateral muscles on either side of the abdomen, the external oblique, internal oblique, and transversus abdominis, listed from lateral to medial aspect. Also seen are the bilateral quadratus lumborum muscles, found adjacent to the transverse processes of the vertebra. The right renal vein is draining the right kidney into the IVC.

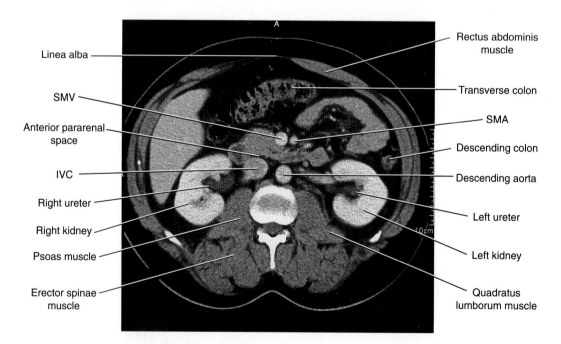

Figure 5-53 On Figure 5-53, extending from right to left anteriorly is a portion of the transverse colon. Note the structures exiting both kidneys, the right and left ureters. The descending colon is still apparent in the left anterior pararenal space. The quadratus lumborum muscles have been relabeled, allowing differentiation from the psoas and erector spinae muscles. The SMV and SMA are still seen.

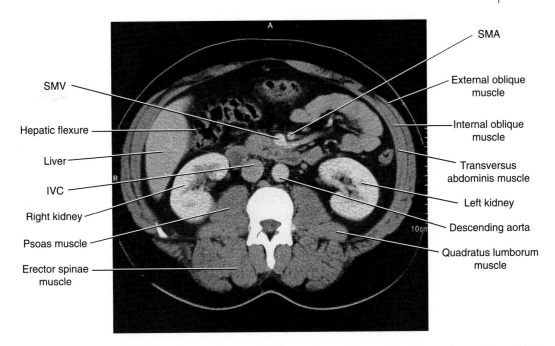

Figure 5-54 Identify the external oblique, internal oblique, and transversus abdominis muscles on Figure 5-54. The hepatic flexure on the right is starting to appear, adjacent to the inferior liver. The kidneys are still evident, as are the IVC and descending aorta. The descending aorta will bifurcate into the right and left common iliac arteries at approximately L4, while the formation of the IVC by the merger of the right and left common iliac veins should appear at approximately L5.

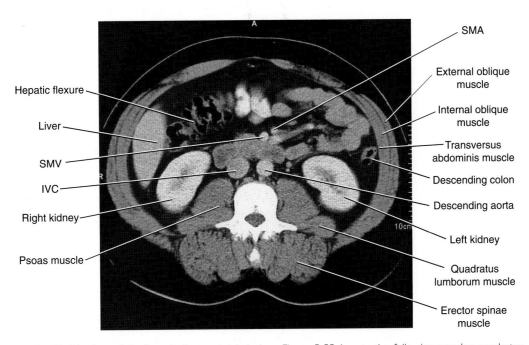

Figure 5-55 The last of the hepatic flexure is labeled on Figure 5-55. Locate the following muscles: quadratus lumborum, erector spinae, psoas, external oblique, internal oblique, and transversus abdominis.

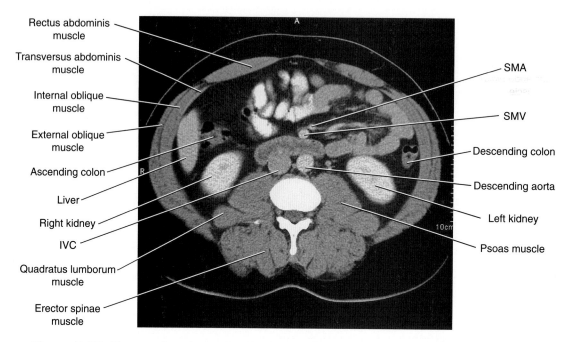

Rectus abdominis muscle

Transversus abdominis muscle

Internal oblique muscle

External oblique muscle

Ascending colon

Liver

Right kidney

IVC

Quadratus lumborum muscle

Erector spinae muscle

SMA

SMV

Descending colon

Descending aorta

Left kidney

Psoas muscle

Figure 5-56 The ascending colon on the right side has just appeared on Figure 5-56. On the left is the descending colon, the continuation of the splenic flexure. Muscles that will continue into the pelvic region include the rectus abdominis, psoas, and erector spinae. Those unique to this level are the quadratus lumborum and lateral muscles. The inferior region of the kidneys is seen bilaterally.

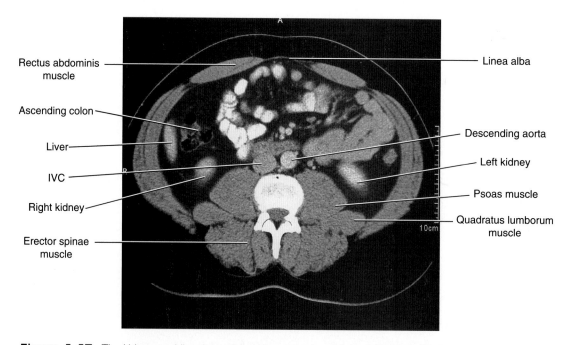

Rectus abdominis muscle

Ascending colon

Liver

IVC

Right kidney

Erector spinae muscle

Linea alba

Descending aorta

Left kidney

Psoas muscle

Quadratus lumborum muscle

Figure 5-57 The kidneys and liver have all but disappeared at this level (Figure 5-57). The IVC and descending aorta are intact but will soon be dividing. The rectus abdominis appears to be gradually becoming foreshortened.

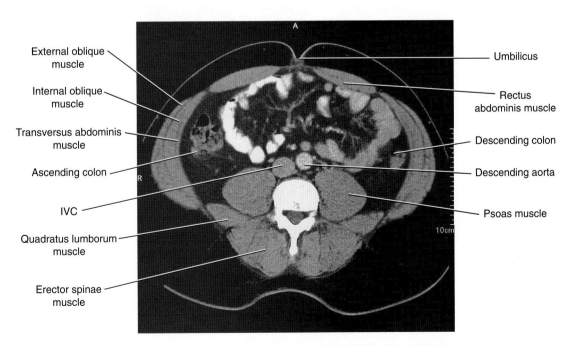

Rectus abdominis muscle

Ascending colon

IVC

Psoas muscle

Erector spinae muscle

External oblique muscle

Internal oblique muscle

Transversus abdominis muscle

Descending colon

Descending aorta

Quadratus lumborum muscle

Figure 5-58 There are few changes between this image (Figure 5-58) and the previous one, although it represents a fairly substantial interslice gap.

External oblique muscle

Internal oblique muscle

Transversus abdominis muscle

Ascending colon

IVC

Quadratus lumborum muscle

Erector spinae muscle

Umbilicus

Rectus abdominis muscle

Descending colon

Descending aorta

Psoas muscle

Figure 5-59 On Figure 5-59, notice along the anterior abdominal wall the midline indentation, the umbilicus. The umbilicus is generally in the vicinity of the upper pelvis, anatomically located at L4/L5. We anticipate seeing the ilia and the bifurcation of the descending aorta soon.

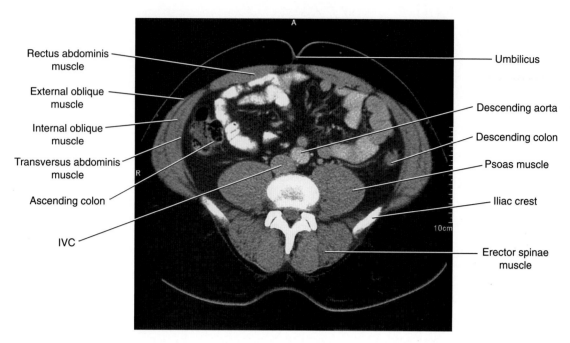

Figure 5-60 On Figure 5-60, the quadratus lumborum muscles have disappeared. However, the superior aspects of the ilia, the iliac crests, are now apparent. Look at the IVC and descending aorta. Which vessel will split first?

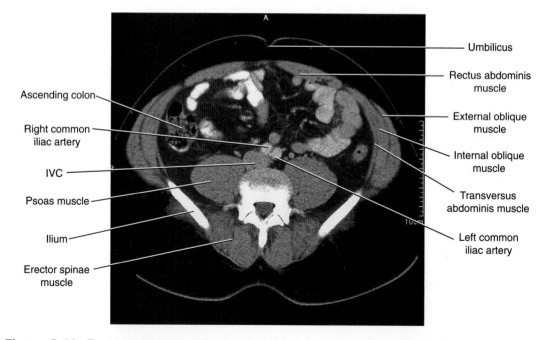

Figure 5-61 The last image in this series (Figure 5-61), with an interslice gap similar to the middle abdominal images, shows the bifurcation of the descending aorta into the right and left common iliac arteries. The erector spinae, psoas, rectus abdominis muscles, as well as the three lateral muscles should easily be located.

This study will be continued as Exam 2 in Chapter 6 on the pelvis.

REVIEW QUESTIONS

1. Which type(s) of contrast medium is/are used for abdominal/pelvic CT?
   a. Barium
   b. Nonionic iodinated
   c. Ionic iodinated
   d. a, b, and c

2. Organize the following branches of the abdominal aorta in the order they present on axial sectional images arranged in descending order:
   a. Celiac artery
   b. IMA
   c. SMA
   d. Renal artery

   _____a,_____
   _____c_____
   _____d_____
   _____b_____

3. Identify the three branches off the celiac axis.

   COMMON hep, l. gastric, splenic

Match the following vessels with the organs they supply.

_C_ 4. SMA

_a_ 5. IMA

_B_ 6. Celiac axis

   a. Left half of transverse colon, descending colon, rectum
   b. Stomach, spleen, liver
   c. Small intestine, cecum, ascending colon, right half of transverse colon

7. Which of the following statements regarding the renal arteries is true?
   (I.) The right renal artery is longer.
   (II.) The left renal artery will usually be the first to branch off the descending aorta.
   a. I
   b. II
   c. Both I and II are true.
   d. Neither I nor II is true.

8. Which of the following vessels is not involved in supplying the liver with blood?
   a. Hepatic artery
   (b.) Hepatic vein
   c. Portal vein
   d. None of the above supplies the liver with blood.
   e. They all supply the liver with blood.

9. Identify the two major vessels that merge to form the portal vein.

   splenic, SMV

10. Which of the following vessel(s) drain(s) into the inferior vena cava?
    (a.) Hepatic veins
    b. Common hepatic artery
    c. Portal vein
    d. a and c
    e. None of the above.

11. On axial CT images, the caudate lobe of the liver can be found anterior to and wrapping around the inferior vena cava.
    a. True
    b. False

12. As seen on axial CT images, what portions of the liver are separated by the falciform ligament?
    (a) Right lobe from left lobe
    b. Caudate lobe from quadrate lobe
    c. Caudate lobe from right lobe
    d. None of the above.

13. Which duct initially drains the bile from the gallbladder?
    (a.) Cystic duct
    b. Hepatic duct
    c. Common bile duct
    d. None of the above.

14. On axial sectional images arranged in descending order, typically the first part of the pancreas to appear is the
    a. head.
    b. body.
    (c.) tail.
    d. they all lie at the same level.

15. Identify the GI organ seen curving around the head of the pancreas on axial CT images.

    duodenum

16. Which vessel is seen posterior to the pancreas on sectional images?
    (a.) Portal vein
    b. Splenic artery
    (c.) Splenic vein
    (d.) a and c
    e. None of the above.

17. On sectional images the esophagus is seen entering the stomach
    a. anteriorly.
    (b.) medially.
    c. laterally.
    (d.) posteriorly.

18. Which of the following statements is true?
    I. The right kidney typically is at a higher level than the left.
    II. The right renal vein is longer than the left.
    a. I
    b. II
    c. I and II
    (d.) Neither I nor II.

19. The left adrenal gland is usually seen at a lower level than the right on sectional images.
    a. True
    (b.) False

Match the organ with its location.

___ 20. Pancreas   a. Anterior pararenal space

___ 21. Kidneys   b. Peritoneal cavity

___ 22. IVC and   c. Perirenal space
        descending aorta
                         d. Posterior pararenal space

___ 23. Transverse colon

24. Which muscle(s) is/are not a constant muscle(s) within the abdominopelvic region?
    a. Psoas
    (b.) Lateral muscles
    c. Rectus abdominis
    d. Erector spinae

25. Which lateral muscle is seen most medially on axial sectional images?
    a. External oblique
    b. Rectus abdominis
    c. Internal oblique
    d. Transversus abdominis

Pelvis

OUTLINE

PELVIC BONY STRUCTURES

The bony **pelvis**, shown on Figure 6-1, is a structure that encloses the pelvic organs and is composed of the **sacrum**, **coccyx**, and two **innominate bones** (**hip bones** or **os coxae**). The two innominate bones form the pelvic **girdle**. Each hip bone is composed of three bones that eventually fuse, the **ilium**, **ischium**, and **pubic** bone. Their point of union, the cup-shaped **acetabulum**, found in the lower, lateral hip, serves as a cavity to contain the head of the **femur**, the upper portion of the lower extremity. The uppermost section of the hip bone is the ilium. Its medial edge joins with the lateral edge of the sacrum to create the **sacroiliac joint**, from which it proceeds to flare outward and in an anterior direction. The flared portion of the ilium is the **ala**. The superior border of the ilium is the **crest** of the ilium, which ends anteriorly and posteriorly as the anterior and posterior superior **iliac spine**, respectively. Inferior to the anterior and posterior superior spines are the anterior and posterior inferior iliac spines. Beneath the posterior inferior iliac spine is a large notch, the **greater sciatic notch**. The inferior thickened section of the ilium, the body, makes up the upper two-fifths of the acetabulum.

The posterior inferior two-fifths of the acetabulum is formed by the body of the ischium. The inferior posterior portion of the ischium is a bony protuberance, the **ischial tuberosity**, upon which the body rests when seated. The **ischial spine** is a posteromedial extension of the ischium while the inferior **ramus** of the ischium extends anteriorly from the ischial tuberosity.

The last of the hip bones, the pubic bone, has two branches extending from the body, the superior and inferior rami. The inferior ramus of the pubic bone articulates with the inferior ramus of the ischial bone. The superior ramus of the pubic bone is involved in making up the remaining one-fifth of the acetabulum. The bodies of the right and left pubic bones join anteriorly midline to form the **symphysis pubis**, a slightly movable joint. The acetabulum and rami of the pubic bone and ischium encircle an opening, the **obturator foramen**. Central to the hip bones is a large aperture, the **pelvic inlet**. The anterior and posterior borders of the pelvic inlet are the superior aspect of the symphysis pubis and the superior anterior rim of the sacrum, respectively. Everything above and/or anterior to the pelvic inlet is the **false pelvis** and everything below

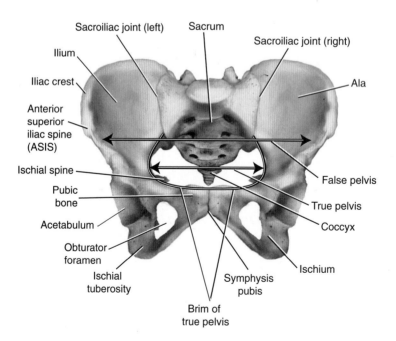

Figure 6-1 Anterior view of the bony pelvis

and/or posterior is the **true pelvis**. Figure 6-2, studied in conjunction with Figure 6-1, allows formulation of a three-dimensional mental model of the structures listed previously.

The sacrum is a triangulated bone made of five fused vertebrae and has a concave anterior surface. The upper broad edge is the **sacral promontory** while the body is the midline anterior surface. There are eight openings on either side of the body bilaterally, the **sacral foramina**, four anterior and four posterior. Lateral to the foramina, bilaterally, are the **lateral masses**. The sacrum articulates bilaterally with the ilia, superiorly with the fifth lumbar vertebra, and inferiorly with the coccyx. In an adult, the coccyx is one or two bones resulting from fusion of four vertebrae. The sacrum and coccyx are isolated on Figure 6-3.

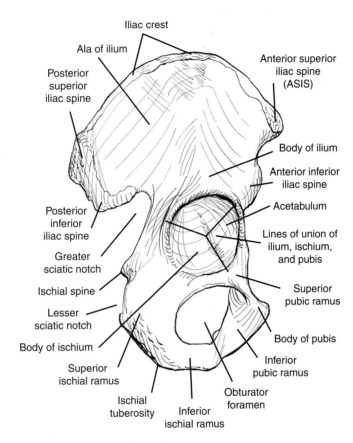

Figure 6-2 Lateral view of the bony pelvis

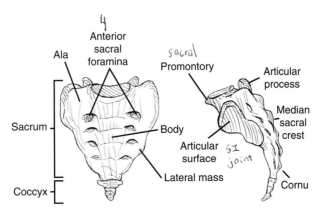

Figure 6-3 Anterior and lateral view of the sacrum

URINARY SYSTEM

In Chapter 5 the structures involved in the urinary system were listed: the bilateral kidneys and ureters and the single **bladder** and **urethra** (see Figure 6-4). Moving from the abdominal into the pelvic region, the right and left ureters continue to head in an anterior and medial direction until they enter the posterolateral aspect of the bladder, the hollow reservoir for urine. A point noted in Chapter 5 was that even with administration of contrast medium the ureters may not be evident on every image because of peristalsis. The bladder is situated posterior to the symphysis pubis and anterior to the rectum in the male, while in the female the **vagina** separates the bladder from the rectum with the **uterus** found along the postero-superior aspect of the bladder. The relationships are seen

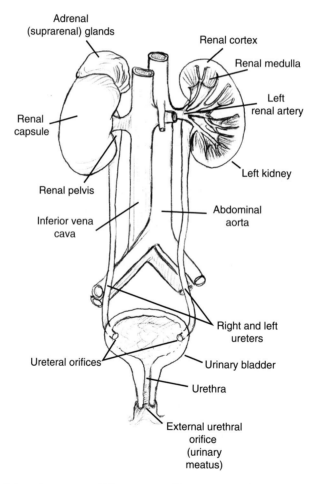

Figure 6-4 Organs of the urinary system: kidneys, ureters, bladder, and urethra

on Figure 6-5 A and B. Because iodinated contrast medium is heavier than urine, with the patient in a supine position the contrast medium may be seen in the posterior bladder on transaxial CT images.

The urine drains from the inferior bladder via the ure-thra, which is short in females, but longer in males as it must travel through the penis. In females the urethra is anterior to the vagina. In males, the urethra is a shared passageway for both urine from the urinary system and **seminal fluid** from the reproductive system.

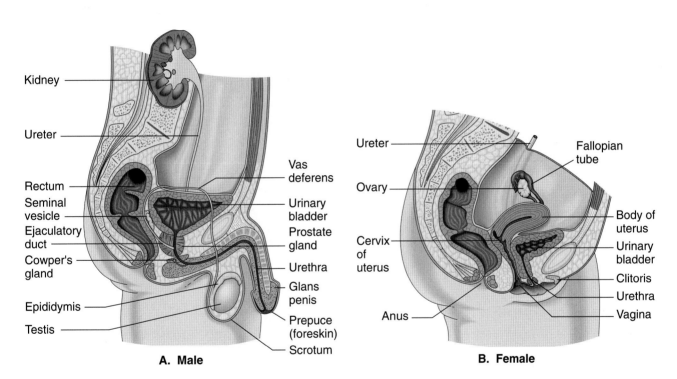

A. Male

Kidney

Ureter

Rectum

Seminal vesicle

Ejaculatory duct

Cowper's gland

Epididymis

Testis

Vas deferens

Urinary bladder

Prostate gland

Urethra

Glans penis

Prepuce (foreskin)

Scrotum

B. Female

Ureter

Ovary

Cervix of uterus

Anus

Fallopian tube

Body of uterus

Urinary bladder

Clitoris

Urethra

Vagina

Figure 6-5 A and B Lateral view of the ureters, bladder, and urethra in males and females

BLOOD VESSELS

Aorta

The aorta commences as the ascending aorta at the superior aspect of the left ventricle, then becomes the arch of the aorta, and, finally, the thoracic and abdominal descending aorta, in that order. The descending aorta is seen to the left of and slightly anterior to the vertebrae. It eventually bifurcates at L4 or approximately the level of the crest into the right and left common iliac arteries. The right and left common iliac arteries each then bifurcate into the **external** and **internal iliac arteries** at the level of the lumbosacral joint, with the external iliac arteries acquiring a new name, the femoral arteries, halfway between the anterior superior iliac spine (ASIS) and the symphysis pubis, when they enter the thighs. The internal iliac arter-

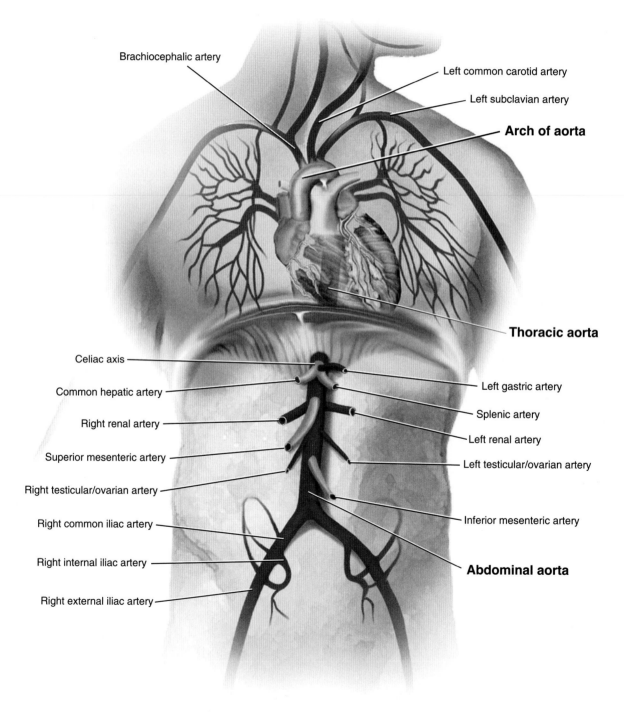

Brachiocephalic artery

Left common carotid artery

Left subclavian artery

Arch of aorta

Thoracic aorta

Celiac axis

Common hepatic artery

Right renal artery

Superior mesenteric artery

Right testicular/ovarian artery

Right common iliac artery

Right internal iliac artery

Right external iliac artery

Left gastric artery

Splenic artery

Left renal artery

Left testicular/ovarian artery

Inferior mesenteric artery

Abdominal aorta

Figure 6-6 Distal branches of the aorta

ies remain within the pelvic area to supply the pelvic (primarily the **gonadal**) organs with freshly oxygenated blood. The bilateral external iliac arteries are anterior to the internal iliac arteries and continue to move more and more anteriorly as they descend. In this region the arteries are anterior to the veins with similar names. Figure 6-6 is a line drawing of vessels discussed in this section while Figure 6-7 is a schematic diagram of the same vessels.

Scheme of Distribution

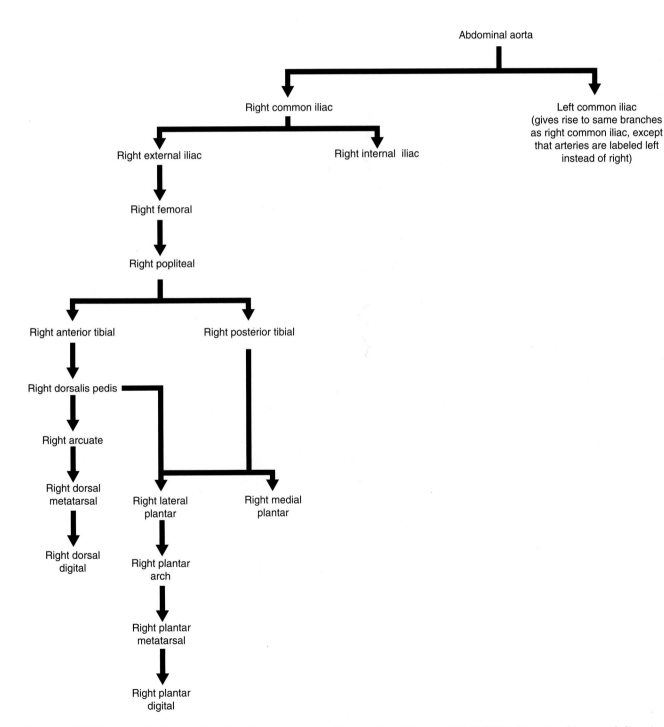

Figure 6-7 A schematic diagram of the branches of the aorta (Tortora, G. and Grabowski, S. R. [2000]. *Principles of Anatomy & Physiology* [9th ed.]. New York: John Wiley & Sons, Inc. This material is used by permission of John Wiley & Sons, Inc.)

Inferior Vena Cava

Returning deoxygenated blood from the lower extremities are the right and left **femoral** veins. Upon entering the anterior pelvic area they become the **external iliac veins**. Within the pelvic area, the external iliac veins join the **internal iliac veins**, found more posteriorly, to form the right and left common iliac veins. Small branches off the common iliac veins are the right and left ascending lumbar veins, which become the azygos and hemiazygos veins, respectively, at a higher level. The inferior vena cava, located slightly to the right of and anterior to the vertebrae, is formed by the merger of the right and left common iliac veins at approximately L5. The inferior vena cava continues to ascend through the abdomen, diaphragm, and the lower mediastinum until it finally enters the inferior aspect of the right atrium (see Figures 6-8 and 6-9).

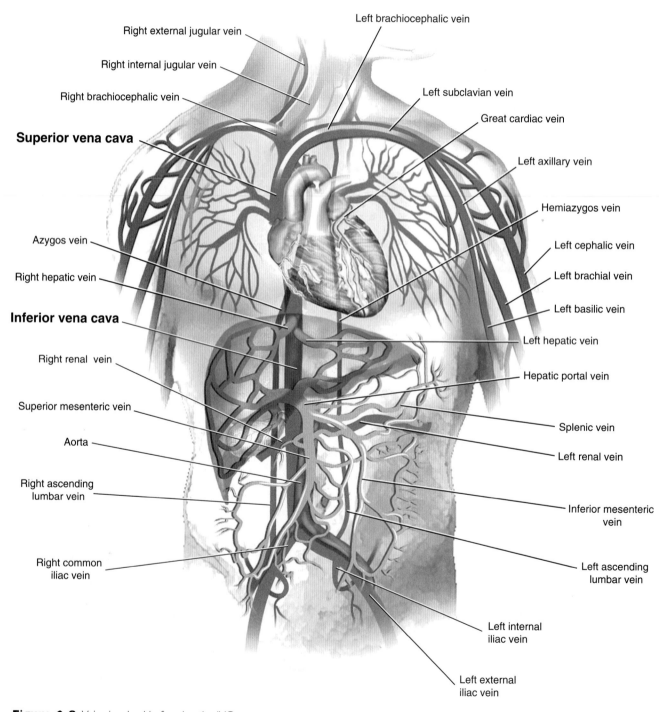

Figure 6-8 Veins involved in forming the IVC

Because of the large number of vessels in the pelvic area, it is helpful to have some sense of their general pattern to properly identify them on sectional images. At approximately the level of the crest are the IVC to the right, and the right and left common iliac arteries to the left. Moving in an inferior direction, the next few sectional images demonstrate the right and left common iliac arteries and the right and left common iliac veins, with the arteries being anterior to the veins. In most cases, the next level, at the upper portion of the sacrum, finds the right and left common iliac arteries and the right and left external and internal iliac veins. Again, arteries are anterior to the veins and the external iliac veins are anterior to the internal iliac veins. Finally, prior to seeing the femoral arteries and veins, the right and left external iliac arteries and veins appear at the level of the sacrum. The same pattern exists: arteries are anterior to veins and external iliac arteries or veins are anterior to the internal iliac arteries or veins.

Scheme of Drainage

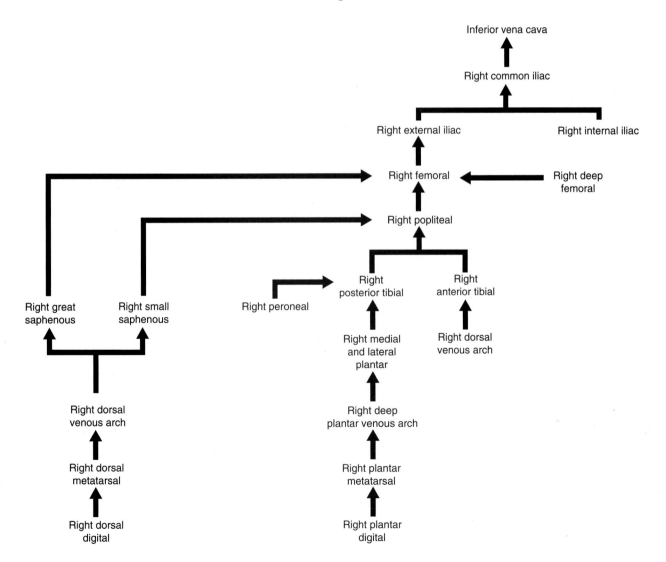

Figure 6-9 A schematic diagram of the veins involved in forming the IVC (Tortora, G. and Grabowski, S. R. [2000]. *Principles of Anatomy & Physiology* [9th ed.]. New York: John Wiley & Sons, Inc. This material is used by permission of John Wiley & Sons, Inc.)

MALE REPRODUCTIVE ORGANS

The male reproductive system is composed of the paired **testis** or **testicles** situated in the **scrotum**, the **epididymis**, **ductus vas deferens**, **seminal vesicles**, **ejaculatory duct**, **prostate gland**, **bulbourethral** or **Cowper's glands**, and urethra, all of which can be seen on Figure 6-10.

Testes/Epididymis

Sperm is manufactured and **testosterone** produced within the testes. The sperm completes its maturation process within the epididymis and travels into the ductus vas deferens.

Ductus Vas Deferens

The bilateral ductus vas deferens ascend within the pelvic cavity anterior to the bladder and then pass along the upper lateral aspect of the bladder and bend to descend on either side of the posterior bladder. They are seen as linear opacities on either side of the posterior bladder on cross-sectional images.

Seminal Vesicles

On either side of the posterior lower bladder are the paired seminal vesicles, whose function is to produce approximately 60% of the fluid in seminal fluid or **semen**. The high levels of fructose in the fluid provide energy for sperm. On transaxial CT images the seminal vesicles appear as oval areas of opacity directly behind the lower bladder. The two ductus vas deferens join with the ducts from the seminal vesicles at the base of the bladder to form the ejaculatory ducts, which empty into the first part of the urethra, the prostatic urethra.

Prostate Gland

The prostatic section of the urethra is encircled by the prostate gland, the largest accessory gland of the male

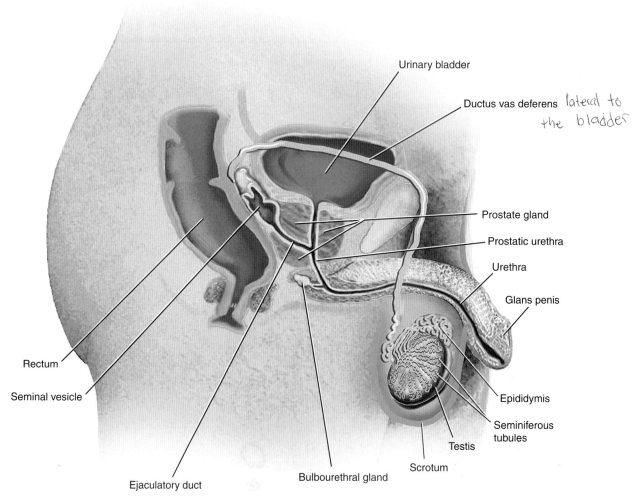

Urinary bladder

Ductus vas deferens *lateral to the bladder*

Prostate gland

Prostatic urethra

Urethra

Glans penis

Epididymis

Seminiferous tubules

Testis

Scrotum

Bulbourethral gland *or Cowper glands*

Ejaculatory duct

Seminal vesicle

Rectum

Figure 6-10 Lateral view of the male reproductive organs

reproductive system. The prostate gland has a dual function: it prevents urine from mixing in with seminal fluid during ejaculation and contributes about 25% of fluid to the seminal fluid. The prostatic secretions aid in the motility and fertility of sperm. The prostate gland is seen posterior to the symphysis pubis on sectional films. Some urine may be visible in the center of the neck of the bladder and/or the first part of the urethra on sectional images.

Bulbourethral/Cowper's Glands

The two pea-sized bulbourethral or Cowper's glands are inferior to the prostate gland and have ducts leading into the urethra. They also contribute to seminal fluid as well as lubricate the end of the penis during intercourse. They are not visible on axial CT images. Figure 6-11 permits visualization of many of these aforementioned structures from a posterior perspective.

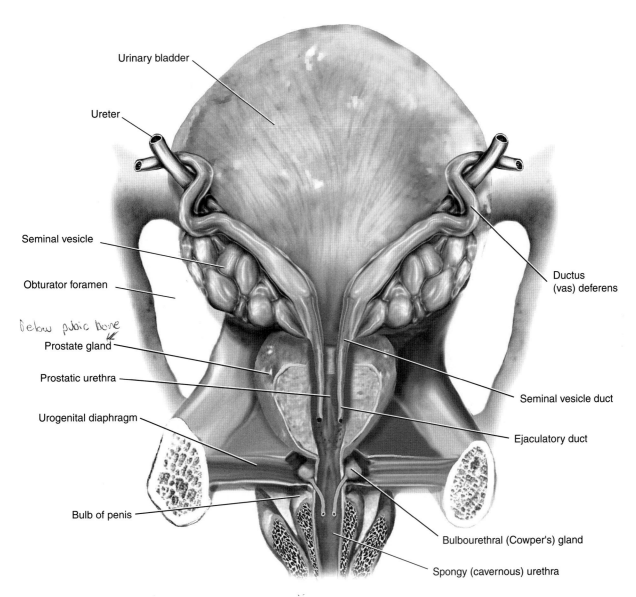

Figure 6-11 Posterior view of the male reproductive organs

FEMALE REPRODUCTIVE ORGANS

The organs involved in the female reproductive system are the **mammary glands** (not relevant to this study of organs in the pelvic region), uterus, **ovaries**, **fallopian** or **uterine tubes** (or **oviducts**), vagina, and **vulva** (or **pudendum**). Consult Figures 6-12 and 6-13 as you study each organ.

Uterus

Similar in size and shape to an inverted pear, the uterus projects up and over the posterior superior bladder. Sperm travel through the uterus to the uterine tubes, with any fertilized ovum eventually gravitating back to the uterus for development. If pregnancy does not occur, it is the sloughing off of the lining of the uterus at the end of a menstrual cycle that is responsible for **menstruation**.

The uterus is divided into regions, the superior dome-shaped fundus, the central body, and the inferior narrowed **cervix**. The cervix is located at approximately the level of the hip. On cross-sectional CT images, the uterus is seen as an irregularly shaped area of opacity anterior to the rectum and appears to indent the posterior bladder at approximately the same level that the ureters enter the posterolateral bladder.

Ovaries

The paired ovaries are lateral to the uterus but their level may vary from individual to individual. Their function is to secrete the female hormones **estrogen** and **progesterone** and to bring to maturation and release the female egg or **ovum**. On axial CT scans they appear as small rounded areas of opacity on either side of the uterus.

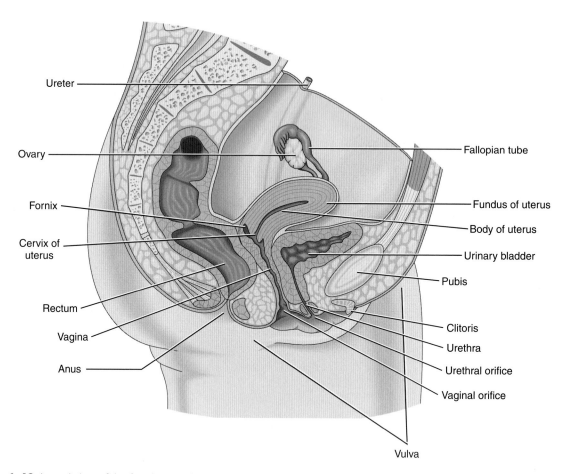

Figure 6-12 Lateral view of the female reproductive organs found in the pelvis

Uterine/Fallopian Tubes

The paired uterine or fallopian tubes (or oviducts) are tubular structures that extend from the superior lateral aspect of the uterus in a lateral direction and terminate in a dilated area called the **infundibulum**. Fingerlike processes called **fimbriae** delineate the edges of the infundibulum. The bilateral fimbriae are adjacent to but do not actually touch the ovaries. The uterine tubes cannot be easily identified on axial CT images.

When a mature egg or ovum is released by an ovary, it enters the infundibulum and travels to approximately the midpoint of the fallopian tube, where fertilization normally occurs. If the egg becomes fertilized, it will migrate to the uterus where it will undergo further development.

By definition, the ovaries and fallopian tubes are considered **adnexa** of the uterus as they are accessories and adjacent to the uterus.

Vagina

The vagina is the receptacle for the penis during intercourse and the passageway for blood flow during menses and the infant during childbirth. Situated between the rectum posteriorly and the bladder anteriorly, the vagina begins at the distal end of the uterus (the cervix). Where the cervix and vagina meet there is a recess, the **fornix**. The distal end of the vagina has an external opening called the **vaginal orifice**. On axial CT images the vagina is posterior to the inferior bladder. Insertion of a tampon into the vagina during sectional imaging allows better visualization.

The vaginal orifice and the distal end of the urethra, the **urethral orifice**, are considered part of the vulva or pudendum, the external female **genitalia**.

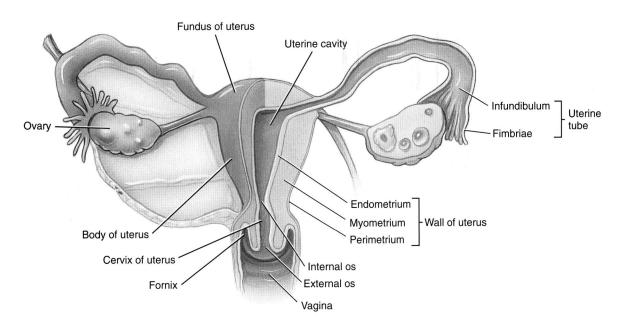

Figure 6-13 Anterior view of the female reproductive organs found in the pelvis

INTESTINES

In reviewing the information on the small and large intestines in Chapter 5 it should be noted that a portion of both intestines are in the pelvic region. While the first segment of the small intestines, the duodenum, begins at approximately L1 when the stomach is empty, the jejunum is in the umbilical region and most of the ileum, the last segment, is in the hypogastric region. The distal portion of the ileum is in the pelvic region.

The junction of the small intestines with the large intestines occurs at the ileocecal valve. The cecum extends 5–7 cm below the ileocecal valve, sitting in the right iliac fossa. The vermiform appendix, averaging 3 inches in length, may be found in any direction from the cecum but commonly is inferior and posterior to it. When the ascending colon meets the transverse colon, the transverse colon may loop down to the level of the pelvic brim. The continuation of the transverse colon is the descending colon, which then becomes the sigmoid colon at the level of the iliac crest. In some individuals the sigmoid colon may extend up into the abdomen but generally is in the left iliac fossa. The final section of the large intestines, the rectum, averaging approximately 8 inches in length, commences at the brim of the true pelvis and ends at the distal coccyx.

In identifying any of the above intestinal structures on sectional images, it is helpful to remember that all but the ascending and descending colon and a portion of the duodenum are in the peritoneal cavity while the exceptions are retroperitoneal. Figure 6-14 is a line drawing showing the small and large intestines.

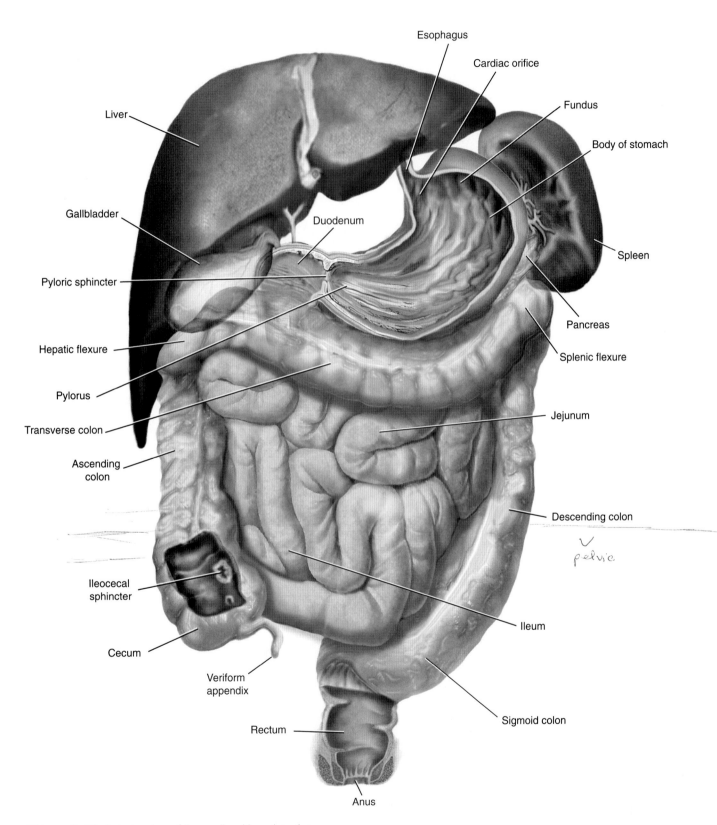

Figure 6-14 Anterior view of the small and large intestines

MUSCLES

There are numerous muscles found in the pelvic region, some of which first appeared in the abdominal region. Those constant through the abdominal and pelvic areas are the rectus abdominis along the anterior abdominal wall, the erector spinae posterior to the vertebrae, and the bilateral psoas muscles. The linea alba remains midline between the rectus abdominis muscles but the muscles taper as they descend, as shown on Figure 6-15. The erector spinae, located posteriorly on either side of the spinous process, disappear at the level of the inferior sacrum. The two psoas muscles still exist within the pelvic region but merge with the bilateral iliacus muscles to become the iliopsoas muscles. The iliopsoas muscles are seen more and more anteriorly and laterally as CT axial cuts descend to the level of the hip (see Figure 6-16).

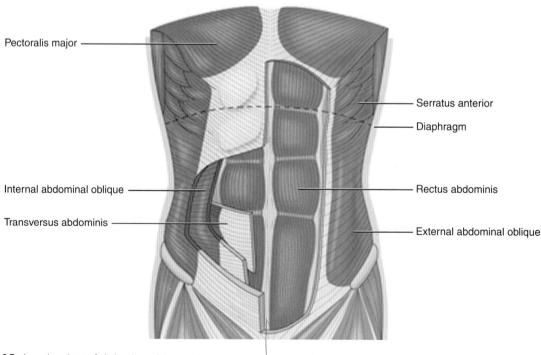

Pectoralis major

Serratus anterior

Diaphragm

Internal abdominal oblique

Rectus abdominis

Transversus abdominis

External abdominal oblique

Figure 6-15 Anterior view of abdominopelvic muscles

linea alba

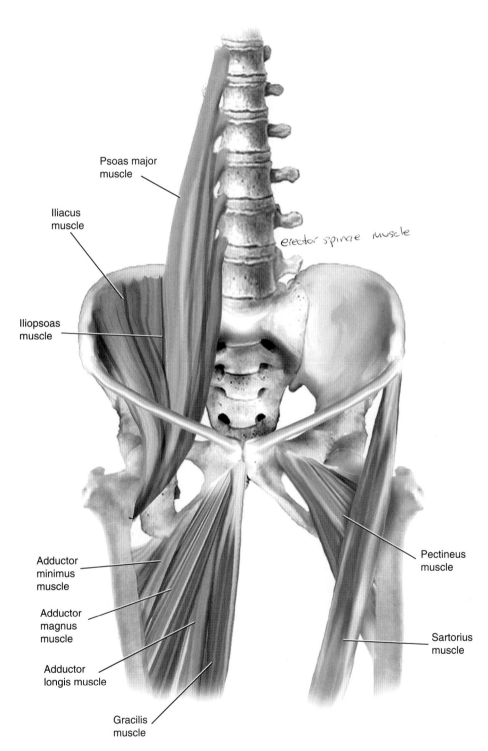

Psoas major muscle

Iliacus muscle

erector spinae muscle

Iliopsoas muscle

Pectineus muscle

Adductor minimus muscle

Adductor magnus muscle

Sartorius muscle

Adductor longis muscle

Gracilis muscle

Figure 6-16 Anterior view of pelvic muscles

Muscles unique to the pelvic region include the bilateral **gluteal**, iliacus, and **piriformis muscles**. There are three gluteal muscles on either side of the posterolateral pelvic region. Separated by a layer of fat, they can easily be differentiated from each other. The order of appearance on descending axial CT images is the gluteal medius, gluteal maximus, and gluteal minimus. Their placement from a posterior to an anterior direction is gluteal maximus, gluteal medius, and gluteal minimus. Their names indicate their relative sizes fully formed and all three taper anteriorly on transaxial CT images. At the level of the hip the only remaining gluteal muscle is the gluteal maximus. The last muscle in the pelvic region is the piriformis, which originates at the anterior sacrum and inserts at the greater trochanter. At higher levels on axial CT images, it appears bilaterally anterior to the inferior sacrum. On lower cuts it extends bilaterally from the lateral aspect of the sacrum

extending behind the ischium to insert onto the greater trochanter. The gluteal muscles and a cut of the piriformis muscles are drawn on Figure 6-17.

At the level of the hip the list of muscles expands to include the gluteal maximus, **sartorius**, iliopsoas, **rectus femoris**, **tensor**, **obturator**, **pectineus**, and **levator ani muscles**. The sartorius is the longest muscle in the human body extending from the ASIS to the proximal medial tibia and is the most anterior of those muscles associated with the hip. It is lateral and anterior to the hip. At the level of the hip the iliopsoas is medial to the sartorius. Immediately posterior to the sartorius is the rectus femoris, which is one of four heads forming the quadriceps femoris. Anterior to the tail of the bilateral gluteal maximus are the tensors. The iliopsoas, sartorius, rectus femoris, and tensor muscles and their relationship with each other are shown on Figure 6-18. The two obturator internus and externus muscles,

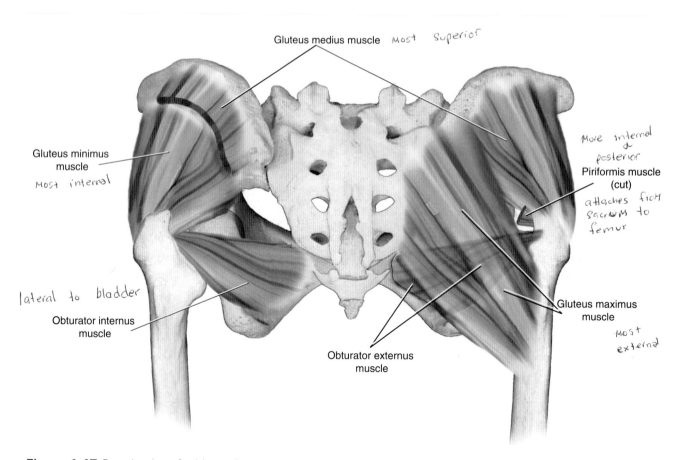

Figure 6-17 Posterior view of pelvic muscles

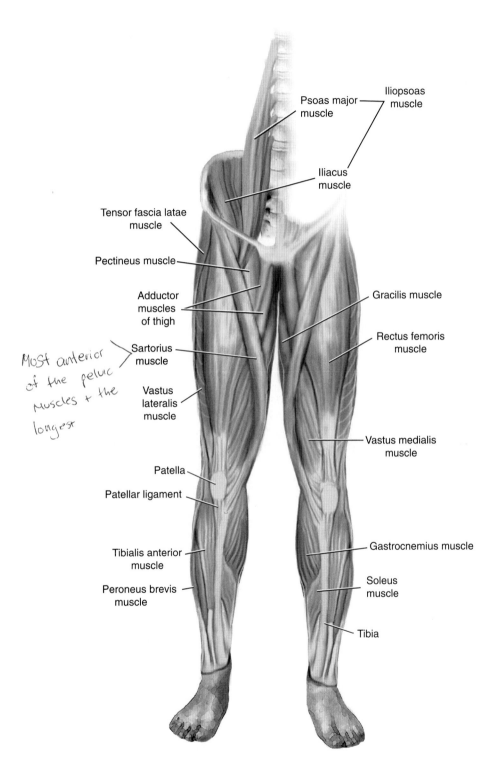

Psoas major muscle

Iliopsoas muscle

Iliacus muscle

Tensor fascia latae muscle

Pectineus muscle

Adductor muscles of thigh

Sartorius muscle

Most anterior of the pelvic muscles + the longest

Vastus lateralis muscle

Patella

Patellar ligament

Tibialis anterior muscle

Peroneus brevis muscle

Gracilis muscle

Rectus femoris muscle

Vastus medialis muscle

Gastrocnemius muscle

Soleus muscle

Tibia

Figure 6-18 Tensor, sartorius, and rectus femoris muscles

seen on Figure 6-17, are anterior and posterior to the bilateral obturator foramina. On axial CT images the obturator foramen is between the symphysis pubis and ischium. The bilateral pectineus muscles are lateral to the rami of the pubic bones. The last muscle, the levator ani, originating at the symphysis pubis and inserting at the coccyx, encircles the rectum and is involved in forming the pelvic floor. Figure 6-19 includes the levator ani.

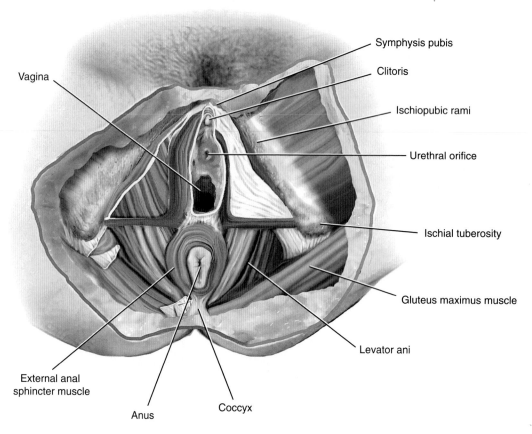

Figure 6-19 Muscles of the pelvic floor seen in a female

CT IMAGES

Exam I

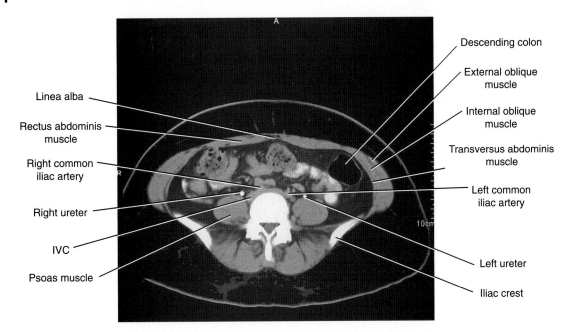

Linea alba
Rectus abdominis muscle
Right common iliac artery
Right ureter
IVC
Psoas muscle

Descending colon
External oblique muscle
Internal oblique muscle
Transversus abdominis muscle
Left common iliac artery
Left ureter
Iliac crest

Figure 6-20 This first image (Figure 6-20) is at the upper level of the pelvis, the iliac crest, and is a continuation of the first series of images for the abdomen (presented in Chapter 5). The right and left common iliac arteries are seen anterior to the IVC. This particular cut is at the level where the right and left common iliac veins are merging to form the IVC. The ureters are seen with a great deal of intensity. They will continue to move anteriorly as we descend through the pelvis, until they enter the bladder posterolaterally. The lateral muscles (external oblique, internal oblique, and transversus abdominis) are evident but will not be constant through the pelvis.

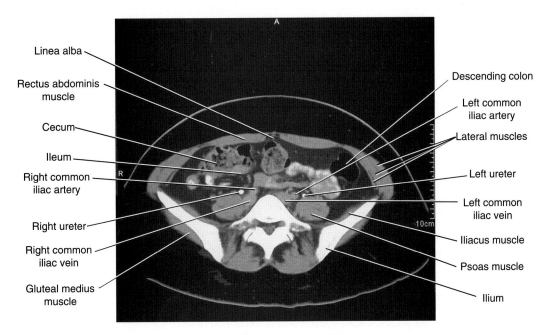

Linea alba
Rectus abdominis muscle
Cecum
Ileum
Right common iliac artery
Right ureter
Right common iliac vein
Gluteal medius muscle

Descending colon
Left common iliac artery
Lateral muscles
Left ureter
Left common iliac vein
Iliacus muscle
Psoas muscle
Ilium

Figure 6-21 On Figure 6-21, the right and left common iliac arteries and veins are now apparent. Remember the rule: arteries are anterior to the veins. Two new pairs of muscles have appeared: the gluteal medius, the first to appear as we descend through the pelvis, and the iliacus, anterior to the ilia. The psoas muscles will eventually merge with the iliacus muscles to form the iliopsoas muscles. The rectus abdominis muscles are seen along the anterior abdominal wall. They will remain constant throughout the pelvic region.

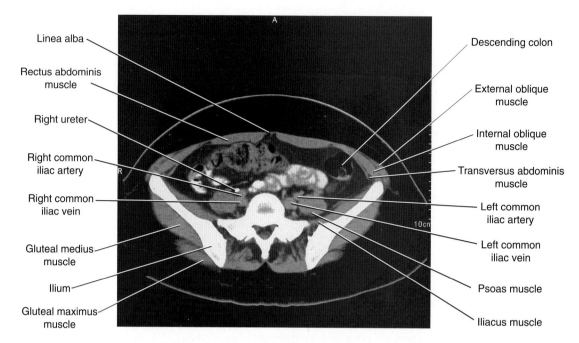

Linea alba

Rectus abdominis muscle

Right ureter

Right common iliac artery

Right common iliac vein

Gluteal medius muscle

Ilium

Gluteal maximus muscle

Descending colon

External oblique muscle

Internal oblique muscle

Transversus abdominis muscle

Left common iliac artery

Left common iliac vein

Psoas muscle

Iliacus muscle

Figure 6-22   The second pair of gluteal muscles, the gluteal maximus, are now seen on Figure 6-22. The gluteal maximus muscles are posterior to the gluteal medius muscles. The gluteal muscles are separated by a layer of fat. Consequently, they can be differentiated from each other. Notice the descending colon on the left. The right ureter can be identified. If an image is obtained while the ureter is undergoing peristalsis it will not be seen.

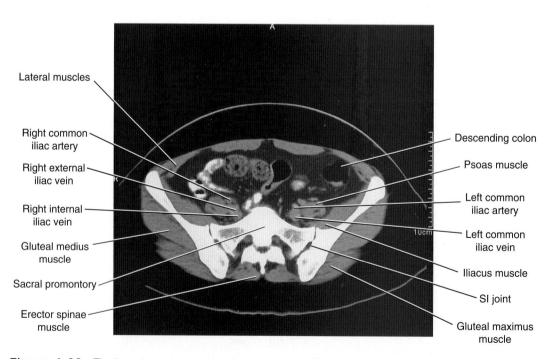

Lateral muscles

Right common iliac artery

Right external iliac vein

Right internal iliac vein

Gluteal medius muscle

Sacral promontory

Erector spinae muscle

Descending colon

Psoas muscle

Left common iliac artery

Left common iliac vein

Iliacus muscle

SI joint

Gluteal maximus muscle

Figure 6-23   The lateral muscles are identified on Figure 6-23, but are not seen as we slice at lower levels. The upper portion of the sacrum, the sacral promontory, along with the sacroiliac (SI) joints, has now appeared. The common iliac arteries and veins are seen, although it appears that this image was obtained where the external and internal iliac veins merged to form the common iliac veins.

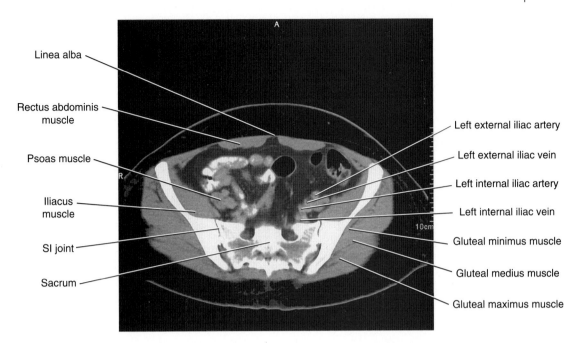

Linea alba

Rectus abdominis muscle

Psoas muscle

Iliacus muscle

SI joint

Sacrum

Left external iliac artery

Left external iliac vein

Left internal iliac artery

Left internal iliac vein

Gluteal minimus muscle

Gluteal medius muscle

Gluteal maximus muscle

Figure 6-24 On Figure 6-24, the psoas and iliacus muscles are adjacent to each other, and will soon merge into the iliopsoas muscles. The three pairs of gluteal muscles are now all identified: the gluteal maximus, medius, and minimus, listed posteriorly to anteriorly. The external and internal arteries and veins are labeled on the left. The two "rules," arteries anterior to veins and external iliac vessels anterior to internal iliac vessels, apply.

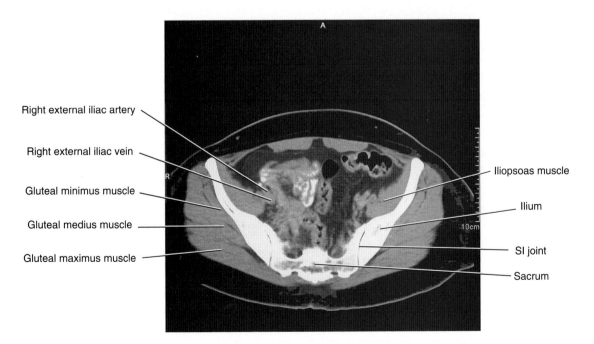

Right external iliac artery

Right external iliac vein

Gluteal minimus muscle

Gluteal medius muscle

Gluteal maximus muscle

Iliopsoas muscle

Ilium

SI joint

Sacrum

Figure 6-25 The iliopsoas muscles now appear as single muscles, bilaterally on Figure 6-25. They will continue to move anteriorly through the lower pelvic region. On the right, identify the external artery and vein, which will also continue to move anteriorly as we image the lower pelvic region. At the level of the symphysis pubis they will acquire new names, the femoral arteries and veins.

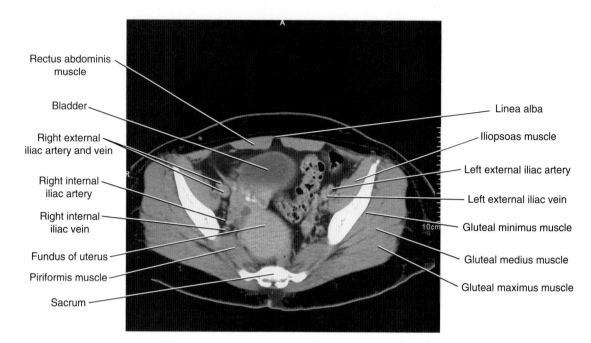

Rectus abdominis
muscle

Bladder

Right external
iliac artery and vein

Right internal
iliac artery

Right internal
iliac vein

Fundus of uterus

Piriformis muscle

Sacrum

Linea alba

Iliopsoas muscle

Left external iliac artery

Left external iliac vein

Gluteal minimus muscle

Gluteal medius muscle

Gluteal maximus muscle

10cm

Figure 6-26   A number of new structures have appeared on Figure 6-26. The first are the piriformis muscles anterior to the sacrum. Also now seen is the bladder. The fundus of the uterus is seen posterior to the bladder. The upper portion of the uterus sits along the posterior superior aspect of the bladder. Some of the external and internal iliac arteries and veins are labeled. Notice that the internal iliac arteries and veins have remained within the posterior pelvic region. The arteries provide the pelvic organs (primarily the gonads) with a source of blood, while the veins drain the same region.

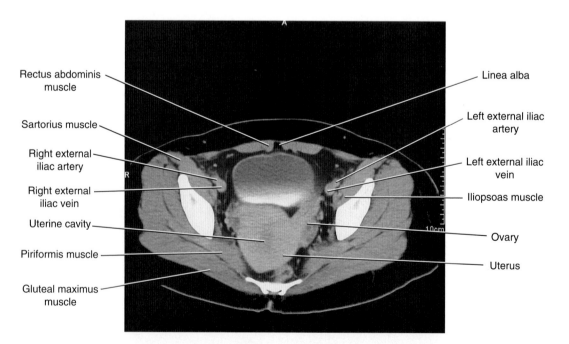

Rectus abdominis
muscle

Sartorius muscle

Right external
iliac artery

Right external
iliac vein

Uterine cavity

Piriformis muscle

Gluteal maximus
muscle

Linea alba

Left external iliac
artery

Left external iliac
vein

Iliopsoas muscle

Ovary

Uterus

10cm

Figure 6-27   On Figure 6-27, the iliopsoas muscles continue to gravitate anteriorly, as do the external arteries and veins. The rectus abdominis muscles appear to be disappearing. The piriformis muscles now extend laterally from the sacrum and are seen anterior to the gluteal maximus muscles. The uterine cavity can be found within the uterus. Adjacent to the uterus, bilaterally, are the ovaries. We see the sartorius muscles at this level. In the lower pelvic region they are the most anterior muscles.

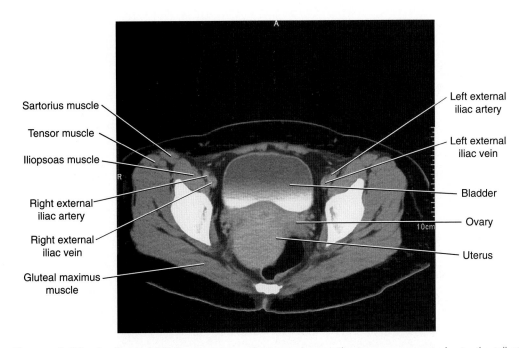

Figure 6-28 On Figure 6-28, the newest muscles appearing are the tensors, seen anterior to the tail of each gluteal maximus muscle. The uterus continues to appear to press against the back of the bladder, an indication that this patient is a female. On a male pelvis, the bladder consistently appears oval in shape. The ovaries are still seen on either side of the bladder.

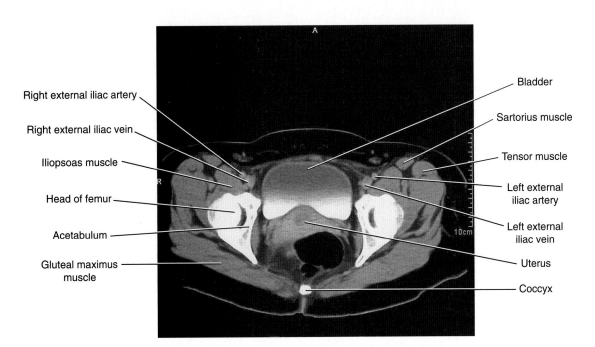

Figure 6-29 Notice how much anteriorly both the iliopsoas muscles and external iliac arteries and veins have moved on Figure 6-29. The only gluteal muscles to appear intact are the gluteal maximus muscles. The head of each femur is identified within the acetabulum. The distal end of the vertebral column, the coccyx, is also labeled.

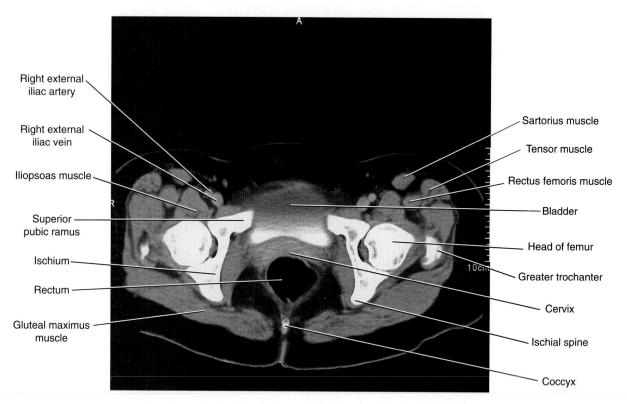

Figure 6-30 On Figure 6-30, on the left, the greater trochanter is seen lateral to the head of the femur. The ischial spines are found posteriorly on each ischium. The cervix is seen posterior to the bladder and anterior to the rectum. The cervix is the most inferior aspect of the uterus. The very tip of the coccyx is identified. The rectus femoris muscles are labeled, as are the superior pubic rami.

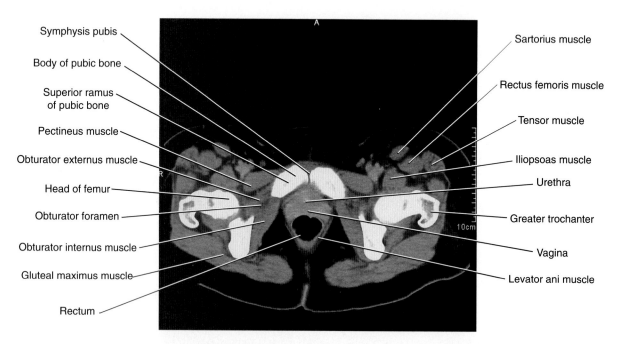

Figure 6-31 The bodies of the pubic bones meet midline to form the symphysis pubis on Figure 6-31. Lateral to the symphysis pubis are the pectineus muscles. The obturator foramen can be identified as the space separating the pubic and ischial bones. The bilateral obturator externus and internus muscles border the obturator foramen anteriorly and posteriorly, respectively. Most posteriorly is the rectum with the levator ani muscles seen on either side. Anterior to the rectum is the vagina and anterior to the vagina is the urethra. Notice the arrangement of the muscles: the sartorius, rectus femoris, and tensor. The greater trochanter is seen lateral to the head of the femur, bilaterally.

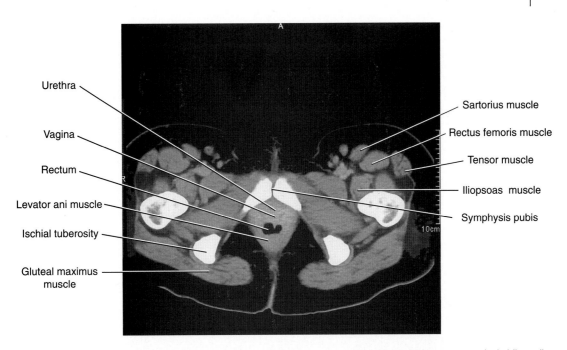

Urethra

Vagina

Rectum

Levator ani muscle

Ischial tuberosity

Gluteal maximus muscle

Sartorius muscle

Rectus femoris muscle

Tensor muscle

Iliopsoas muscle

Symphysis pubis

10cm

Figure 6-32 On Figure 6-32, the inferior aspect of the ischium, the ischial tuberosity, is seen posteriorly, bilaterally. The iliopsoas muscles continue to be seen anterior to the actual hip joint, bilaterally. Even at this level, the gluteal maximus muscles remain. The levator ani muscles straddle the rectum. The urethra is anterior to the vagina.

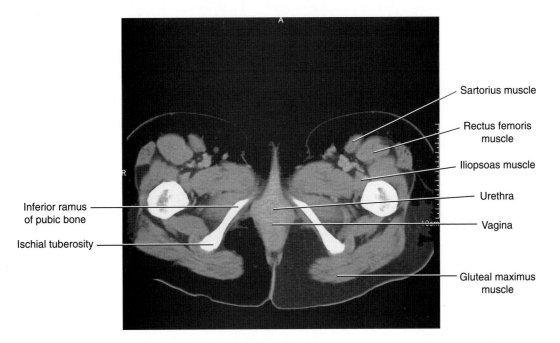

Inferior ramus of pubic bone

Ischial tuberosity

Sartorius muscle

Rectus femoris muscle

Iliopsoas muscle

Urethra

Vagina

Gluteal maximus muscle

Figure 6-33 On this last image of E xam 1 (Figure 6-33), the inferior rami of the pubic bones are labeled as are the muscles found at this level.

Exam 2

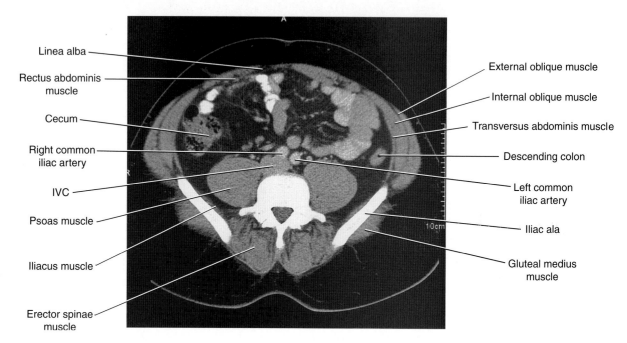

Figure 6-34   This second exam is a continuation of the study presented as Exam 2 in Chapter 5. The first image (Figure 6-34) shows the descending aorta having already divided into the right and left common iliac arteries. The right and left common iliac veins are merging to form the inferior vena cava. The first of the three gluteal muscles, the gluteal medius, has appeared. Also new, but barely visible, are the bilateral iliacus muscles, medial to the ilia. The three lateral muscles, external and internal obliques and transversus abdominis, are still present but will not remain constant through the pelvic region. The rectus abdominis muscles, separated by the linea alba, will. The cecum, the originating point of the large intestines, is evident on the right.

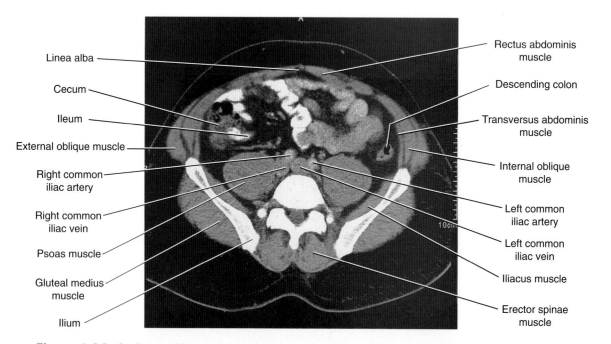

Figure 6-35   On Figure 6-35, both the right and left common iliac arteries are now apparent while the formation of the IVC is occurring with the merger of the right and left common iliac veins. Remember the rule: arteries are anterior to veins. More of the iliacus muscles are seen. They will eventually merge with the psoas muscles to form the iliopsoas muscles. The distal ileum is emptying into the cecum. The descending colon is seen on the left. The three lateral muscles can still be differentiated from each other.

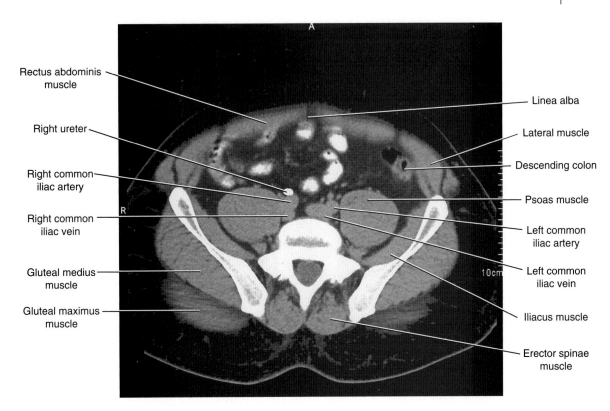

Rectus abdominis muscle

Right ureter

Right common iliac artery

Right common iliac vein

Gluteal medius muscle

Gluteal maximus muscle

Linea alba

Lateral muscle

Descending colon

Psoas muscle

Left common iliac artery

Left common iliac vein

Iliacus muscle

Erector spinae muscle

10cm

Figure 6-36 The right ureter is seen with a great deal of intensity on Figure 6-36. As a reminder, the ureters are not apparent on images taken during peristalsis. A second gluteal muscle is also shown, the gluteal maximus. The gluteal maximus is the most posterior of the three gluteal muscles. The remnants of the three lateral muscles are labeled.

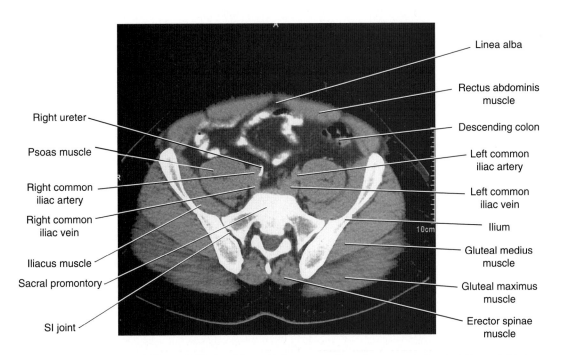

Right ureter

Psoas muscle

Right common iliac artery

Right common iliac vein

Iliacus muscle

Sacral promontory

SI joint

Linea alba

Rectus abdominis muscle

Descending colon

Left common iliac artery

Left common iliac vein

Ilium

Gluteal medius muscle

Gluteal maximus muscle

Erector spinae muscle

10cm

Figure 6-37 At this level (Figure 6-37), the right and left common iliac veins appear to be stretching out. It is here that the external and internal iliac veins join to form the common iliac veins. The psoas muscles are moving closer to the iliacus muscles and are now much more anterior than when first identified. The upper portion of the sacrum, the sacral promontory, is demonstrated along with the SI joints.

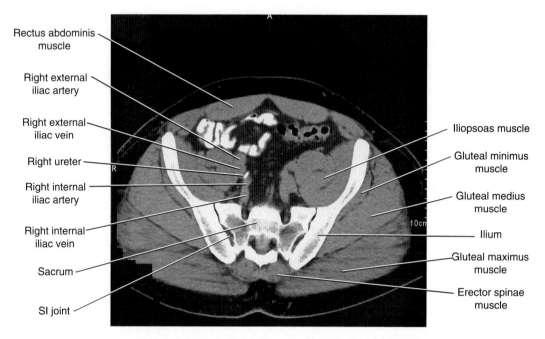

Rectus abdominis muscle

Right external iliac artery

Right external iliac vein

Right ureter

Right internal iliac artery

Right internal iliac vein

Sacrum

SI joint

Iliopsoas muscle

Gluteal minimus muscle

Gluteal medius muscle

Ilium

Gluteal maximus muscle

Erector spinae muscle

Figure 6-38 On Figure 6-38, the merger of the psoas and iliacus muscles appears complete. The last (and most anterior) of the gluteal muscles, the gluteal minimus, is now seen. The gluteal muscles are separated from each other by a layer of fat, allowing easy identification. On the right, the four iliac vessels can be identified: the external and internal iliac arteries and veins. The external vessels are anterior to the internal vessels and the arteries are anterior to the veins. The internal iliac vessels remain within the pelvic cavity while the externals will continue to gravitate anteriorly. Eventually, at the level of the symphysis pubis, they will acquire a new name, the femoral arteries and veins.

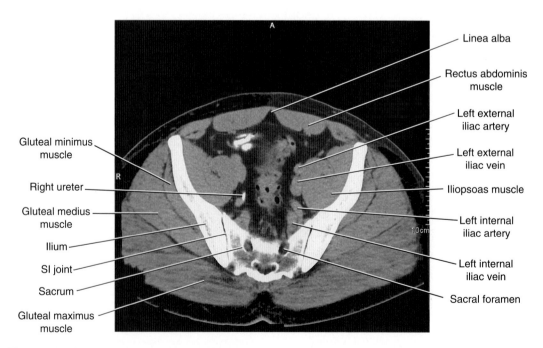

Linea alba

Rectus abdominis muscle

Left external iliac artery

Left external iliac vein

Iliopsoas muscle

Left internal iliac artery

Left internal iliac vein

Sacral foramen

Gluteal minimus muscle

Right ureter

Gluteal medius muscle

Ilium

SI joint

Sacrum

Gluteal maximus muscle

Figure 6-39 For the first time the sacral foramina are identified on Figure 6-39. The iliopsoas muscles and external iliac arteries and veins continue to gravitate anteriorly, as expected. In this image it is obvious that the gluteal muscles acquire their names by their sizes.

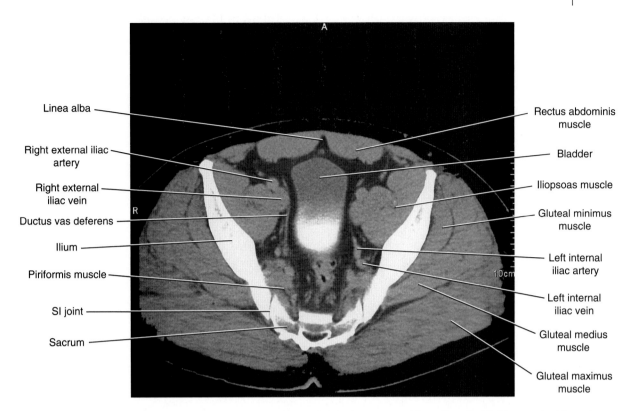

Figure 6-40 On Figure 6-40, a new structure, the bladder, has appeared. Lateral to the bladder are the bilateral ductus vas deferens. Once leaving the scrotum they ascend anteriorly to the bladder, pass along the sides of the upper bladder and descend behind it. Also apparent is a new muscle, the piriformis, anterior to the sacrum. We continue to see the external and internal iliac arteries and veins.

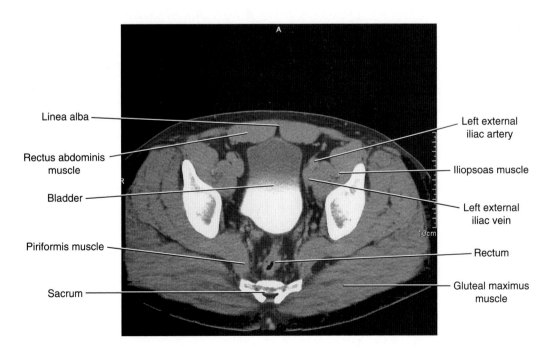

Figure 6-41 This image (Figure 6-41) is at the level of the distal sacrum. Anterior to the sacrum is the rectum. The piriformis muscles stretch out laterally to the sacrum, passing anterior to the gluteal maximus muscles. Notice the anterior position of the iliopsoas muscles.

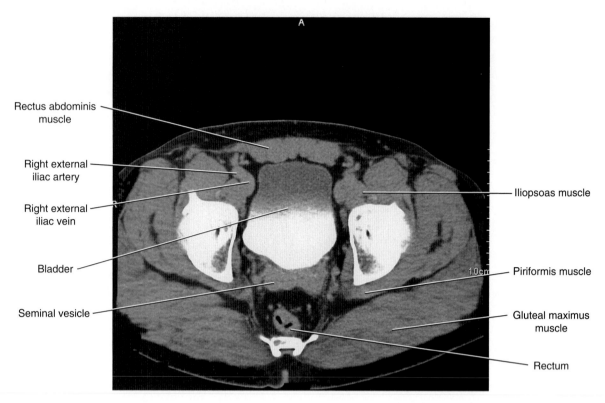

Rectus abdominis muscle

Right external iliac artery

Right external iliac vein

Bladder

Seminal vesicle

Iliopsoas muscle

Piriformis muscle

Gluteal maximus muscle

Rectum

Figure 6-42   On Figure 6-42, posterior to the bladder are the seminal vesicles, which produce the bulk of the fluidic semen. On this image, the linea alba separating the bilateral rectus abdominis muscles is not apparent.

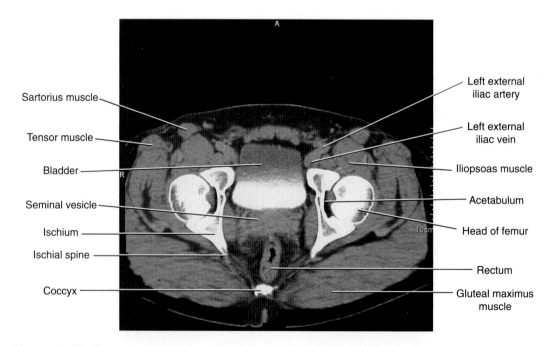

Sartorius muscle

Tensor muscle

Bladder

Seminal vesicle

Ischium

Ischial spine

Coccyx

Left external iliac artery

Left external iliac vein

Iliopsoas muscle

Acetabulum

Head of femur

Rectum

Gluteal maximus muscle

Figure 6-43   The coccyx, the distal portion of the vertebral column, is seen posterior to the rectum on Figure 6-43. Also new is the appearance of the heads of the femora within the acetabula. The ischial spines are identified on the posterior aspect of the ischia. Two new muscles are also identified, the bilateral sartorius, which are the most anterior muscles in the lower pelvic region, and the tensor muscles.

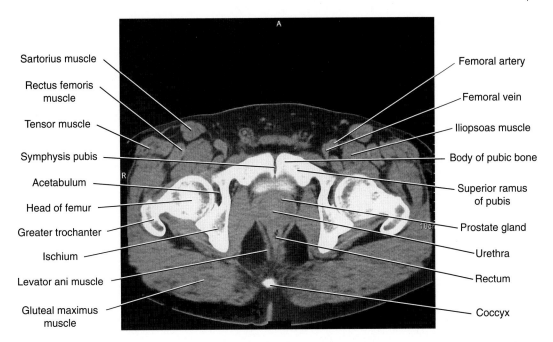

Sartorius muscle
Rectus femoris muscle
Tensor muscle
Symphysis pubis
Acetabulum
Head of femur
Greater trochanter
Ischium
Levator ani muscle
Gluteal maximus muscle

Femoral artery
Femoral vein
Iliopsoas muscle
Body of pubic bone
Superior ramus of pubis
Prostate gland
Urethra
Rectum
Coccyx

Figure 6-44 This image (Figure 6-44) was obtained inferior to the bladder. Two new structures are seen: the urethra and the prostate gland, which encircles the first part of the urethra. The symphysis pubis, involving the bodies of the pubic bones, is also now seen. At the level of the symphysis pubis the external iliac arteries and veins acquire new names: the femoral arteries and veins. The greater trochanters are seen along the lateral aspect of the femoral heads and the last segment of the coccyx is labeled. Newly identified anteriorly are another pair of muscles, the rectus femoris, while the levator ani muscles are seen posteriorly on either side of the rectum.

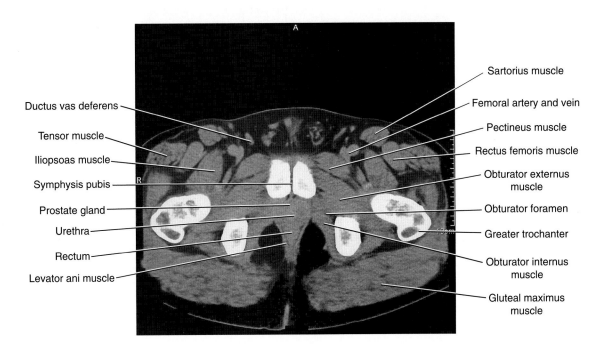

Ductus vas deferens
Tensor muscle
Iliopsoas muscle
Symphysis pubis
Prostate gland
Urethra
Rectum
Levator ani muscle

Sartorius muscle
Femoral artery and vein
Pectineus muscle
Rectus femoris muscle
Obturator externus muscle
Obturator foramen
Greater trochanter
Obturator internus muscle
Gluteal maximus muscle

Figure 6-45 New to this image (Figure 6-45) are the obturator foramina. Associated with the obturator foramina are the obturator externus and internus muscles. The levator ani muscles are again seen on either side of the rectum. Lateral to each side of the symphysis pubis are the pectineus muscles. Anterior to the pectineus muscles are the ductus vas deferens. The urethra continues to descend. It will eventually pass through the penis.

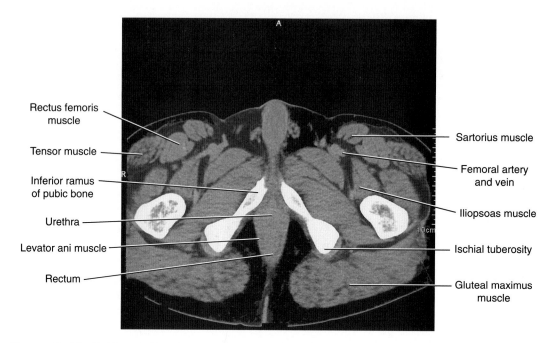

Figure 6-46 On Figure 6-46, at the level of the inferior pelvis, we see the ischial tuberosities as well as the inferior rami of the pubic bones. The urethra is anterior to the rectum. The gluteal maximus muscles are still apparent. On the left, the femoral artery and vein are labeled.

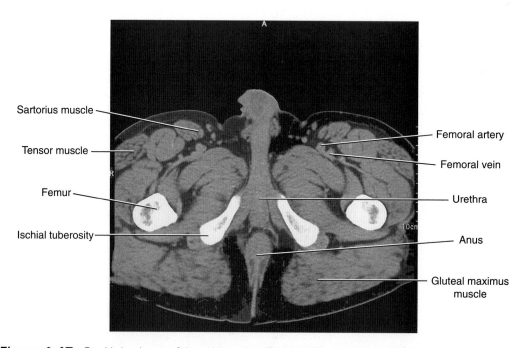

Figure 6-47 On this last image of the pelvic region (Figure 6-47), the distal end of the gastrointestinal system, the anus, is labeled. The inferior portion of each ischium, the ischial tuberosities, are still identifiable. When a person is sitting in an upright position, the ischial tuberosities, protected by the gluteal maximus muscles, absorb the weight of the upper body. The femoral arteries and veins continue into the femoral region.

REVIEW QUESTIONS

1. On axial CT images arranged in descending order the first portion of the hip bone to appear is the
   a. ilium.
   b. ischium.
   c. pubis.
   d. They are all on the same plane.

2. As they descend from the kidneys the ureters head
   a. posterior and lateral.
   b. posterior and medial.
   c. anterior and lateral.
   d. anterior and medial. *(circled)*

3. Which of the following statements regarding the male urethra is true?
   I. The male urethra is longer than the female urethra.
   II. The male urethra is a common passageway for urine and semen.
   III. The prostate gland is found surrounding the first part of the urethra.
   a. I
   b. II
   c. III
   d. I and II
   e. I, II, and III *(circled)*

4. On axial CT images the ureters are seen entering the bladder
   a. midline.
   b. posterolaterally. *(circled)*
   c. anteriorly and laterally.
   d. along the lateral borders.

5. The bifurcation of the aorta into the right and left common iliac arteries occurs at
   a. L1.
   b. L2.
   c. L3.
   d. L4. *(circled)*
   e. L5.

6. Generally speaking, in the pelvic area, arteries are posterior to the veins with a similar name.
   a. True *(circled)*
   b. False

7. The vessels becoming the femoral arteries are the
   a. common iliac arteries.
   b. external iliac arteries. *(circled)*   at the inguinal canal
   c. internal iliac arteries.
   d. None of the above.

8. The IVC is formed at L5 by the right and left common iliac veins.
   a. True *(circled)*
   b. False

Identify the function of the following:

9. Seminal vesicles _____

_____

10. Prostate gland _____

_____

11. Bulbourethral glands _____

_____

12. On axial CT images, the seminal vesicles are found in a male pelvis
    a. anterior to the bladder.
    b. superior to the bladder.
    c. posterior to the bladder.
    d. They are not found in the male pelvis.

13. As seen on sectional images, the prostate gland is
    a. superior to the bladder.
    b. lateral to the bladder.
    c. posterior to the bladder.
    d. inferior to the bladder.

14. Define the term adnexa.
    _____ lateral to the uterus _____

_____

15. The fundus of the uterus is located
    a. superiorly.
    b. centrally.
    c. inferiorly.
    d. There is no fundus of the uterus.

16. The part of the intestines not in the pelvic region as defined in this textbook (at or below the level of the crest) is the
    a. ileum.
    b. cecum.
    c. duodenum.
    d. sigmoid.

17. Looking at CT axial images in descending order the first gluteal muscle to appear is the
    a. gluteal maximus.
    b. gluteal medius.
    c. gluteal minimus.
    d. They all appear at the same time.

18. The gluteal muscle seen most anteriorly on axial sectional images is the
    a. minimus.
    b. medius.
    c. maximus.
    d. None is more anterior than the other.

19. The longest muscle in the body is the
    a. rectus femoris.
    b. iliopsoas.
    c. sartorius.
    d. tensor.

20. The muscles seen anterior to the sacrum on axial CT
    images are the
    a. iliacus.
    b. piriformis.
    c. pectineus.
    d. quadratus lumborum.

Vertebral Column

OUTLINE

VERTEBRAE

The spine is composed of 33 **vertebrae** in a child, 26 in an adult. It is divided into five regions, as shown on Figure 7-1. Listed superiorly to inferiorly, along with the number of vertebrae, they are: cervical (7), thoracic (12), lumbar (5), sacral (5 fused), and coccygeal (4 which have fused into 1 or 2). The first three regions have movable or true vertebrae and the last two fixed or false vertebrae. At birth, in the sitting position, an infant's vertebral column forms a convex arch dorsally and a concave arch anteriorly. An exaggeration of this type of curvature is **kyphosis**. Sec-

ondary curvatures that develop with certain developmental markers are identified on Figure 7-1 B. The first is an anterior convexity in the cervical region as an infant becomes capable of lifting his or her head. The second is a convexity in the lumbar region as a child learns to walk upright. The term **lordosis** applies to these normal curvatures or an exaggeration. The variation in curvatures strengthens the spine, helps maintain balance when the body is upright, and cushions the spine when the individual is walking. The vertebrae get increasingly larger as they descend from the cervical to the lumbar region, which allows them to carry more weight.

Vertebral column

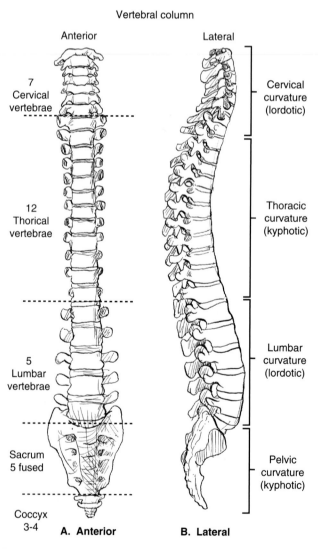

Anterior

7
Cervical
vertebrae

12
Thorical
vertebrae

5
Lumbar
vertebrae

Sacrum
5 fused

Coccyx
3-4

A. Anterior

Lateral

Cervical
curvature
(lordotic)

Thoracic
curvature
(kyphotic)

Lumbar
curvature
(lordotic)

Pelvic
curvature
(kyphotic)

B. Lateral

Figure 7-1 A and B Anterior and lateral view of vertebral column

Typical Vertebra

A typical vertebra, such as a lumbar vertebra, is an irregularly shaped bone, best studied in conjunction with Figure 7-2. The main portion, the body, is located anteriorly. The body has compact bone on the superior and inferior surfaces, but the central portion of the body contains bone marrow, fat, and water. Extending from either side of the body in a posterolateral direction are two processes, the **pedicles**. Directed posteromedially from each of the pedicles is a **lamina**. With normal anatomy, the laminae unite midline. The two pedicles and two laminae construct the **vertebral** or **neural arch**. A **vertebral foramen** (formed by the vertebral arch and body) in the lumbar region tends to be more triangular. With all the vertebrae in place, the collective vertebral foramina comprise the vertebral or **spinal canal**, which has the spinal cord passing through it. Superior and inferior to each of the pedicles is a concavity, the **vertebral notch**. As a result of articulation of two adjacent vertebrae, openings are formed by the bilateral superior and inferior vertebral notches, the **intervertebral foramina**, through which exit nerves from the spinal cord.

There are seven processes attached to the arch. The bilateral **transverse processes** project laterally from the union of the pedicles and laminae. A **spinous process** extends posteriorly from the midline union of the laminae. Heading in a superior direction are bilateral **superior articulating processes**, and in an inferior and slightly more medial direction, bilateral **inferior articulating processes**.

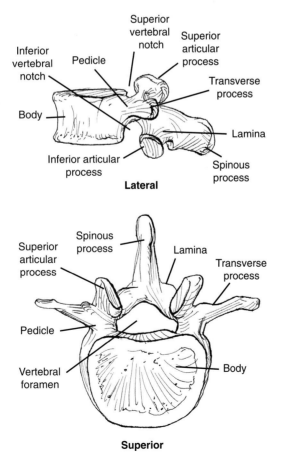

Figure 7-2 Lateral and superior view of typical vertebra

Every vertebra other than the first and last articulates with the one above and below. Figure 7-3 is an example of a typical articulation. The bodies are separated by **intervertebral disks** (the composition to be discussed shortly). This joint is an example of **amphiarthrosis**, or a slightly movable joint. The bilateral superior articulating processes of one vertebra articulate with the bilateral inferior articulating processes of the vertebra above it, forming the **zygoapophyseal joints** or **apophyseal joints**. When seen on axial CT images, the inferior articulating processes are seen medial to the superior articulating processes.

Atypical Vertebrae

Atypical vertebrae are found in both the cervical and thoracic regions. In particular, the first two vertebrae of the cervical region are unique (see Figure 7-4 A and B). The first vertebra, C1 or the **atlas**, has bilateral superior articulating processes with depressions for articulation with the occipital condyles of the skull. Replacing the spinous process is a posterior arch. Off the neural arch are bilateral **lateral masses**. Projecting from the lateral masses are transverse processes that contain transverse foramina. The vertebral arteries, studied in Chapters 1 and 3, pass through the transverse foramina. Instead of a body there is an anterior arch. C2, or the **axis**, is another notable atypical vertebra. It has an additional structure projecting from the upper surface of the body, the **odontoid process** or **dens**. The odontoid process is the remnant of the body of C1, which, through the course of evolution, has fused onto C2. It is the articulation of the odontoid process with C1 that allows the head to pivot on its axis. C2 and the remaining cervical vertebrae also have bilateral transverse foramina accommodating the vertebral arteries. Lastly, with the exception of C1 and C7, the spinous processes of the cervical vertebrae may be bifid, or split in two. The seventh cervical vertebra, the **vertebra prominens**, has a very prominent palpable spinous process. The vertebral canal

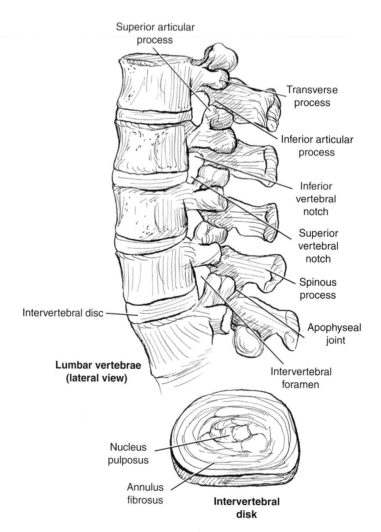

Figure 7-3 Lateral view of articulating vertebrae and superior view of intervertebral disk

is widest in the cervical region because of the size of the spinal cord in that region.

A thoracic vertebra more closely resembles a typical vertebra than the first few cervical vertebrae but there are costal facets or demifacets on all the bodies and transverse processes of T1–T12 for articulation with the heads and tubercles of the ribs, respectively.

The sacrum and coccyx were discussed in Chapter 6 along with the other bony pelvic structures.

INTERVERTEBRAL DISKS

The intervertebral disks, which are fibrocartilaginous, assume the same shape as the bodies of the vertebrae and have articulating cartilage on the superior and inferior sur-faces. Figure 7-3 demonstrates the outermost disk, the **annulus fibrosus**, and the innermost core, the **nucleus pulposus**, from a superior perspective. The disks are very elastic initially, but start to degenerate by the second decade of life. With continued degeneration, the nucleus pulposus eventually may rupture through the annulus fibrosus. Although there is a natural inclination to rupture directly posteriorly, with possible impingement on the spinal cord itself, there is a ligament, discussed later in this chapter, that generally prevents this. Instead, the disk more often ruptures in a posterolateral direction, limiting the impingement to the nerves exiting the spinal cord. The most common location for this occurrence is in the lumbar region where the disks bear the most weight and are sub-jected to more bending.

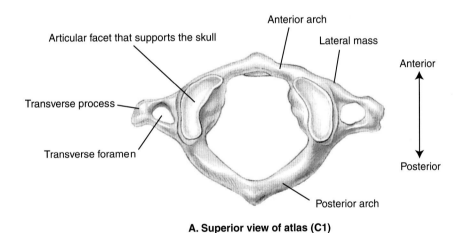

A. Superior view of atlas (C1)

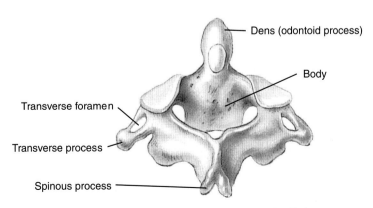

B. Posterior-superior view of axis (C2)

Figure 7-4 A and B Superior view of Cl (atlas) and posterosuperior view of C2 (axis)

SPINAL CORD

The spinal cord, as seen on Figure 7-5, originates at the base of the brain, and is a continuation of the medulla oblongata once it passes through the foramen magnum. Thicker in the cervical and lumbar regions, it extends to approximately L1/L2 in adults, passing through the verte- bral canal. In children, the spinal cord fills the entire spinal canal but does not keep pace with the growth of the verte- bral column with continued development. Remaining within the vertebral canal are hairlike nerve fibers, the **cauda equina** (horse's tail), which extend from the tapered end of the spinal cord, the **conus medullaris**. Unlike the

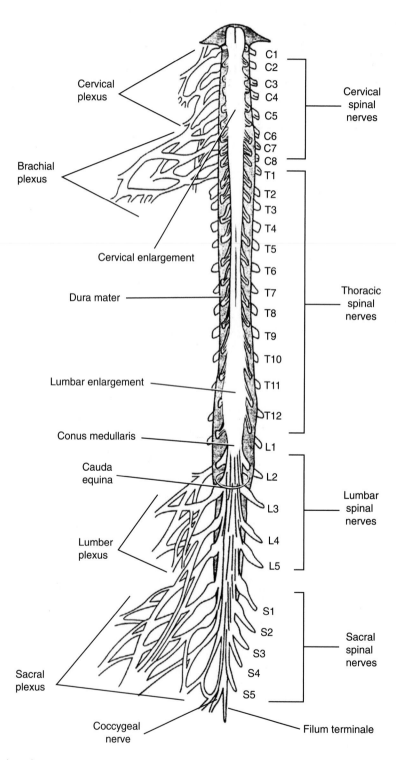

Figure 7-5 Spinal cord

brain, which has external gray matter surrounding central white matter, the spinal cord is composed of gray matter in the center, assuming the shape of an H on an axial CT image (see Figure 7-6), surrounded by white matter. There is more gray matter in the cervical and lumbar regions. Sensory or ascending tracts conducting nerve impulses to the brain, and motor or descending tracts conducting nerve impulses from the brain, travel within the white matter. In the center of the gray matter is the central canal, a continuation of the fourth ventricle of the brain. There are 31 pairs of **spinal nerves** that attach to the spinal cord. The point of attachment is the nerve root, with the root divided into an anterior or ventral portion and posterior or dorsal portion. The anterior portion has passing through it motor fibers while the posterior portion contains sensory fibers. Thus, a spinal nerve can be classified as a **mixed nerve**. The number of spinal nerves approximately matches the number of vertebrae in each region with the exception of the cervical region, which has eight, and the coccygeal region, which has one.

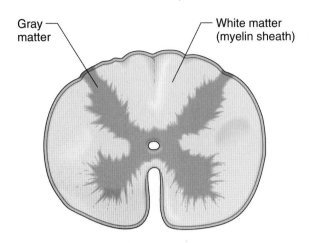

Figure 7-6 Cross-section of the spinal cord

MENINGES

The meninges encasing the brain also envelop the spinal cord. The three meninges, as described in Chapter 1, are the outermost tough fibrous dura mater, the arachnoid, and the innermost pia mater. Cerebrospinal fluid circulates between the arachnoid and pia mater. There is an extension of the pia mater from the conus medullaris, the **filium terminale**, which serves to anchor the spinal cord to the coccyx.

LIGAMENTS

Five important ligaments are associated with the vertebral column: the **anterior longitudinal ligament**, **posterior longitudinal ligament**, **ligamentum flava**, **ligamentum nuchae**, and **supraspinous ligament**. The anterior longitudinal ligament (**ALL**), thicker in the thoracic region, is anterior to the bodies and extends from C2 to the sacrum. It is best seen on a sagittal MRI of the spine. The posterior longitudinal ligament (**PLL**) lies inside the vertebral canal posterior to the bodies and also extends from C2 to the sacrum. It is this ligament that prevents herniation of the intervertebral disks in a direct posterior direction. The ligamentum flava runs between the medial laminae on either side of the spinous process. The ligamentum nuchae passes along the tips of the spinous processes from C7 to the occipital bone, while the supraspinous ligament continues along the same path from C7 to the sacrum.

Whether looking at axial CT images or sagittal MR images of the spine, it is important to remember that the vertebrae themselves are irregular in shape and thus will not all be seen on any one image. MRI is the best modality to demonstrate the intervertebral disks, spinal cord, and ligaments because of its superior ability to differentiate structures with very low inherent soft tissue differences. Although cortical bone will not give off a signal, the cancellous bone found in the bodies of the vertebrae will. The administration of gadolinium chelate preceding MRI allows for better visualization of lesions within the vertebral bodies. CT is the preferred modality to demonstrate fractures of the actual vertebrae. On CT axial images, the nucleus pulposus of the intervertebral disks appears more translucent than the annulus fibrosus.

MUSCLES

The muscles of the spine are quite complex and are more appropriately discussed and labeled in each chapter. Because the intent of this book is to introduce the reader to the fundamentals of sectional anatomy, the simplest classification has been chosen to label the muscles in the cervical and lumbar region: the erector spinae. This classification could also be applied to the thoracic region. A student at the intermediate level would subdivide these muscles into three general categories: the lateral or iliocostalis group, the intermediate or longissimus group, and the medial or spinalis group. The advanced sectional anatomist would specify exact muscle names, depending upon which group and which level of the spine was being discussed. The muscles associated with the sacrum and coccyx have also been labeled in the chapter on the pelvis, Chapter 6.

CT IMAGES

Exam I

Figures 7-7 through 7-12 are CT images demonstrating a section of the cervical spine. They were not imaged using bone windowing, to more clearly demonstrate anatomy.

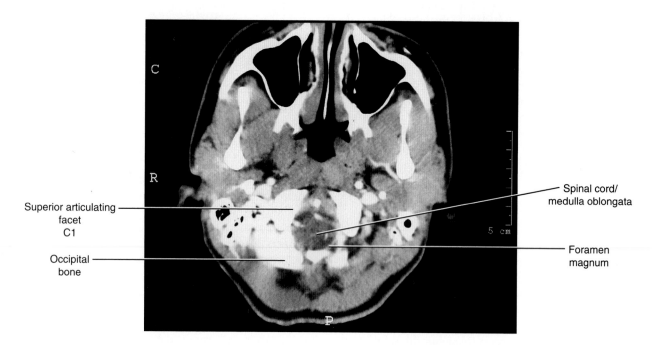

Figure 7-7 This first image (Figure 7-7) is at the level where CI (the atlas) is articulating with the occipital bone. Labeled are the superior articulating facets of CI. As the medulla oblongata passes through the foramen magnum of the occipital bone it acquires a new name, the spinal cord. The spinal cord will eventually terminate at L1/L2.

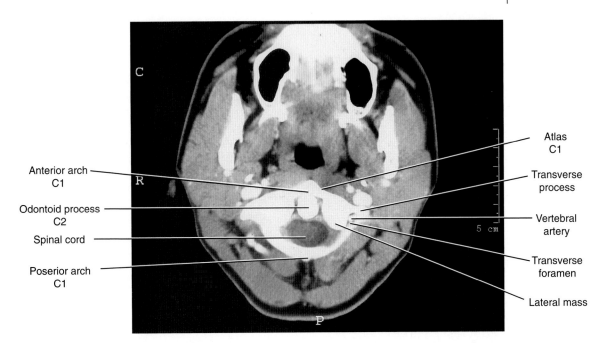

Figure 7-8 Figure 7-8 allows identification of the different parts of C1. There is no body, but instead an anterior arch. Nor is there a spinous process, but instead a posterior arch. Extending from the bilateral lateral masses are the transverse processes. Passing through the transverse foramina of the transverse processes are the vertebral arteries, bilaterally. The odontoid process of C2 is articulating with C1, allowing for rotation of the head.

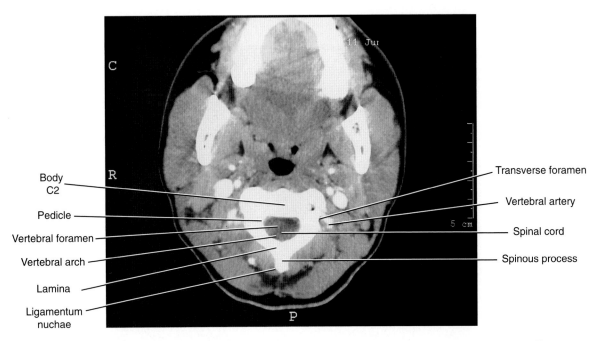

Figure 7-9 Unlike C1, C2 (the axis) has a body anteriorly and a spinous process posteriorly, shown on Figure 7-9. The vertebral arch is formed by the pedicles and laminae while the vertebral foramen is formed by the vertebral arch and body. The vertebral foramen is widest in the cervical region. The ligamentum nuchae runs along the tips of the spinous processes in the cervical region.

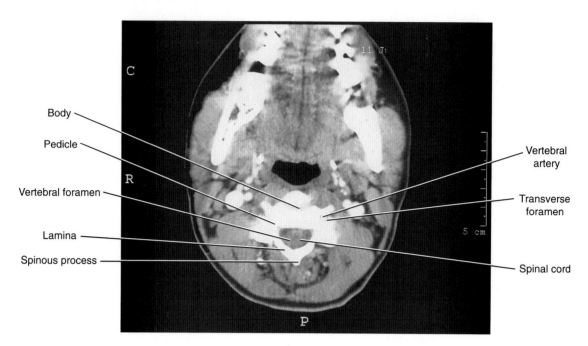

Figure 7-10   Figure 7-10 again shows the spinal cord passing through the vertebral foramen and the bilateral vertebral arteries passing through the transverse foramina.

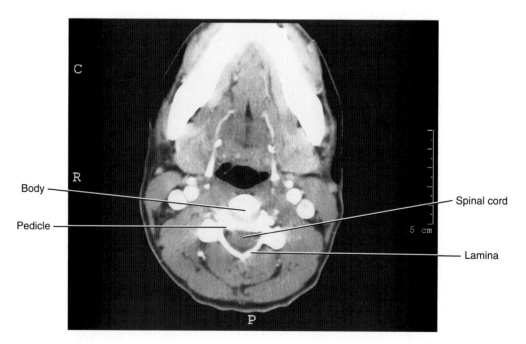

Figure 7-11   On Figure 7-11, the entire vertebra is not visible on a single slice because the vertebrae are irregularly shaped bones. The spinous process is missing on this image.

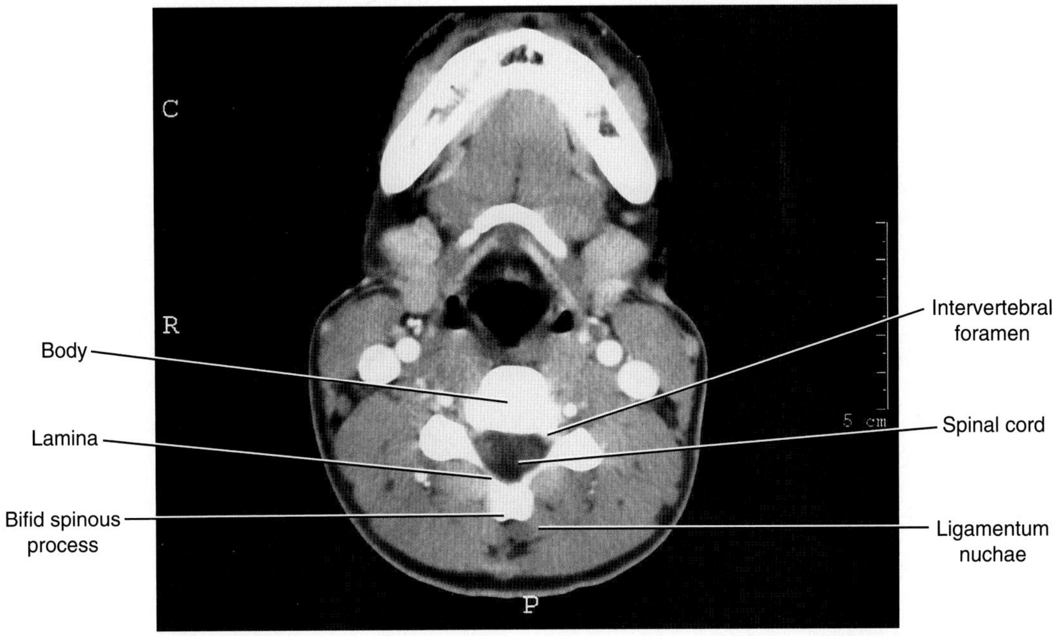

Figure 7-12 The last image of this limited series (Figure 7-12) shows an incomplete bifid spinous process and a segment of the intervertebral foramen. The spinal nerves exit from the spinal cord and pass through the bilateral intervertebral foramina.

Exam 2

Figures 7-13 through 7-18 are CT images of a segment of the lumbar spine. Again, bone windowing was not utilized.

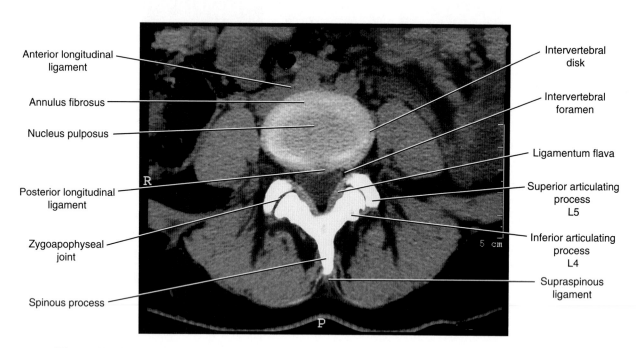

Figure 7-13   Figure 7-13 shows the intervertebral disk between L4 and L5. Intervertebral disks assume the same shape as the associated vertebral bodies. With a herniation the nucleus pulposus generally ruptures posterolaterally as the posterior longitudinal ligament tends to prevent it from rupturing directly posteriorly. This results in compression of the nerve roots exiting through the intervertebral foramina. Note the presence of the other ligaments. The lumbar region is the most common site of herniated disks.

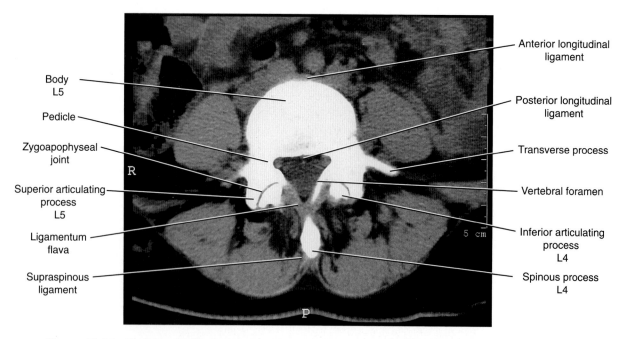

Figure 7-14   On Figure 7-14, notice the more triangulated appearance of the vertebral foramen as compared to the cervical region. The inferior articulating processes of L4 are articulating with the superior articulating processes of L5 bilaterally to form the zygoapophyseal joints.

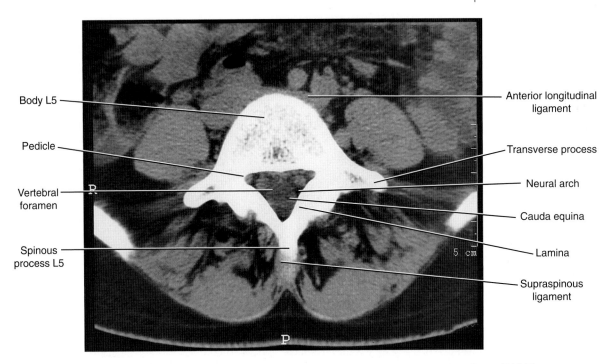

Body L5

Pedicle

Vertebral
foramen

Spinous
process L5

Anterior longitudinal
ligament

Transverse process

Neural arch

Cauda equina

Lamina

Supraspinous
ligament

Figure 7-15   The bilateral pedicles and laminae are forming the vertebral or neural arch on Figure 7-15. These same structures, along with the body, form the vertebral foramen. The spinal cord terminates at L1/L2 but the cauda equina remains within the vertebral foramen.

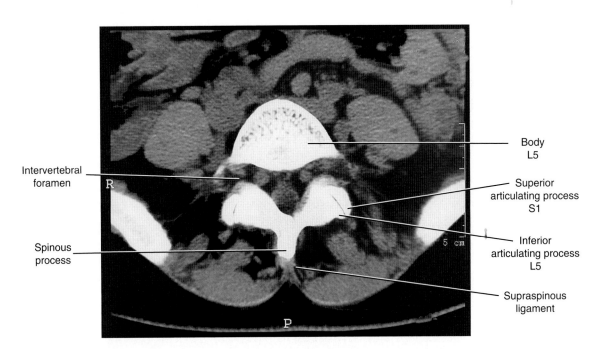

Intervertebral
foramen

Spinous
process

Body
L5

Superior
articulating process
S1

Inferior
articulating process
L5

Supraspinous
ligament

Figure 7-16   Figure 7-16 demonstrates the superior articulating process of S1 and the inferior articulating process of L5. Also labeled are the intervertebral foramina between L5 and S1.

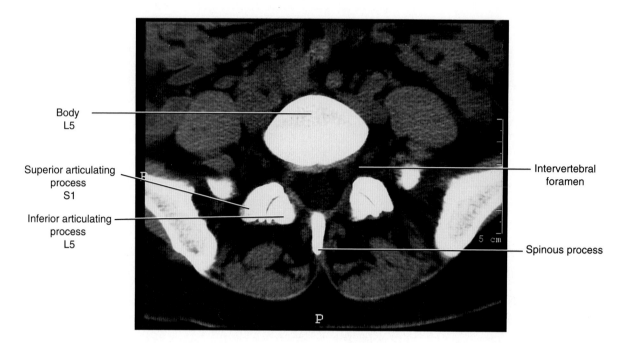

Body
L5

Intervertebral
foramen

Superior articulating
process
S1

Inferior articulating
process
L5

Spinous process

Figure 7-17 The last of the body and spinous process of L5 are shown on Figure 7-17. Still apparent are the bilateral intervertebral foramina.

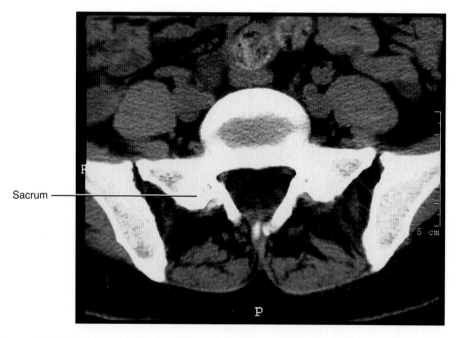

Sacrum

Figure 7-18 This image (Figure 7-18) is at the level of the sacrum. For more images of the sacrum review Chapter 6.

MR IMAGES

Exam 1

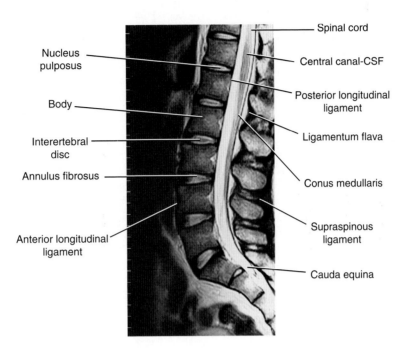

Nucleus pulposus

Body

Interertebral disc

Annulus fibrosus

Anterior longitudinal ligament

Spinal cord

Central canal-CSF

Posterior longitudinal ligament

Ligamentum flava

Conus medullaris

Supraspinous ligament

Cauda equina

Figure 7-19 Figure 7-19, which is a straight midsagittal cut, demonstrates all the ligaments found in the lumbar region: the ALL, PLL, ligamentum flava, and supraspinous ligament. The cauda equina extends from the tapered end of the spinal cord, the conus medullaris. Typically the spinal cord terminates at L1/L2. The nucleus pulposus and annulus fibrosus of the intervertebral disk can be distinguished.

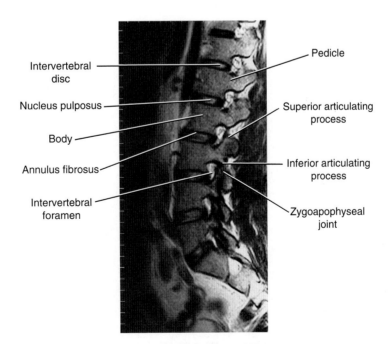

Intervertebral disc

Nucleus pulposus

Body

Annulus fibrosus

Intervertebral foramen

Pedicle

Superior articulating process

Inferior articulating process

Zygoapophyseal joint

Figure 7-20 This sagittal image (Figure 7-20) is off-centered, thereby allowing you to identify the superior and inferior articulating processes and their articulation, the zygoapophyseal joints. Labeled are the intervertebral foramina and the pedicles. The 31 pairs of spinal nerves exit the spinal cord and pass through the bilateral intervertebral foramina along the length of the spinal cord.

Exam 2

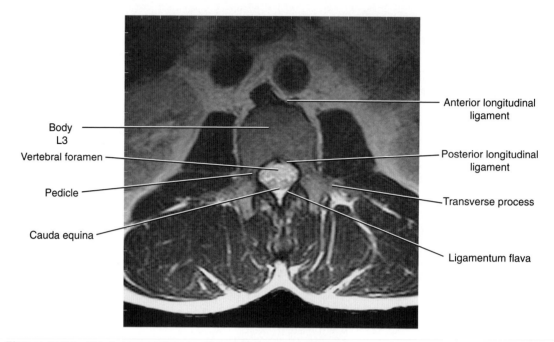

Body
L3

Vertebral foramen

Pedicle

Cauda equina

Anterior longitudinal
ligament

Posterior longitudinal
ligament

Transverse process

Ligamentum flava

Figure 7-21   This first axial MR image (Figure 7-21) is of L3. Within the vertebral foramen is the cauda equina, the collection of hairlike nerve fibers that extend from the conus medullaris. The conus medullaris, the tapered end of the spinal cord, is typically located at L1/L2.

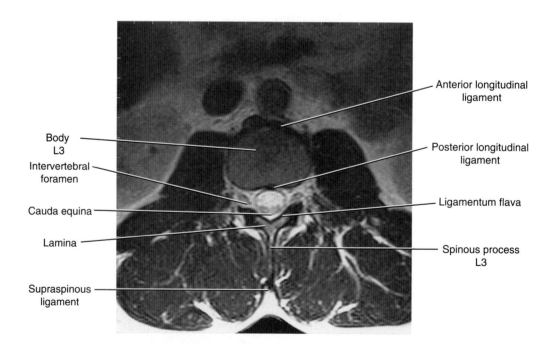

Body
L3

Intervertebral
foramen

Cauda equina

Lamina

Supraspinous
ligament

Anterior longitudinal
ligament

Posterior longitudinal
ligament

Ligamentum flava

Spinous process
L3

Figure 7-22   More of L3 is shown on Figure 7-22, including the spinous process and bilateral lamina. Also seen bilaterally are the intervertebral foramina through which pass the spinal nerves.

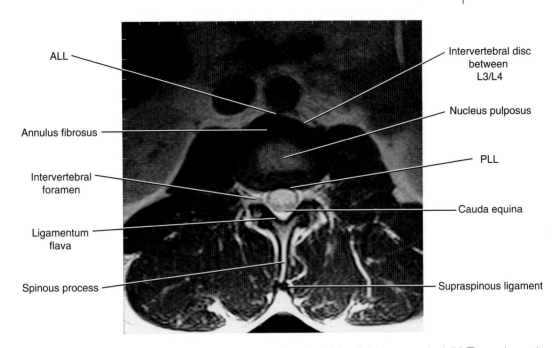

ALL

Annulus fibrosus

Intervertebral
foramen

Ligamentum
flava

Spinous process

Intervertebral disc
between
L3/L4

Nucleus pulposus

PLL

Cauda equina

Supraspinous ligament

Figure 7-23 Figure 7-23 is an image between L3 and L4, in the vicinity of the intervertebral disk. The nucleus pulposus and annulus fibrosus are distinct.

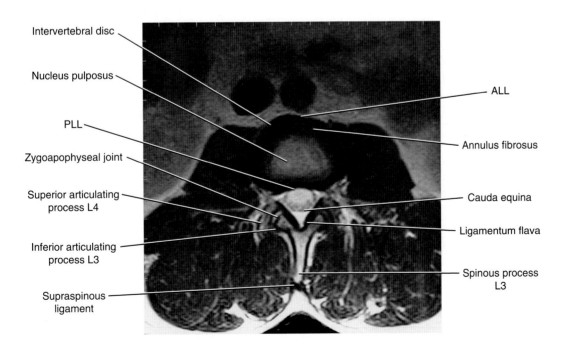

Intervertebral disc

Nucleus pulposus

PLL

Zygoapophyseal joint

Superior articulating
process L4

Inferior articulating
process L3

Supraspinous
ligament

ALL

Annulus fibrosus

Cauda equina

Ligamentum flava

Spinous process
L3

Figure 7-24 Still at the level of the intervertebral disk, parts of both L3 (the inferior articulating process) and L4 (the superior articulating process) are identified on Figure 7-24.

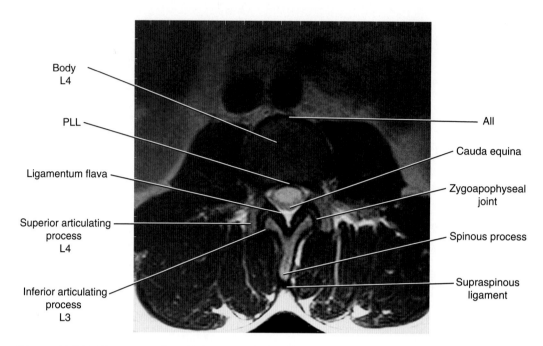

Body
L4

PLL

Ligamentum flava

Superior articulating
process
L4

Inferior articulating
process
L3

All

Cauda equina

Zygoapophyseal
joint

Spinous process

Supraspinous
ligament

Figure 7-25   The zygoapophyseal joints are easily identified on Figure 7-25, as are the ligaments.

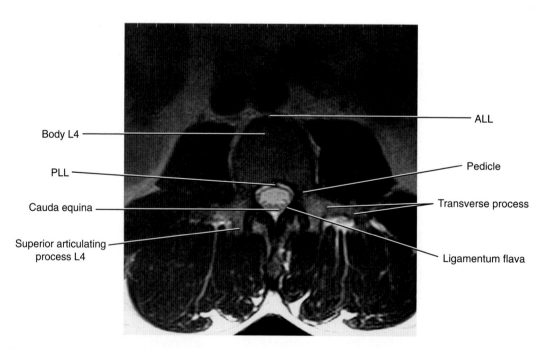

Body L4

PLL

Cauda equina

Superior articulating
process L4

ALL

Pedicle

Transverse process

Ligamentum flava

Figure 7-26   The bulk of L4 is seen on this last image (Figure 7-26). Subsequent images would demonstrate structures already identified on L3 for the remaining lumbar vertebrae, and the sacrum, which is unique.

REVIEW QUESTIONS

1. On axial CT images, the inferior articulating processes of a vertebra are more medial than the superior articulating processes.
   a. True
   b. False

2. The odontoid process is associated with (the)
   a. C1.
   b. atlas.
   c. axis.
   d. vertebra prominens.

3. Where in the spine would you typically find bifid spinous processes?
   a. C spine
   b. T spine
   c. LS spine
   d. All of the above.

4. Which vertebra/ae has no body?

   _____

   _____

5. The portion of an intervertebral disk that ruptures is the
   a. annulus fibrosus.
   b. nucleus pulposus.
   c. Both a and b.
   d. Neither a or b.

6. In what direction would an intervertebral disk most likely rupture?
   a. Anteriorly
   b. Posteriorly
   c. Laterally
   d. Anterolaterally
   e. Posterolaterally

7. The spinal cord ends at
   a. L4/L5.
   b. L3/L4.
   c. L2/L3.
   d. L1/L2.

8. The tapered end of the spinal cord is the
   a. cauda equina.
   b. conus medullaris.
   c. filium terminale.
   d. None of the above.

9. On sagittal MR images, which ligament in the cervical region would be seen most posteriorly?
   a. Anterior longitudinal ligament
   b. Posterior longitudinal ligament
   c. Ligament flava
   d. Ligamentum nuchae
   e. Supraspinous ligament

10. On sagittal MR images, which ligament is seen running between the laminae of the vertebrae on either side of the spinous process?
    a. Ligamentum flava
    b. Anterior longitudinal ligament
    c. Posterior longitudinal ligament
    d. Ligamentum nuchae
    e. Supraspinous ligament

Upper Extremity

OUTLINE

SKELETAL ANATOMY

There are 206 bones in the adult human skeleton, 80 considered part of the **axial skeleton** and 126 considered part of the **appendicular skeleton**. The axial skeleton is composed of the skull (8 cranial and 14 facial bones), 3 auditory ossicles, hyoid bone, sternum, 24 ribs, and the bones of the vertebral column. The appendicular skeleton includes the bones of the shoulder and pelvic girdles and the bones of the upper and lower extremity. The bilateral **shoulder girdles** are constructed by the **scapulae** and **clavicles**, while the bilateral pelvic girdles are formed by the innominate bones. The bones of the upper extremity are the **humerus**, **radius**, **ulna**, 8 **carpal bones**, 5 **metacarpal bones**, and 14 **phalanges**, all demonstrated on Figure 8-1, along with the shoulder girdle. The total number of bones in the bilateral upper extremities and shoulder girdles is 64.

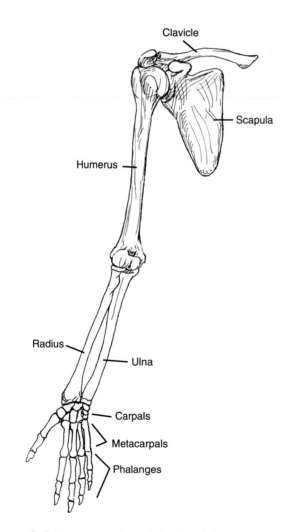

Figure 8-1 Upper extremity and shoulder girdle

Shoulder Girdle

Scapula

The bilateral scapulae are primarily located posteriorly and have numerous significant anatomic markings, all of which are identified on Figure 8-2 A and B. Triangular in shape, the base of the triangle is located superiorly and identified as the superior border. The medial aspect of the superior border is the superior angle. The medial border is the vertebral border; the lateral border is the axillary border. The apex of the triangle is the inferior angle. Along the lateral aspect of the superior border is a notch, the suprascapular notch, and lateral to the notch is a bony process, the coracoid process. The lateral edge of the superior border forms the glenoid fossa or cavity in which sits the humerus to form the **shoulder joint**. Above and below the glenoid fossa are the supra- and infraglenoid tubercles. Immediately adjacent to the glenoid fossa is a constricted region, the neck. On the anterior surface of the scapula is the subscapular fossa, forming a shallow depression. Projecting from the posterior surface, inferior to the superior border at approximately the one-third mark, is a crest of bone termed the spine or spinous process. Above and below the spine are hollowed areas, the supraspinous and infraspinous fossae. The spine projects beyond the lateral border, swinging anteriorly to form a bony prominence, the acromion.

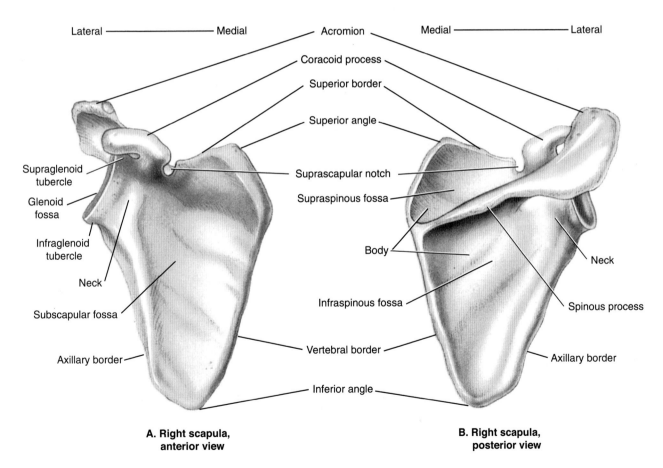

A. Right scapula, anterior view

B. Right scapula, posterior view

Figure 8-2 Right scapula, (A) anterior view (B) posterior view

Clavicle

The clavicle, drawn on Figure 8-3, is an S-shaped bone, having four points of interest: the shaft or body, the lateral or acromial end, the medial or sternal end, and a small tubercle close to the acromial end and seen on the inferior posterior aspect, the conoid tubercle. The articulation of the acromial end of the clavicle with the acromion of the scapula is the acromioclavicular or AC joint, while the articulation of the sternal end of the clavicle with the medial aspect of the manubrium of the sternum is the sternoclavicular or SC joint.

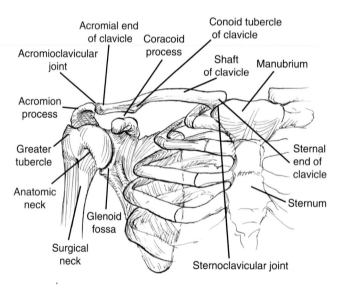

Figure 8-3 The clavicle and its articulations

Humerus

In anatomic terms the **arm** is that portion of the skeleton between the shoulder joint and elbow joint consisting of one bone, the humerus. The humerus is the longest bone of the upper extremity. The head of the humerus, located proximally and medially, articulates with the glenoid fossa of the scapula. Immediately adjacent to the head is a constricted portion, the anatomic neck. The greater tubercle is also proximal, but lateral, while the lesser tubercle is found on the anterior proximal aspect of the humerus, midline. The intertubercular or bicipital groove separates the greater and lesser tubercles. Distal to the tubercles is another constricted region, the surgical neck. Figure 8-4 A and B is a line drawing of the humerus from anterior and posterior perspectives.

The main shaft of the humerus is the diaphysis. At approximately midshaft along the lateral border is the deltoid tuberosity. On the distal aspect of the humerus are the lateral and medial condyles and epicondyles; on the anterior distal humerus are the capitulum, medial to the lateral epicondyle, and the trochlea, lateral to the medial epicondyle. Also found anteriorly are the radial and coronoid fossae, with the radial fossa immediately proximal to the capitulum, accommodating the proximal radius, and the coronoid fossa proximal to the trochlea, accommodating the proximal anterior ulna.

On the posterior distal humerus is a depression, the olecranon fossa, accommodating the posterior proximal ulna to form the **elbow joint**.

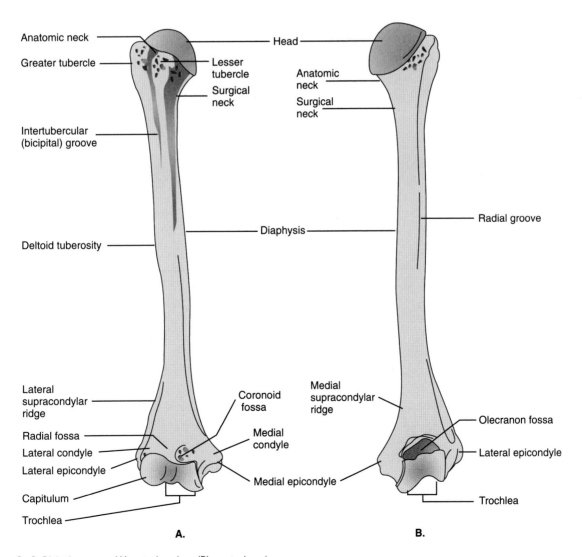

Figure 8-4 Right humerus, (A) anterior view (B) posterior view

Forearm

The **forearm**, that part of the upper extremity between the elbow and wrist, is composed of the radius, located laterally, and the ulna, located medially.

Radius

The radius has a head proximally, a neck inferior to the head, and a radial tuberosity, inferior and medial to the neck. The shaft or diaphysis is centrally located. Along the lateral distal aspect of the radius is the styloid process while the ulnar notch, accommodating the ulna, is seen on the distal medial aspect of the radius. Figure 8-5 is a line drawing of the radius and ulnar, seen from anterior and posterior perspectives.

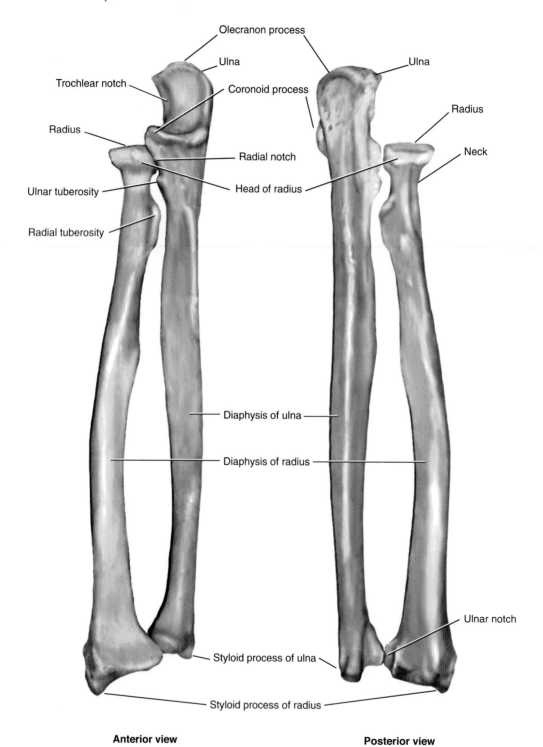

Anterior view   Posterior view

Figure 8-5 Radius and ulna

Ulna

Structures of interest on the proximal ulna include the olecranon process, found posteriorly, the coronoid process, found anteriorly, and the concavity situated between the olecranon and coronoid processes, the trochlear or semi-lunar notch. The ulnar tuberosity is just distal to the coronoid process on the anterior proximal ulna. Slightly distal and lateral to the coronoid process is the radial notch, in which sits the radius.

The main shaft of the ulna is the diaphysis. On the medial aspect of the distal ulna is the styloid process. All anatomic landmarks described are evident on Figure 8-5.

Hand

The **hand**, shown on Figure 8-6, is composed of the 8 carpal bones, 5 metacarpal bones, and 14 phalanges. The **wrist** can be divided into a proximal and distal row of carpal bones. Starting on the lateral aspect of the wrist, the proximal row includes the scaphoid, lunate, triquetrum, and pisiform. The distal row, listed laterally to medially, includes the trapezium, trapezoid, capitate, and hamate.

Articulating with the distal row of carpal bones are the metacarpals I through V, numbered starting on the lateral or thumb side, forming the palm of the hand. The bases of the metacarpals are proximal and the heads are distal.

There are 14 phalanges: a proximal and distal phalanx associated with the thumb, and a proximal, middle, and distal phalanx associated with each remaining finger.

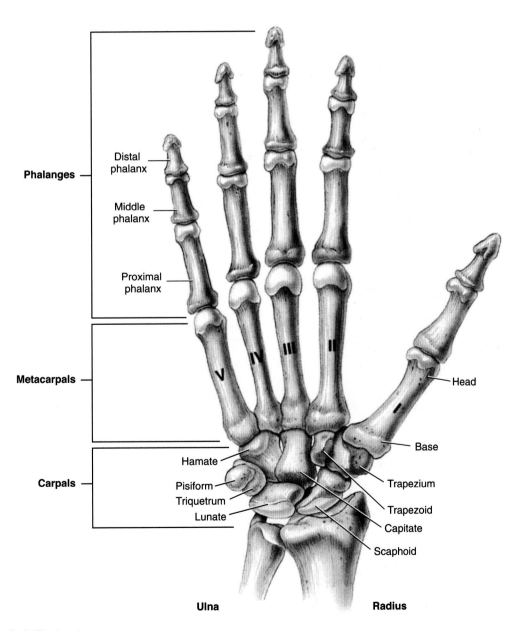

Figure 8-6 The hand

MUSCLES

Muscles That Move the Humerus

A review of the general information about muscles in Chapter 3 is suggested before studying the muscles of the upper and lower extremities. There are nine muscles involved in the shoulder joint, with seven scapular muscles originating on the scapula and two axial muscles originating on the axial skeleton. The scapular muscles are the deltoid, subscapularis, supraspinatus, infraspinatus, teres major, teres minor, and coracobrachialis. The two axial muscles are the pectoralis major and latissimus dorsi. All are identified on Figure 8-7 A and B with the exception of the subscapularis and supraspinatus, which are seen on Figure 8-8.

The deltoid muscle surrounds the shoulder joint; it originates from the acromial end of the clavicle and the acromion and spine of the scapula, and inserts on the deltoid tuberosity of the humerus. The subscapularis, supraspinatus, and infraspinatus acquire their names from the point of origin relevant to the scapula, with the points of insertion being the lesser tubercle of the humerus for the subscapularis and the greater tubercle for the supra-

and infraspinatus. The teres major originates on the inferior angle of the scapula and inserts on the intertubercular groove of the humerus, while the teres minor originates on the axillary border of the scapula and inserts on the greater tubercle of the humerus. The remaining scapular muscle, the coracobrachialis, originates on the coracoid process of the scapula and inserts on the medial aspect of the middle humeral shaft. The scapular muscles of the shoulder are summarized in Table 8-1.

The pectoralis major muscle originates on the medial inferior clavicle, sternum, and costal cartilages of the first or second to sixth or seventh ribs and inserts on the intertubercular groove of the humerus. The other axial muscle, the latissimus dorsi, originates from the spinous processes of T6–L5, the iliac and sacral crests, and ribs 9–12, and inserts on the bicipital groove of the humerus. The axial muscles of the shoulder are summarized in Table 8-2.

Rotator Cuff

The tendons of four muscles nearly enclose the shoulder joint and form a cuff. The muscles are the subscapularis, supra- and infraspinatus, and teres minor. Rotator cuff injuries most commonly involve the supraspinatus muscle.

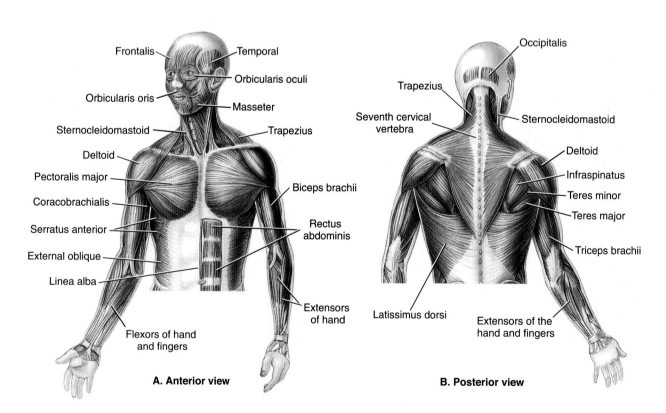

Figure 8-7 Muscles of the upper extremity, (A) anterior view (B) posterior view

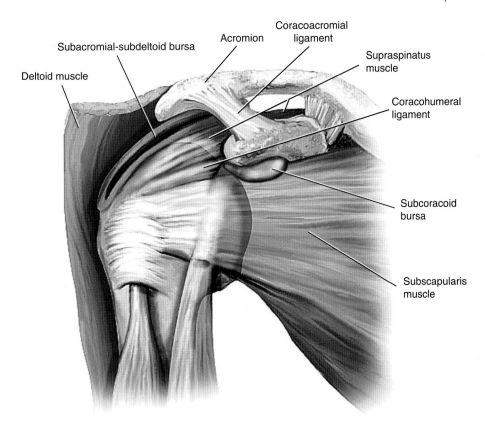

Figure 8-8 Deep muscles of the shoulder joint, anterior view

TABLE 8-1 SCAPULAR MUSCLES OF THE SHOULDER

Muscle	Origin	Insertion
Coracobrachialis	Coracoid process of scapula	Medial aspect of middle humeral shaft
Deltoid	Acromial end of clavicle, acromion of scapula, scapular spine	Humeral deltoid tuberosity
Infraspinatus	Infraspinatus fossa of scapula	Greater tubercle of humerus
Subscapularis	Subscapular fossa of scapula	Lesser tubercle of humerus
Supraspinatus	Supraspinatus fossa of scapula	Greater tubercle of humerus
Teres major	Inferior angle of scapula	Intertubercular groove of humerus
Teres minor	Axillary border of scapula	Greater tubercle of humerus

TABLE 8-2 AXIAL MUSCLES OF THE SHOULDER

Muscle	Origin	Insertion
Latissimus dorsi	Spinous processes of T6–L5, iliac and sacral crests, ribs 9–12	Bicipital groove of humerus
Pectoralis major	Medial inferior clavicle, sternum, costal cartilages (1st or 2nd to 6th or 7th ribs)	Intertubercular groove of humerus

Muscles That Move the Radius and Ulna

The muscles that move the radius and ulna can be categorized as either those involved in flexing or extending the forearm or those involved in supination or pronation. Muscles that allow for flexion of the forearm are the biceps brachii, the brachialis, and the brachioradialis or supinator longus; all are located anteriorly. The triceps brachii, located posteriorly, allows for forearm extension. The pronator quadratus and pronator teres, both anterior muscles, permit pronation of the forearm; the supinator permits supination. The anconeus, a posterior muscle, is involved in extension of the forearm and pronation of the ulna. Figure 8-9 A and B is a line drawing of these muscles, with the pronator quadratus and supinator identified on Figure 8-10.

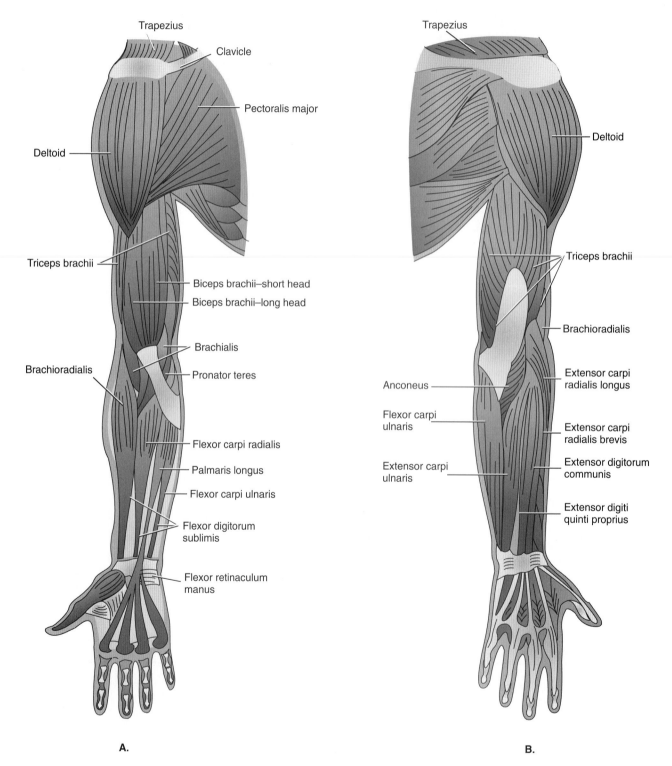

A.

B.

Figure 8-9 Muscles that move the forearm, (A) anterior view (B) posterior view

The biceps brachii, a large muscle covering the humerus anteriorly, originates on the supraglenoid tubercle and the coracoid process of the scapula and inserts on the radial tuberosity. The brachialis, situated deep to the biceps brachii on the lower anterior humerus, originates on the anterior distal humerus and inserts on the ulnar tuberos-ity and coronoid process of the ulna. The brachioradialis or supinator longus originates superior to the lateral epicondyle of the distal humerus and inserts just above the radial styloid process. Table 8-3 summarizes the flexor muscles of the forearm.

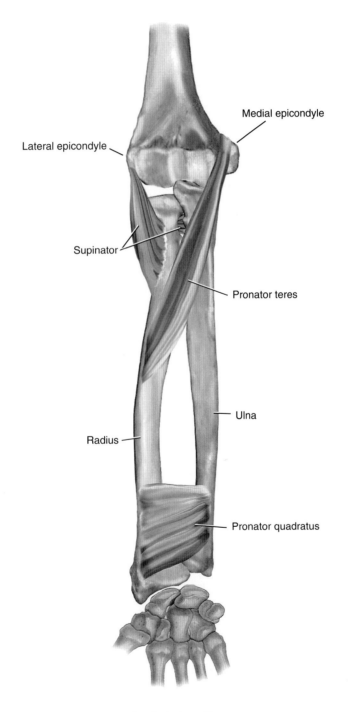

Supinated position

Figure 8-10 Deep muscles that move the forearm, anterior view

The triceps brachii originates inferior to the infraglenoid tubercle and the lateral and posterior humeral surface and inserts on the olecranon process of the ulna. The extensor muscles of the forearm are summarized in Table 8-4.

The pronator quadratus originates on the distal shaft of the ulna and inserts on the distal anterior shaft of the radius. The pronator teres originates superior to the medial epicondyle of the humerus and inferior and medial to the coronoid process of the ulna and inserts on the middle of the lateral aspect of the radius. The pronator muscles of the forearm are summarized in Table 8-5.

The supinator originates on the lateral condyle of the humerus and the proximal lateral ulna and inserts on the proximal lateral radius. Table 8-6 summarizes the supinator muscles of the forearm.

The anconeus (see Figure 8-9 B), a short muscle running transversely on the posterior elbow joint, originates on the posterior lateral condyle of the humerus and inserts just below the olecranon process of the ulna and the upper one-quarter of the posterior shaft of the ulna.

Muscles That Move the Hand

To avoid overwhelming the beginning student with the extensive list of muscles involved in moving the hand, this book groups them according to compartments. The anterior compartment muscles originate on the distal medial humerus and insert on the carpals, metacarpals, and phalanges. If listed, they would be further subdivided into superficial and deep groups; all serve as flexors.

The posterior compartment muscles originate on the distal lateral humerus and insert onto the metacarpals and phalanges. They, too, can be subdivided into superficial and deep groups but their function is to serve as extensors. Refer to Figure 8-9 A and B for these flexor and extensor muscles.

TABLE 8-3 FLEXOR MUSCLES OF THE FOREARM

Muscle	Origin	Insertion
Biceps brachii	Supraglenoid tubercle and coracoid process of scapula	Radial tuberosity
Brachialis	Anterior distal humerus	Ulnar tuberosity and coronoid process of ulna
Brachioradialis	Superior to lateral epicondyle of humerus	Just above radial styloid process

TABLE 8-4 EXTENSOR MUSCLES OF THE FOREARM

Muscle	Origin	Insertion
Anconeus	Posterior lateral condyle of humerus	Just below olecranon process of ulna and upper ¼ posterior ulnar shaft
Triceps brachii	Inferior to infraglenoid tubercle of scapula, lateral and posterior humeral surface	Olecranon process of ulna

TABLE 8-5 PRONATOR MUSCLES OF THE FOREARM

Muscle	Origin	Insertion
Anconeus	Posterior lateral condyle of humerus	Just below olecranon process of ulna and upper ¼ posterior ulnar shaft
Pronator quadratus	Distal ulnar shaft	Distal anterior radial shaft
Pronator teres	Superior to medial humeral epicondyle, inferior and medial to coronoid process of ulna	Middle of lateral aspect of radius

TABLE 8-6 SUPINATOR MUSCLES OF THE FOREARM

Muscle	Origin	Insertion
Supinator	Lateral humeral condyle, proximal lateral ulna	Proximal lateral radius

SHOULDER JOINT

The shoulder or **glenohumeral joint** is a **diarthrodial** or **synovial joint** and, as such, is freely movable. More specifically, it is a **ball and socket joint** formed by the head of the humerus and the glenoid fossa of the scapula, both having **articular cartilage** on the surface. The joint is enclosed by an **articular capsule**, composed of a fibrous joint capsule lined with a **synovial membrane**. The synovial membrane secretes **synovial fluid**, lubricating the joint. The articular capsule extends from the glenoid cavity of the scapula to the anatomic neck of the humerus.

Ligaments

The glenoid **labrum** is a rim of fibrocartilage extending beyond the edge of the glenoid cavity. The shoulder joint is strengthened by three **ligaments** or bands of fibrous tissue: the coracohumeral, glenohumeral, and transverse humeral, labeled on Figure 8-11. The coracohumeral ligament extends from the coracoid process of the scapula to the greater tubercle of the humerus. The glenohumeral ligament, composed of three fibrous bands, helps to form the glenoid labrum. It extends from the glenoid cavity of the scapula to the lesser tuberosity and upper bicipital groove of the humerus. The transverse humeral ligament passes from the greater tubercle of the humerus to the lesser tubercle of the humerus. The coracoacromial ligament along with the coracoid process and acromion of the scapula form a protective arch over the shoulder.

Bursae

A number of **bursae** help cushion the shoulder joint: the subacromial, subcoracoid, subdeltoid, and subscapular, is shown on Figure 8-11. A bursa is a sac of synovial fluid lined by a synovial membrane. The subdeltoid and subacromial bursae are joined together.

CT and MR images for the upper and lower extremities have been selectively chosen to demonstrate the three major joints of each extremity from multiple planes.

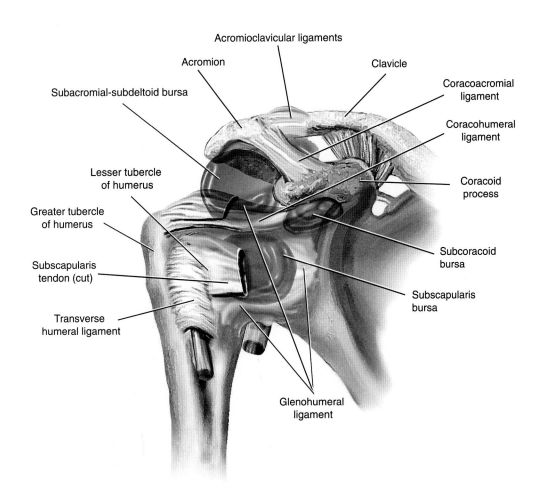

Figure 8-11 Ligaments and bursae of the shoulder, anterior view

CT Images of the Shoulder

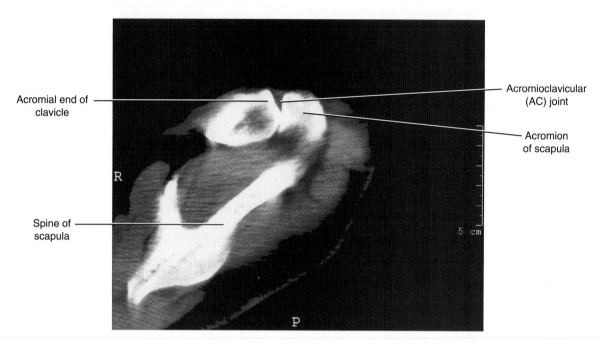

Acromial end of clavicle

Acromioclavicular (AC) joint

Acromion of scapula

Spine of scapula

R

P

5 cm

Figure 8-12   Figure 8-12 is a CT axial image above the level of the shoulder joint. Labeled is the acromioclavicular joint, involving the acromion of the scapula and the acromial or lateral end of the clavicle. Because of its curvature only a portion of the clavicle is seen on a single axial slice.

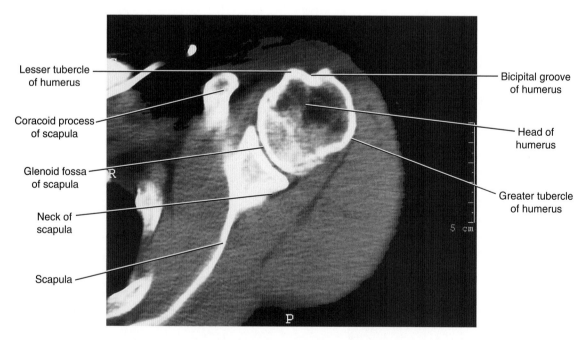

Lesser tubercle of humerus

Coracoid process of scapula

Glenoid fossa of scapula

Neck of scapula

Scapula

Bicipital groove of humerus

Head of humerus

Greater tubercle of humerus

R

P

5 cm

Figure 8-13   Figure 8-13 is at the level of the shoulder joint where the head of the humerus articulates with the glenoid fossa of the scapula, forming a ball and socket diarthrodial joint. The ball and socket joint provides the most mobility of any type of joint.

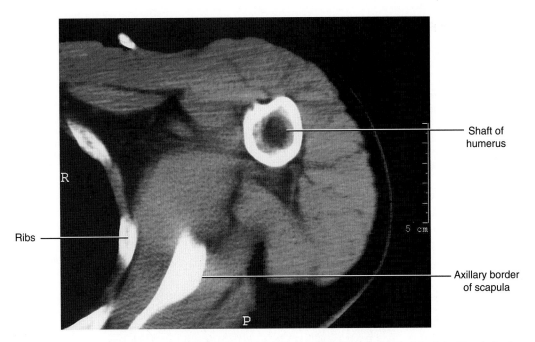

Shaft of
humerus

Ribs

Axillary border
of scapula

Figure 8-14 The last CT axial image of the shoulder joint, Figure 8-14, is below the level of the joint. The shaft of the humerus is seen, as is the axillary border of the scapula.

MR Images of the Shoulder

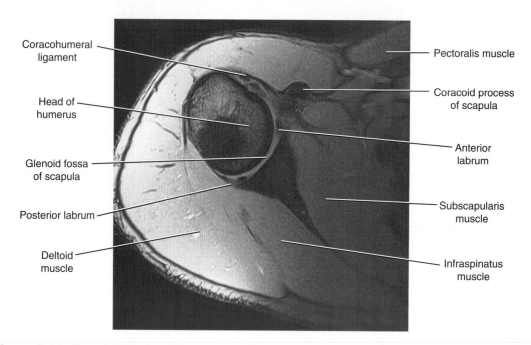

Coracohumeral ligament

Head of humerus

Glenoid fossa of scapula

Posterior labrum

Deltoid muscle

Pectoralis muscle

Coracoid process of scapula

Anterior labrum

Subscapularis muscle

Infraspinatus muscle

Figure 8-15   Figure 8-15 is a single MR axial image of the shoulder joint. Demonstrated again is the ball and socket joint formed by the head of the humerus within the glenoid fossa of the scapula. Notice the anterior and posterior labrum deepening the cavity formed by the glenoid fossa. The deltoid muscle is the most significant muscle in this region and is seen surrounding the shoulder.

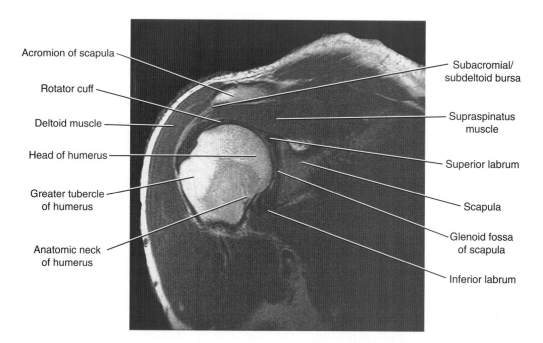

Acromion of scapula

Rotator cuff

Deltoid muscle

Head of humerus

Greater tubercle of humerus

Anatomic neck of humerus

Subacromial/ subdeltoid bursa

Supraspinatus muscle

Superior labrum

Scapula

Glenoid fossa of scapula

Inferior labrum

Figure 8-16   The next image, Figure 8-16, offers the opportunity to look at a sectional image of the shoulder joint from a coronal perspective. Once again, you see the head of the humerus articulating within the glenoid fossa of the scapula, but on this image the superior and inferior labrum are noted. The deltoid muscle is lateral to the head of the humerus and the rotator cuff, involving the infra- and supraspinatus and teres minor muscle tendons, can be seen. Notice also the subacromial-subdeltoid bursae.

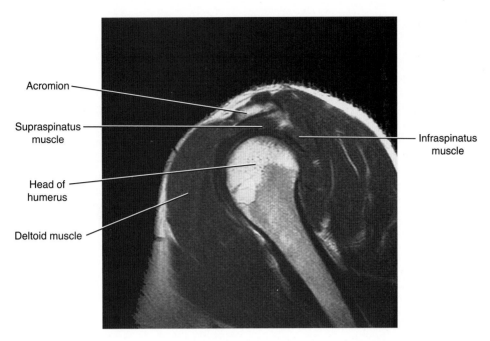

Acromion

Supraspinatus muscle

Head of humerus

Deltoid muscle

Infraspinatus muscle

Figure 8-17 The last image of the shoulder, Figure 8-17, is from a sagittal perspective. You may recall that the coracoacromial ligament, coracoid process, and acromion of the scapula form a protective arch over the shoulder. This image shows the involvement of the acromion in the formation of that arch over the shoulder. Finally, note the size of the deltoid muscle.

ELBOW JOINT

The elbow joint is a synovial or diarthrodial joint involving the distal humerus, and proximal radius and ulna. The articulation between the humerus, radius, and ulna is a **hinge joint**, allowing for flexion of the forearm anteriorly and extension. The articulation between the proximal radius and ulna is a **pivot joint**, which allows for pronation and supination of the forearm.

The articular capsule is attached proximally to the distal humerus on the superior borders of the coronoid and radial fossae anteriorly and the olecranon fossa posteriorly. Distally, the points of attachment are the circumference of the head of the radius with a fold between the radius and the coronoid process and trochlear notch of the ulna, seemingly forming two separate joints: the humeral/radial and humeral/ulnar joints.

Ligaments

Three ligaments bind the elbow joint: the annular ligament of the radius, the radial collateral or external, and the ulnar collateral or internal. The annular ligament partially encircles the radial head, attaching the radius to the proximal lateral ulna. The radial collateral extends from the lateral epicondyle of the humerus to the superior radius and lateral proximal ulna. The ulna collateral extends from the medial epicondyle of the humerus to the coronoid and olecranon processes of the ulna. Figure 8-18 shows the ligaments discussed.

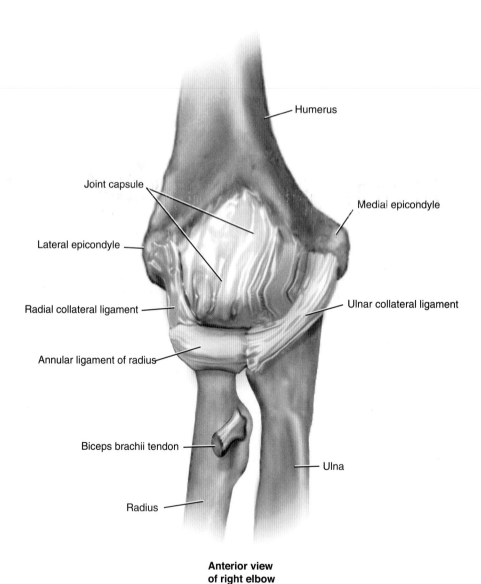

Anterior view
of right elbow

Figure 8-18 Ligaments of the elbow, anterior view

Bursa

The subcutaneous olecranon bursa cushions the posterior elbow (see Figure 8-19).

Fat Pads

There are three fat pads associated with the elbow, all situated over the fossae of the humerus: the coronoid, radial, and olecranon. The largest is over the olecranon fossa.

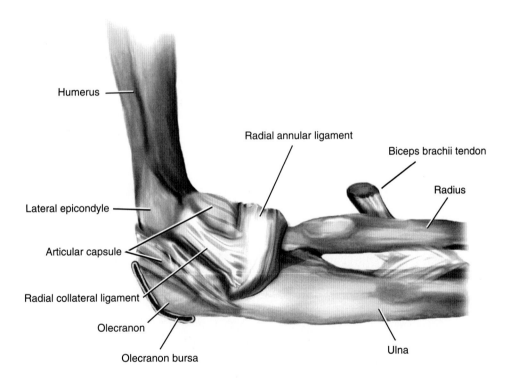

Lateral aspect

Figure 8-19 Lateral view of the elbow

CT Images of the Elbow

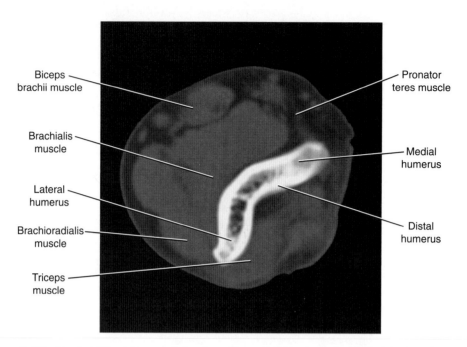

Figure 8-20 The first CT axial image of the elbow (Figure 8-20) is above the level of the joint. Shown is the distal humerus, the triceps muscle along the posterior aspect of the humerus, the superficial anterior muscle, the biceps brachii, and the deep muscles found on the anterior distal humerus, the brachioradialis, brachialis, and pronator teres, listed laterally to medially.

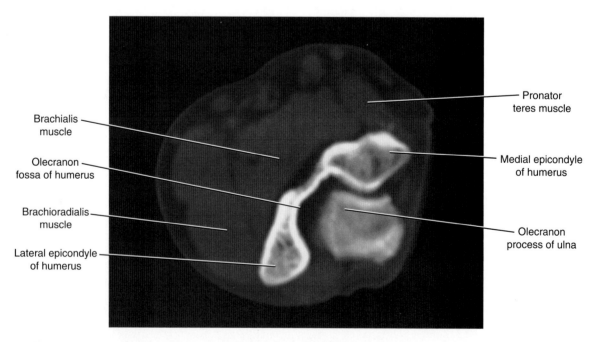

Figure 8-21 Figure 8-21 moves into the vicinity of the elbow joint, a hinge-type synovial joint formed by the articulation of the distal humerus and proximal radius and ulna. Identified are the lateral and medial humeral epicondyles and the olecranon process of the ulna within the olecranon fossa of the distal humerus.

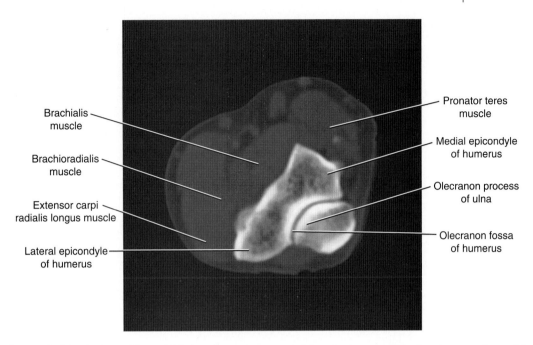

Brachialis muscle

Brachioradialis muscle

Extensor carpi radialis longus muscle

Lateral epicondyle of humerus

Pronator teres muscle

Medial epicondyle of humerus

Olecranon process of ulna

Olecranon fossa of humerus

Figure 8-22 Again, on Figure 8-22, the olecranon process of the ulna is seen within the olecranon fossa of the distal humerus. The largest muscles at this level are the brachioradialis and extensor carpi radialis longus seen along the lateral border.

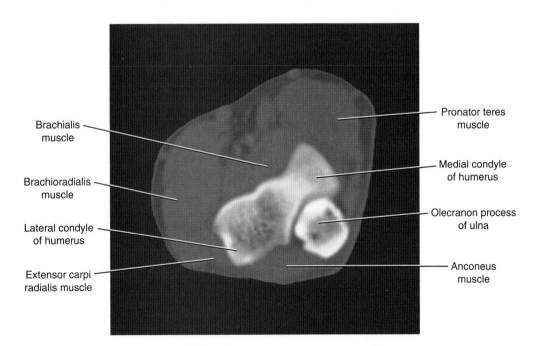

Brachialis muscle

Brachioradialis muscle

Lateral condyle of humerus

Extensor carpi radialis muscle

Pronator teres muscle

Medial condyle of humerus

Olecranon process of ulna

Anconeus muscle

Figure 8-23 Figure 8-23 is the last image in this series to demonstrate the articulation of the distal humerus and proximal ulna. Notice the presence of the anconeus muscle, which runs transversely on the posterior elbow between the posterior lateral condyle of the humerus and the proximal posterior ulna.

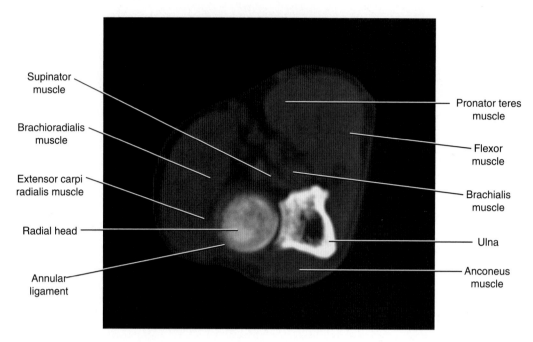

Supinator muscle

Brachioradialis muscle

Extensor carpi radialis muscle

Radial head

Annular ligament

Pronator teres muscle

Flexor muscle

Brachialis muscle

Ulna

Anconeus muscle

Figure 8-24 Moving out of the vicinity of the distal humerus, Figure 8-24 demonstrates the proximal head of the radius and the proximal ulna. The articulation of the proximal radius with the ulna is a pivot-type joint. Notice the anular ligament partially encircling the radial head and attaching it to the proximal lateral ulna.

MR Images of the Elbow

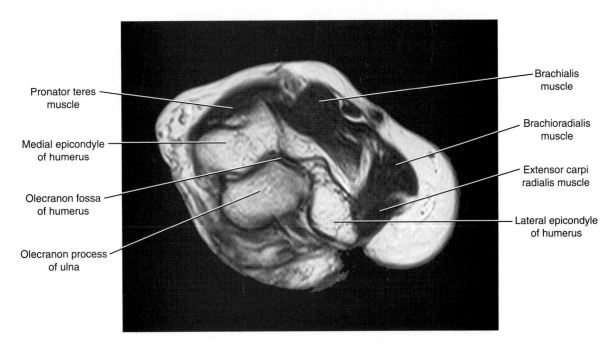

Pronator teres muscle

Medial epicondyle of humerus

Olecranon fossa of humerus

Olecranon process of ulna

Brachialis muscle

Brachioradialis muscle

Extensor carpi radialis muscle

Lateral epicondyle of humerus

Figure 8-25 A single axial MR image of the elbow joint has been chosen on Figure 8-25 to demonstrate some of the anatomy seen on the CT axial images. Evident are the olecranon process of the proximal ulna within the olecranon fossa of the distal posterior humerus and the medial and lateral epicondyles of the humerus.

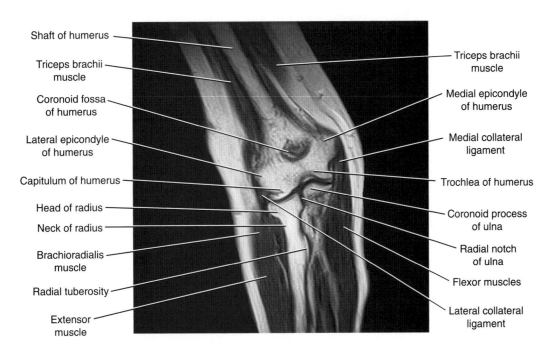

Shaft of humerus

Triceps brachii muscle

Coronoid fossa of humerus

Lateral epicondyle of humerus

Capitulum of humerus

Head of radius

Neck of radius

Brachioradialis muscle

Radial tuberosity

Extensor muscle

Triceps brachii muscle

Medial epicondyle of humerus

Medial collateral ligament

Trochlea of humerus

Coronoid process of ulna

Radial notch of ulna

Flexor muscles

Lateral collateral ligament

Figure 8-26 Figure 8-26 is the first of two MR images of the elbow from a coronal perspective. This image is a more anterior cut clearly showing the head, neck, and radial tuberosity of the radius. The coronoid process of the ulna and coronoid fossa of the distal humerus are seen, along with the medial and lateral epicondyles of the humerus. Also labeled are the trochlea, lateral to the medial epicondyle, and the capitulum, medial to the lateral epicondyle. Along the lateral border is a segment of the extensor carpi radialis longus muscle; along the medial border are the flexor muscles.

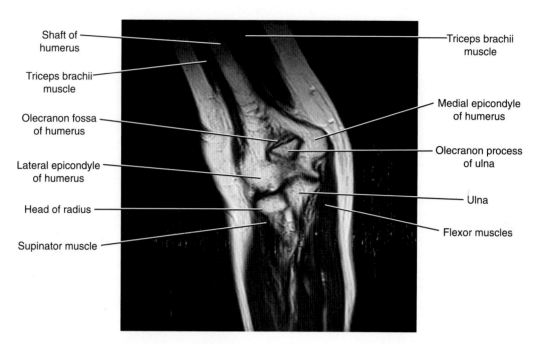

Shaft of humerus

Triceps brachii muscle

Olecranon fossa of humerus

Lateral epicondyle of humerus

Head of radius

Supinator muscle

Triceps brachii muscle

Medial epicondyle of humerus

Olecranon process of ulna

Ulna

Flexor muscles

Figure 8-27 The second coronal image, shown on Figure 8-27, is a more posterior cut showing the olecranon process of the ulna within the olecranon fossa of the distal humerus. As this image is more posterior, the triceps brachii muscle can be identified superior to the elbow joint.

WRIST JOINT

The wrist is that region between the forearm and the hand. Articulations exist between the radius, ulna, and carpal bones, between the carpal bones themselves, and between the carpal bones and metacarpals. The joint between the radius and scaphoid, lunate, and triquetrum is a synovial or diarthrodial joint, specifically a **condyloid joint**. The cavity of the condyloid joint is formed by the distal radius and the fibrocartilage on its undersurface, while the scaphoid, lunate, and triquetrum collectively form a convex shape, or the condyle. In the wrist area the muscles of the forearm have narrowed into tendons going to the hand with the flexor tendons located anteriorly on the palmar side and the extensor tendons located posteriorly.

Ligaments

Ligaments found in the wrist include the dorsal carpal or posterior, palmar carpal or anterior, radial collateral or external, ulnar collateral or internal, and the flexor **retinaculum** manus or carpal transverse. The dorsal carpal ligaments, passing from the posterior distal radius and ulna to the scaphoid, lunate, and triquetrum and between the

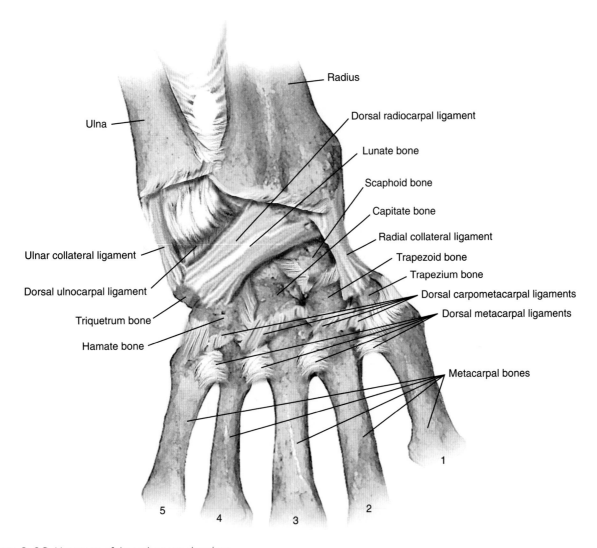

Radius
Dorsal radiocarpal ligament
Lunate bone
Scaphoid bone
Capitate bone
Radial collateral ligament
Trapezoid bone
Trapezium bone
Dorsal carpometacarpal ligaments
Dorsal metacarpal ligaments
Metacarpal bones

Ulna
Ulnar collateral ligament
Dorsal ulnocarpal ligament
Triquetrum bone
Hamate bone

1
2
3
4
5

Figure 8-28 Ligaments of the wrist, posterior view

first and second rows of carpal bones, are drawn on Figure 8-28. The palmar carpal ligaments, as shown on Figure 8-29, extend from the distal radius and ulna to the anterior aspect of the scaphoid, lunate, triquetrum, and capitate. The radial collateral ligament joins the radial styloid process with the scaphoid and trapezium, while the ulnar collateral ligament connects the ulnar styloid process with the triquetrum and pisiform. Both the radial and ulnar collateral ligaments are identified on Figures 8-28 and 8-29.

The remaining ligament, the flexor retinaculum manus, labeled on Figure 8-9 A, is a thick band of fascia passing across the anterior wrist, and forming a canal, the carpal tunnel. It connects the hamate and pisiform with the trapezium and scaphoid. The flexor muscle tendons pass through the canal along with the median nerve, found midline. Carpal tunnel syndrome results in pain or numbness of the hand caused by compression of the median nerve by the flexor muscle tendons as it passes through the carpal tunnel.

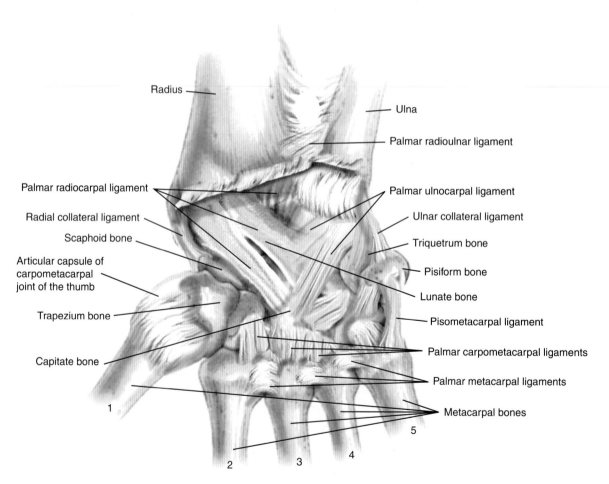

Figure 8-29 Ligaments of the wrist, anterior view

CT Images of the Wrist

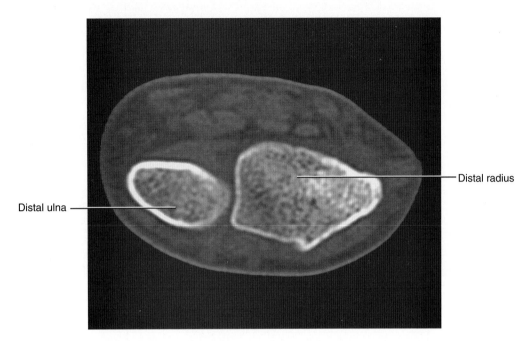

Figure 8-30   Figure 8-30, the first of three axial CT images of the wrist, shows the distal radius and ulna. It is the articulation of the distal radius and ulna with the scaphoid, lunate, and triquetrum of the wrist that forms the wrist joint, a condyloid synovial joint.

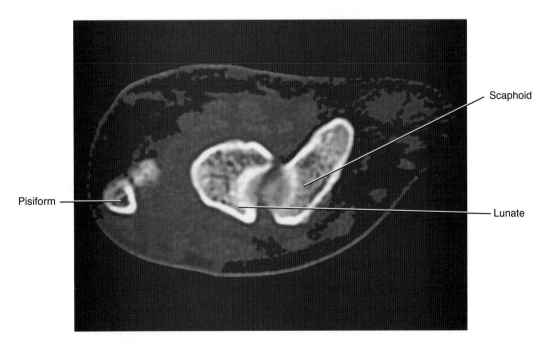

Figure 8-31   The second CT axial image of the wrist joint, Figure 8-31, allows identification of three of the four carpal bones in the proximal row: the scaphoid, lunate, and pisiform, with the scaphoid being most lateral. Because the carpal bones are not arranged in straight linear rows, it is difficult to isolate a single row of carpal bones on axial images.

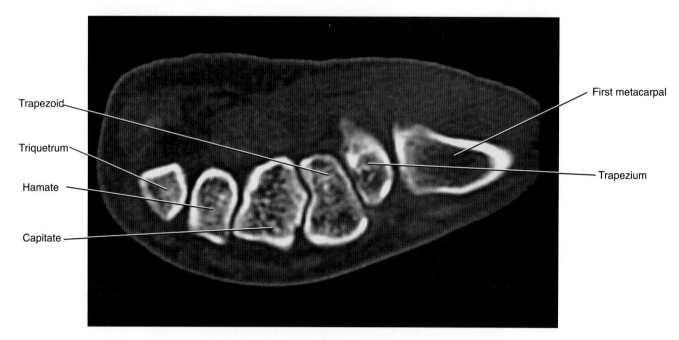

Figure 8-32   The last CT axial image of the wrist, Figure 8-32, identifies all the carpal bones in the distal row (the trapezium, trapezoid, capitate, and hamate) but also shows a bone in the proximal row, the triquetrum.

MR Images of the Wrist

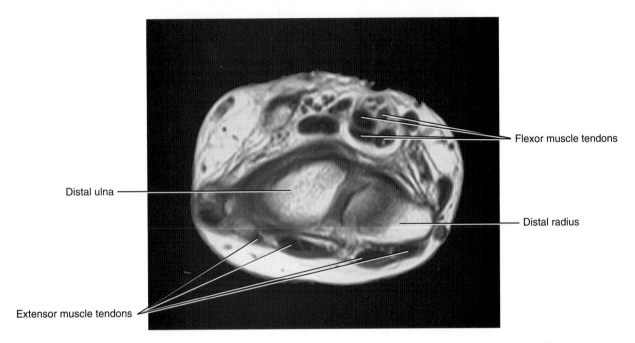

Figure 8-33 Figure 8-33 is an axial MR image of the wrist at the level of the distal radius and ulna. The flexor muscle tendons are located anteriorly while the extensor muscle tendons are seen posteriorly.

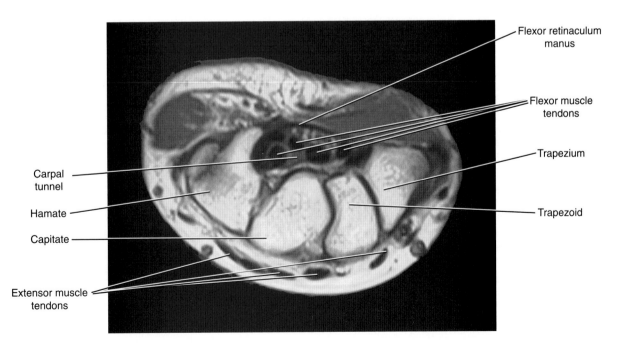

Figure 8-34 Figure 8-34 shows the four carpal bones of the distal row, the trapezium, trapezoid, capitate, and hamate. Identified is the flexor retinaculum manus, the ligament involved in forming the carpal tunnel. Passing through the tunnel are the flexor muscle tendons and the median nerve. Compression of the median nerve by the flexor muscle tendons results in carpal tunnel syndrome.

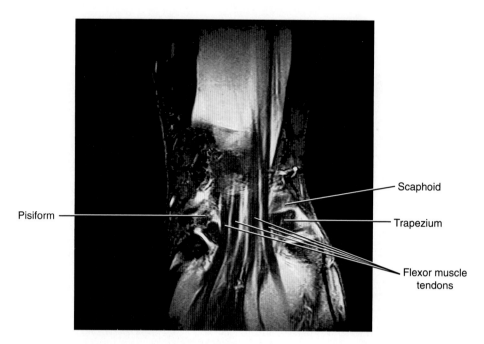

Pisiform

Scaphoid

Trapezium

Flexor muscle
tendons

Figure 8-35 Figures 8-35 and 8-36 are two coronal MR images of the wrist, with Figure 8-35 being more anterior. Seen on Figure 8-35 are the flexor muscle tendons in the carpal tunnel, and three of the carpal bones, the scaphoid and pisiform in the proximal row and the trapezium in the distal row.

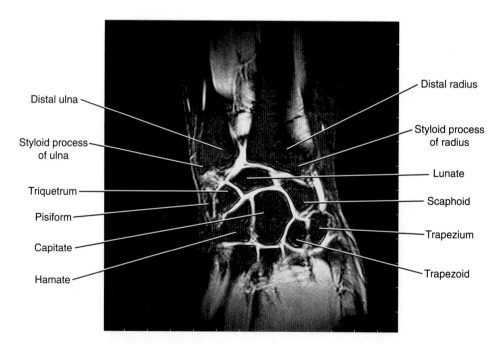

Distal ulna

Styloid process
of ulna

Triquetrum

Pisiform

Capitate

Hamate

Distal radius

Styloid process
of radius

Lunate

Scaphoid

Trapezium

Trapezoid

Figure 8-36 Figure 8-36 shows all the carpal bones. From this perspective one can appreciate why it is difficult to isolate a single row of carpal bones on one axial image. This particular image allows visualization of articulation of the distal radius and ulna with the scaphoid, lunate, and triquetrum, to form the wrist joint.

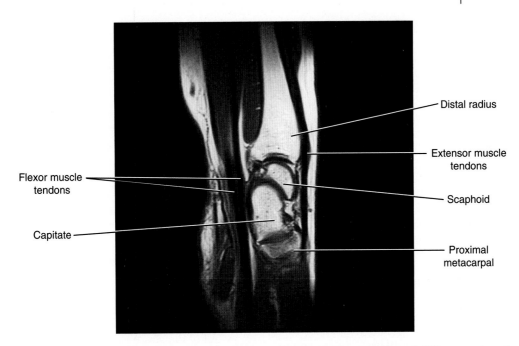

Figure 8-37   The final two sectional images are sagittal MR images of the wrist. Figure 8-37 is a more lateral sagittal image and shows the radius and scaphoid. The flexor muscle tendons are anterior while the extensor muscle tendons are posterior.

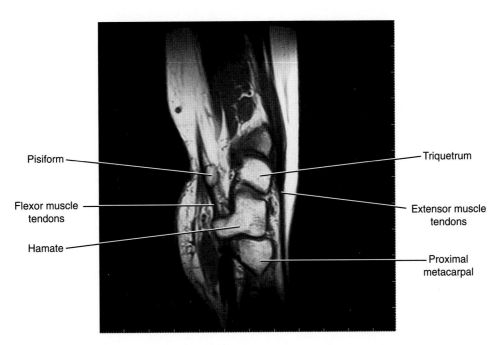

Figure 8-38   Figure 8-38 demonstrates the medial carpal bones, the pisiform and hamate. Note the presence of the flexor muscle tendons anteriorly and the extensor muscle tendons posteriorly.

REVIEW QUESTIONS

1. The subscapular fossa is a
   a. depression on the anterior surface of the scapula.
   b. point beneath the glenoid fossa.
   c. point beneath the inferior angle of the scapula.
   d. depression on the posterior surface of the scapula.

2. On a coronal sectional image of the shoulder the greater tubercle of the humerus is
   a. along the medial edge of the proximal humerus.
   b. midline on the anterior proximal humerus.
   c. along the lateral edge of the proximal humerus.
   d. The greater tubercle is not seen on a coronal sectional image of the shoulder; it is on the distal humerus.

3. On a coronal sectional image of the elbow joint the radial fossa is
   a. medial to the lateral epicondyle.
   b. proximal to the capitulum.
   c. on an image of the anterior surface of the humerus.
   d. a, b, and c

4. On axial CT images of the elbow the head of the radius is seen lateral to the ulna.
   a. True
   b. False

Indicate whether the following muscles move the (a) humerus, (b) radius and ulna, or (c) hand.

____ 5. Brachioradialis

____ 6. Deltoid

____ 7. Flexor

____ 8. Supinator

9. List the muscles involved in forming the rotator cuff of the shoulder joint.

   _____

   _____

   _____

   _____

Match the following ligaments with the joint they are associated with.

____ 10. Transverse humeral   a. Shoulder

____ 11. Flexor retinaculum manus   b. Elbow

____ 12. Anular ligament of the radius   c. Wrist

13. The joint having fat pads is the
    a. shoulder.
    b. elbow.
    c. wrist.
    d. None of the above.
    e. All of the above.

14. On axial, coronal, and sagittal images of the wrist which of the following is *not* found anteriorly?
    a. Carpal tunnel
    b. Flexor tendons
    c. Median nerve
    d. Extensor tendons

15. On axial and coronal images of the shoulder joint which muscle is seen surrounding the shoulder?
    a. Teres major
    b. Coracobrachialis
    c. Deltoid
    d. Pectoralis major

Lower Extremity

SKELETAL ANATOMY OF THE LOWER EXTREMITY

Of the 206 bones in the adult human skeleton, 126 are considered part of the appendicular skeleton. Included in the appendicular skeleton are the bilateral lower extremities and pelvic girdles. The lower extremity, as seen on Figure 9-1, is made of the **femur**, **patella**, **fibula**, **tibia**, 7 **tarsal bones**, 5 **metatarsals**, and 14 phalanges. The bilateral pelvic girdles are composed of the 2 innominate or hip bones.

Pelvic Girdle

The innominate or hip bone was discussed in Chapter 6. A review is suggested before continuing in this chapter.

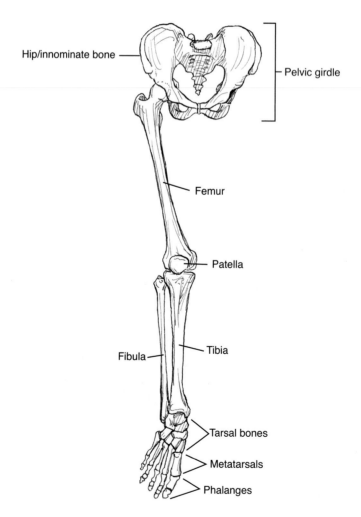

Figure 9-1 Pelvis and lower limb

Femur

The femur (**thigh**) (see Figure 9-2 A and B) is the longest, heaviest, and strongest bone in the human body. The medial proximal aspect of the femur, the head, articulates with the acetabulum of the hip bone to form the **hip joint**. On the head is a small pit, the fovea capitis, which provides a point of attachment for a ligament. Immediately adjacent to the head is a constricted region, the neck. On the lateral proximal femur there is a large tuberosity, the greater trochanter. The lesser trochanter is on the posteromedial proximal femur, inferior to the greater trochanter. Anteriorly, the intertrochanteric line connects the greater and lesser trochanters. Posteriorly, between the greater and lesser trochanter is a bridge of bone, the intertrochanteric crest.

The main shaft of the femur is the diaphysis. The linea aspera is a ridge of bone running longitudinally in the middle third of the posterior femur. Distally on the femur are the medial and lateral condyles and epicondyles. Superior to the medial epicondyle is the adductor tubercle. The anterior inferior surface of the femur, the patellar surface, is concave to accommodate the patella. Posteriorly and inferiorly a large depression exists, the intercondylar fossa.

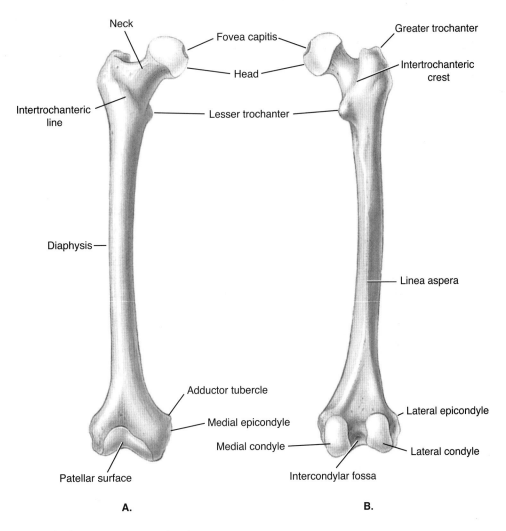

Figure 9-2 Femur, (A) anterior view (B) posterior view

Patella

The patella is a triangularly shaped bone, as drawn on Figure 9-3 A and B, and is located anterior to the distal femur. It is most commonly categorized as a sesamoid bone because it is imbedded in a tendon, and is the largest sesamoid bone in the body. The base, the wider part, is superior and the more pointed end, the apex, is inferior. The posterior surface has a ridge running lengthwise with facets on either side for articulation with the femoral condyles.

Fibula

The fibula, drawn on Figure 9-4 A and B, is a long slender bone found laterally in the lower leg. The proximal fibula is the head; beneath the head is a constricted region, the neck. Jutting superiorly from the head of the fibula laterally is a pointed eminence, the apex or styloid process.

The main shaft of the fibula is the diaphysis. Distally the fibula terminates in the lateral malleolus. The medial surface of the lateral malleolus has an articulating facet for the talus.

Tibia

The tibia, located medially to the fibula, is the larger weight-bearing bone of the lower leg. On the proximal tibia are the medial and lateral condyles. On the superior surface of the tibia the medial and lateral intercondylar tubercles form the intercondyloid eminence. On either side of the intercondyloid eminence are the tibial plateaus. On the anterior surface of the proximal tibia there is a palpable secondary site of ossification, the tibial tuberosity.

The main shaft of the tibia is the diaphysis, which has along its anterior border a ridge, the anterior crest. The distal medial aspect of the tibia is a bony projection, the medial malleolus. The inferior tibia and inner surface of the medial malleolus have articulating surfaces for articulation with the talus. On the lateral distal tibia is the fibular notch, in which fits the fibula. All the above landmarks are identified on Figure 9-4 A and B.

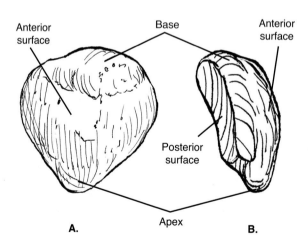

Figure 9-3 Patella, (A) anterior view (B) lateral view

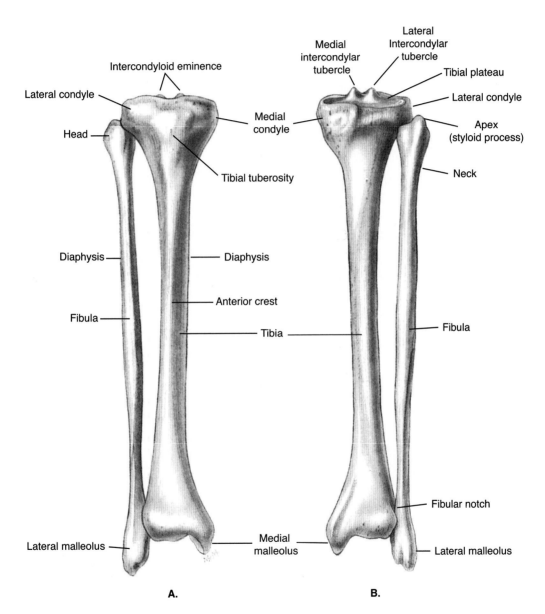

Figure 9-4 Tibia, fibula, (A) anterior view (B) posterior view

Foot

The **foot**, drawn on Figure 9-5 A and B, is that part of the lower extremity distal to the tibia and fibula. It is composed of the 7 tarsal bones, 5 metatarsals, and 14 phalanges.

Tarsal Bones

There are 7 tarsal bones: the talus or astragalus, calcaneus or os calcis, cuboid, navicular, and first, second, and third cuneiforms (medial, intermediate, and lateral). The talus is the most superior of the tarsal bones and through its articulation with the tibia and fibula the **ankle** or **mortise joint** is formed. The superior surface of the talus that articulates with the tibia is the trochlea; the anterior surface that articulates with the navicular is the head; the posterior process is located on the posterior talus. The lateral process extends inferiorly on the lateral aspect,

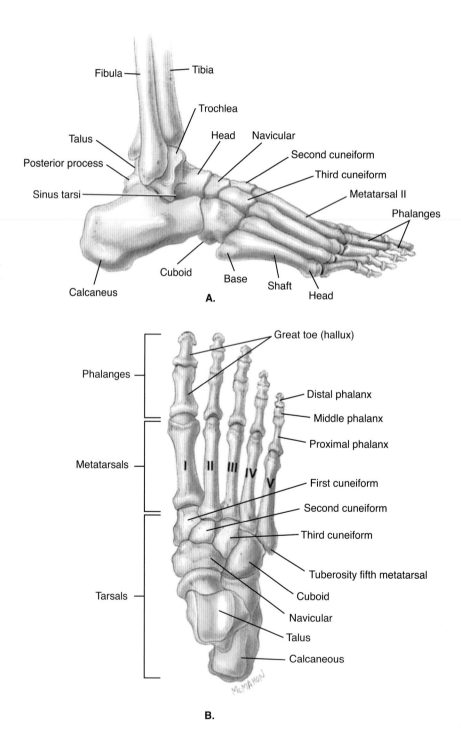

Figure 9-5 Right ankle and foot, (A) lateral view (B) superior view

approximately halfway between the head and posterior process.

Inferior to the talus is the largest tarsal bone, the calcaneus (isolated on Figure 9-6), a multidimensional bone. The articulation of the talus and calcaneus forms the subtalar joint. The anterior half of the superior calcaneus has three facets for articulation with the talus: the anterior, middle, and posterior articulating surfaces. The middle talar articulating surface rests on a ledge of bone that projects medially, the sustentaculum tali. On the posterior calcaneus is a large roughened mass of bone, the tuberosity. On either side of the tuberosity are the medial and lateral processes. On the lateral calcaneus, just inferior to the posterior talar articular surface, is the peroneal or trochlear process. The anterior calcaneus has an articular surface for the cuboid bone. Between the talus and calcaneus is a tunnel, the sinus tarsi, identified on Figure 9-5.

The cuboid bone, located laterally on the foot, is anterior to the calcaneus; the navicular or scaphoid bone, located medially on the foot, is anterior to the talus. Medial to the cuboid and anterior to the navicular are the first or medial, second or intermediate, and third or lateral cuneiform bones.

Metatarsals

There are 5 metatarsals, numbered I–V, starting on the medial foot. The bases, articulating with the 3 cuneiforms and cuboid bones, are proximal, and the heads, articulating with the phalanges, are distal. The fifth metatarsal has a tuberosity extending from the base.

Phalanges

There are 14 phalanges on the foot, 2 on the great or big toe (hallux) located medially, a proximal and distal, and 3 on each remaining toe, a proximal, middle, and distal. The proximal phalanges articulate with the heads of the metatarsals. All tarsal, metatarsal, and phalangeal associations are drawn on Figure 9-5 A and B.

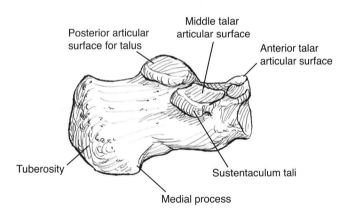

Figure 9-6 Calcaneus, medial aspect

MUSCLES

Muscles That Move the Femur

Although the list of muscles that move the femur is extensive, the muscles involved can be grouped as being anterior, posterior, medial, or lateral, thereby making their localization on sectional images somewhat simpler. In general, the muscles in each group share a similar action with respect to movement of the femur. The muscles, their points of origination, and their points of insertion are most concisely identified in a table format. Many of the muscles illustrated on Figures 9-7 and 9-8 A and B and described in Tables 9-1 through 9-4 were previously discussed in Chapter 6, as most originate on the pelvic girdle. The majority insert on the femur. The only muscle not seen on either line drawing is the obturator externus. It should be noted that the rectus femoris is one of four heads of the quadriceps femoris, with all four heads having the same point of insertion via a single tendon, unlike the hamstring muscles, which are actually three separate muscles.

Muscles That Move the Lower Leg

Some of the muscles that move the femur also move the lower leg and are seen on Figures 9-7 and 9-8 A and B. They are the gracilis, hamstrings, quadriceps femoris (which includes the rectus femoris), and sartorius. The gracilis, hamstrings, and sartorius flex the leg at the knee joint while the quadriceps femoris extends the leg at the knee (see Tables 9-5 and 9-6).

Heads of the quadriceps femoris not discussed previously include the vastus lateralis, vastus medialis, and vastus intermedius. The vastus lateralis originates on the anterior inferior root of the greater trochanter and superior linea aspera of the femur; the vastus medialis originates on the lower anterior intertrochanteric line and the linea aspera of the femur; the vastus intermedius originates on the anterior and lateral femoral shaft. All of these heads, along with the rectus femoris, merge to form the quadriceps femoris muscle, which then inserts onto the patella and tibial tuberosity via a single tendon. Figure 9-7 demonstrates the vastus lateralis and vastus medialis. The vastus intermedius lies under the rectus femoris.

TABLE 9-1 MUSCLES THAT MOVE THE FEMUR: ANTERIOR GROUP

Muscle	Origin	Insertion
Iliopsoas	Iliac fossa, transverse processes and bodies of lumbar vertebrae	Lesser trochanter
Sartorius	ASIS	Superior anterior medial tibial shaft
Rectus femoris	Anterior inferior iliac spine, superior to posterior acetabulum	Patella, tibial tuberosity

*These muscles flex the thigh at the hip joint.

TABLE 9-2 MUSCLES THAT MOVE THE FEMUR: POSTERIOR GROUP

Muscle	Origin	Insertion
Hamstrings		
a. Biceps femoris	Long head—inferior ischial tuberosity	Head of fibula
b. Semimembranosus	Superior ischial tuberosity	Medial tibial condyle
c. Semitendinosus	Inferior ischial tuberosity	Proximal medial tibial shaft
Inferior gemellus	Superior ischial tuberosity	Greater trochanter
Obturator externus	Outer obturator foramen, pubis, ischium	Medial inferior greater trochanter
Obturator internus	Inner obturator foramen	Greater trochanter
Piriformis	Anterior sacrum	Greater trochanter
Quadratus femoris	Superior external ischial tuberosity	Superior to middle of intertrochanteric crest
Superior gemellus	Ischial spine	Greater trochanter

*These muscles rotate the leg laterally.

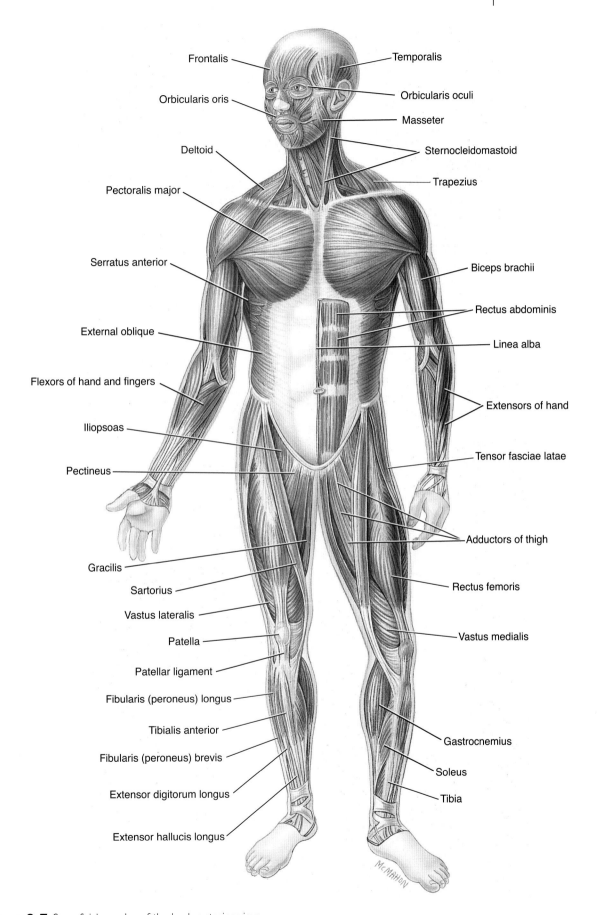

Figure 9-7 Superficial muscles of the body, anterior view

TABLE 9-3 MUSCLES THAT MOVE THE FEMUR: MEDIAL GROUP

Muscle	Origin	Insertion
Adductors		
a. Brevis	Inferior pubic ramus	Linea aspera
b. Longus	Superior pubic ramus, symphysis pubis	Linea aspera
c. Magnus	Inferior pubic and ischial rami to ischial tuberosity	Linea aspera
Gracilis	Pubic arch and symphysis	Medial aspect of superior anterior tibial shaft
Pectineus	Superior pubic ramus	Between lesser trochanter and linea aspera

*These muscles adduct the thigh at the hip joint.

TABLE 9-4 MUSCLES THAT MOVE THE FEMUR: LATERAL GROUP

Muscle	Origin	Insertion
Gluteal maximus	Iliac crest, sacrum, coccyx	Superior linea aspera
Gluteal medius	Ilium	Greater trochanter
Gluteal minimus	Ilium	Greater trochanter
Tensor	Iliac crest	Lateral femur and tibial condyle

*These muscles are abductors.

TABLE 9-5 MUSCLES THAT MOVE THE LOWER LEG: FLEXORS

Muscle	Origin	Insertion
Gracilis	Pubic arch and symphysis	Medial aspect of superior anterior tibial shaft
Hamstrings		
a. Biceps femoris	Long head—inferior ischial tuberosity	Head of fibula
b. Semimembranosus	Superior ischial tuberosity	Medial tibial codyle
c. Semitendinosus	Inferior ischial tuberosity	Proximal medial tibial shaft
Sartorius	ASIS	Superior anterior medial tibial shaft

*These muscles flex the leg at the knee joint.

Muscles That Move the Foot

The muscles of the lower leg can be divided into anterior, posterior, and lateral or peroneal compartments.

The anterior compartment, visible on Figure 9-7, includes the extensor digitorum longus, extensor hallucis longus, and tibialis anterior (see Table 9-7). The extensor digitorum longus originates on the lateral tibial condyle and anterior fibula and inserts onto the middle and distal phalanges of the second through fifth digits. The extensor hallucis longus originates on the anterior fibula and inserts onto the distal phalanx of the great toe. The tibialis anterior originates on the lateral tibial condyle and lateral shaft and inserts onto the first cuneiform and metatarsal.

The posterior compartment, drawn on Figure 9-8 A and B and summarized in Table 9-8, includes the gastrocnemius, plantaris, and soleus superficially, and, at a deeper level, the flexor digitorum longus, flexor hallucis longus, popliteus, and tibialis posterior. The gastrocnemius originates on the lateral and medial femoral condyles and articular knee capsule. The plantaris originates on the femur above the lateral condyle. The soleus, lying underneath the gastrocnemius, originates on the posterior fibular head. All three insert onto the calcaneus with the gastrocnemius and soleus forming a single tendon, the Achilles. The plantaris inserts alongside the medial aspect of the Achilles.

The flexor digitorum longus originates on the posterior tibia and inserts onto the second through the fifth distal phalanges. The flexor hallucis longus originates on the lower two-thirds of the posterior fibula and inserts onto the distal phalanx of the great toe. The popliteus originates on the lateral femoral condyle and inserts onto the proxi-mal tibia, while the tibialis posterior originates on the posterior tibia and fibula and inserts onto the navicular, 3 cuneiforms, cuboid, and the second through fourth metatarsals.

The lateral or peroneal compartment includes the per-oneus brevis and longus. The peroneus brevis originates on the fibular shaft and inserts onto the base of the fifth metatarsal; the peroneus longus originates on the fibular head and shaft and inserts onto the first cuneiform and metatarsal (see Table 9-9).

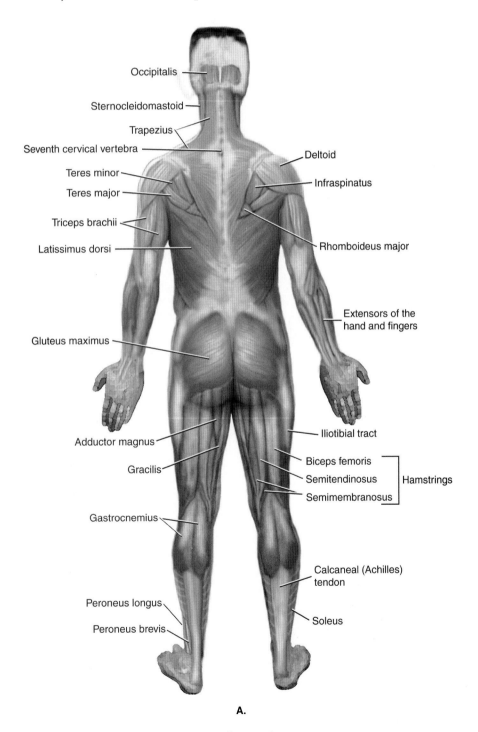

A.

Figure 9-8 (A) Superficial muscles of the body, posterior view *(continues)*

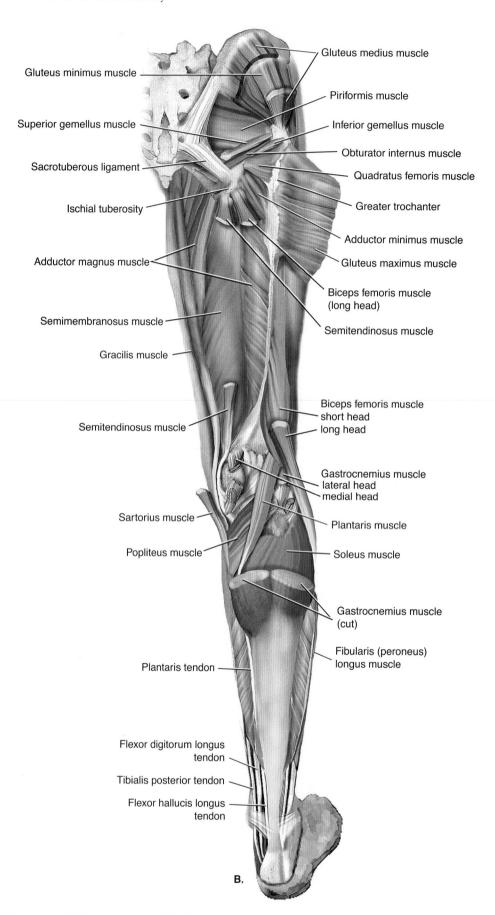

Gluteus medius muscle

Gluteus minimus muscle

Piriformis muscle

Superior gemellus muscle

Inferior gemellus muscle

Obturator internus muscle

Sacrotuberous ligament

Quadratus femoris muscle

Ischial tuberosity

Greater trochanter

Adductor minimus muscle

Adductor magnus muscle

Gluteus maximus muscle

Biceps femoris muscle
(long head)

Semimembranosus muscle

Semitendinosus muscle

Gracilis muscle

Biceps femoris muscle
short head
long head

Semitendinosus muscle

Gastrocnemius muscle
lateral head
medial head

Sartorius muscle

Plantaris muscle

Popliteus muscle

Soleus muscle

Gastrocnemius muscle
(cut)

Fibularis (peroneus)
longus muscle

Plantaris tendon

Flexor digitorum longus
tendon

Tibialis posterior tendon

Flexor hallucis longus
tendon

B.

Figure 9-8 (continued) (B) deep muscles of the leg, posterior view

TABLE 9-6 MUSCLES THAT MOVE THE LOWER LEG: EXTENSORS

Muscle	Origin	Insertion
Quadriceps femoris		
a. Vastus intermedius	Anterior and lateral femoral shaft	Patella, tibial tuberosity
b. Vastus lateralis	Anterior inferior root of greater trochanter, superior linea aspera of femur	Patella, tibial tuberosity
c. Vastus medialis	Linea aspera of femur, lower anterior intertrochanteric line	Patella, tibial tuberosity
d. Rectus femoris	Anterior inferior iliac spine, superior to posterior acetabulum	Patella, tibial tuberosity

*These muscles extend the leg at the knee joint.

TABLE 9-7 MUSCLES THAT MOVE THE FOOT: ANTERIOR COMPARTMENT

Muscle	Origin	Insertion
Extensor digitorum longus	Lateral tibial condyle, anterior fibula	Middle and distal phalanges, second–fifth digits
Extensor hallucis longus	Anterior fibula	Distal phalanx great toe
Tibialis anterior	Lateral tibial condyle and shaft	First cuneiform and metatarsal

TABLE 9-8 MUSCLES THAT MOVE THE FOOT: POSTERIOR COMPARTMENT

Muscle	Origin	Insertion
Flexor digitorum longus	Posterior tibia	Second–fifth distal phalanges
Flexor hallucis longus	Lower ⅔ of posterior fibula	Distal phalanx great toe
Gastrocnemius	Lateral and medial femoral condyles, articular knee capsule	Calcaneus
Plantaris	Femur—above lateral condyle	Calcaneus
Popliteus	Lateral femoral condyle	Proximal tibia
Soleus	Posterior fibular head	Calcaneus
Tibialis posterior	Posterior tibia and fibula	Navicular, 3 cuneiforms, cuboid, second–fourth metatarsals

TABLE 9-9 MUSCLES THAT MOVE THE FOOT: LATERAL OR PERONEAL COMPARTMENT

Muscle	Origin	Insertion
Peroneus brevis	Fibular shaft	Base of fifth metatarsal
Peroneus longus	Fibular head and shaft	First cuneiform and metatarsal

HIP JOINT

The hip joint is a synovial or diarthrodial joint, and, similar to the shoulder, a ball and socket joint. It is formed by the femoral head and acetabulum of the hip bone. The head of the femur and the acetabulum have surfaces covered with articulating cartilage, although the covering is incomplete on the acetabulum. On the inferior acetabulum is an indentation, the acetabular or cotyloid notch. Above the acetabular notch, just inferior to the center of the acetabulum, is the acetabular fossa, which contains a fat pad covered with a synovial membrane. The acetabular fossa has no articulating cartilage nor does it articulate with the head of the femur.

The articular capsule, one of the strongest structures of the body, connects the acetabular rim with the femoral neck. Lined with a synovial membrane, it has a unique construction, having inner circular fibers (the zona orbicularis) encircling the femoral neck, as well as longitudinal fibers strengthened by ligaments.

Ligaments

The ligaments reinforcing the articular capsule are the iliofemoral, ischiofemoral, and pubofemoral, all identified on Figure 9-9 A and B. Particularly strong is the iliofemoral ligament. It extends from the anterior inferior iliac spine of the ilium to the intertrochanteric line of the femur. The

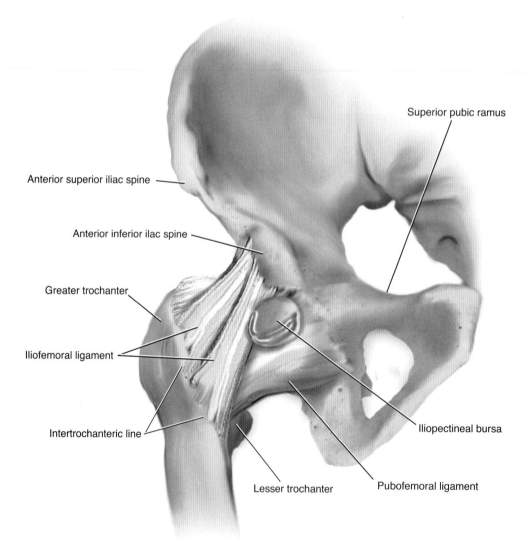

A.

Figure 9-9 Ligaments of the hip, (A) anterior view *(continues)*

ischiofemoral ligament passes from a point immediately inferior to that part of the acetabulum formed by the ischium to the neck of the femur. The pubofemoral ligament extends from the rim of that part of the acetabulum formed by the pubic bone to the neck of the femur.

Other ligaments involved in the hip joint are the acetabular labrum or cotyloid ligament, ligament of the head of the femur or ligamentum teres femoris, and transverse ligament. The acetabular labrum is a rim of fibrocartilage around the margin of the acetabulum, thereby increasing its depth. Because the diameter of the acetabular rim is smaller than the head of the femur, dislocations of the hip joint are uncommon. The ligament of the head of the

femur is a triangulated flat band connecting the fovea capitis of the head of the femur by its apex with the acetabular or cotyloid notch by its base. The transverse ligament is a continuation of the cotyloid ligament across the acetabular notch; thus, it is in contact with both the cotyloid ligament and the ligamentum teres femoris. Refer to Figure 9-10 to locate these structures.

Bursa

Over a gap existing between the proximal iliofemoral and pubofemoral ligaments is the iliopectineal bursa, as seen on Figure 9-9 A.

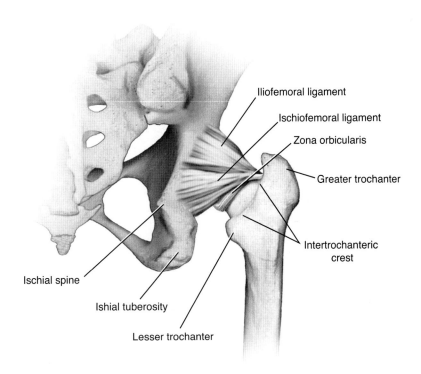

B.

Figure 9-9 *(continued)* (B) posterior view

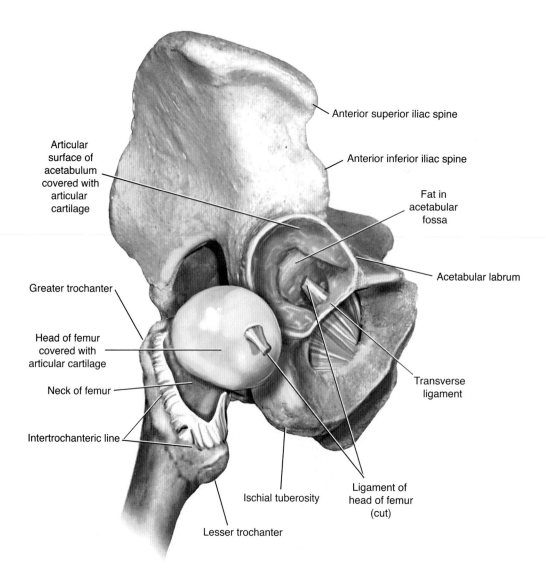

Anterior superior iliac spine

Anterior inferior iliac spine

Fat in acetabular fossa

Articular surface of acetabulum covered with articular cartilage

Acetabular labrum

Greater trochanter

Head of femur covered with articular cartilage

Neck of femur

Intertrochanteric line

Transverse ligament

Ischial tuberosity

Ligament of head of femur (cut)

Lesser trochanter

Figure 9-10 Right hip, lateral view

CT Images of the Hip

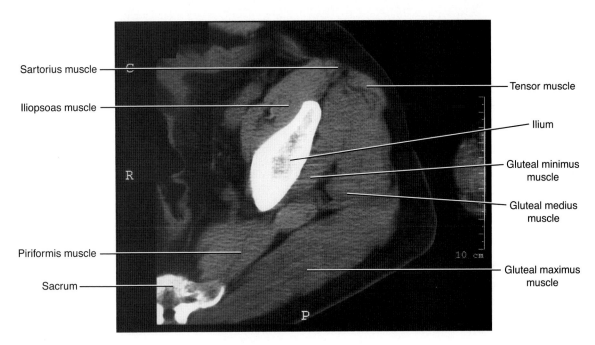

Sartorius muscle

Iliopsoas muscle

Piriformis muscle

Sacrum

Tensor muscle

Ilium

Gluteal minimus muscle

Gluteal medius muscle

10 cm

Gluteal maximus muscle

Figure 9-11 Figure 9-11 is an axial CT image just above the level of the hip joint. Chapter 6 noted that the upper two-fifths of the acetabulum is formed by the body of the ilium.

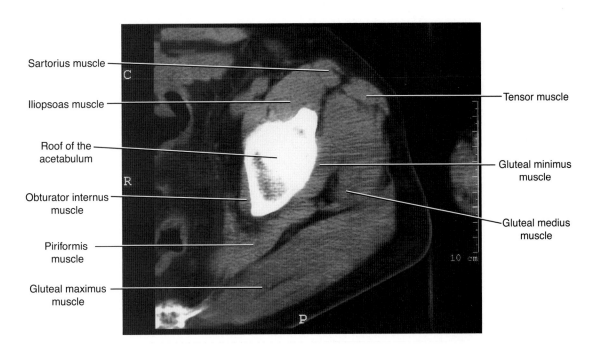

Sartorius muscle

Iliopsoas muscle

Roof of the acetabulum

Obturator internus muscle

Piriformis muscle

Gluteal maximus muscle

Tensor muscle

Gluteal minimus muscle

Gluteal medius muscle

10 cm

Figure 9-12 Figure 9-12 demonstrates the roof of the acetabulum. The iliopsoas and sartorius muscles, in the anterior group of muscles that move the femur, are involved in flexing the thigh at the hip joint. The gluteal muscles, along with the tensor muscle, are part of the lateral group and act as abductors. The obturator internus and pyriformis laterally rotate the femur.

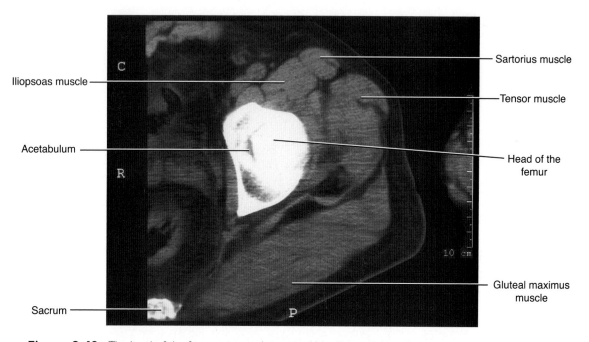

Iliopsoas muscle

Acetabulum

Sacrum

Sartorius muscle

Tensor muscle

Head of the femur

Gluteal maximus muscle

Figure 9-13   The head of the femur can now be seen within the acetabulum on Figure 9-13. The hip joint is a diarthrodial joint, specifically, a ball and socket joint. This type of joint offers the most mobility.

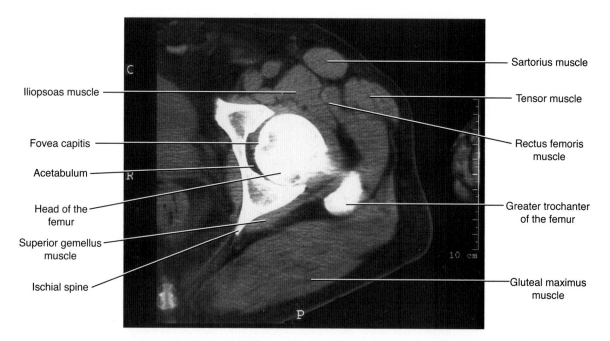

Iliopsoas muscle

Fovea capitis

Acetabulum

Head of the femur

Superior gemellus muscle

Ischial spine

Sartorius muscle

Tensor muscle

Rectus femoris muscle

Greater trochanter of the femur

Gluteal maximus muscle

Figure 9-14   On Figure 9-14, the fovea capitis can be seen. The ligament of the head of the femur passes from the fovea capitis to the acetabular notch, anchoring the femur to the acetabulum. Because the diameter of the rim of the acetabulum is smaller than the diameter of the head of the femur, dislocations of the hip are less common than dislocations of the shoulder joint. The superior gemellus muscle is seen arising from the ischial spine.

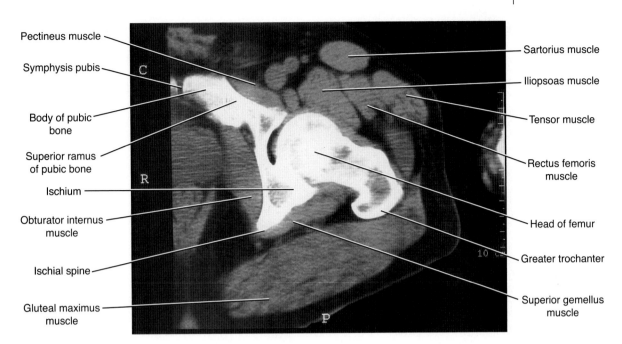

Pectineus muscle

Symphysis pubis

Body of pubic bone

Superior ramus of pubic bone

Ischium

Obturator internus muscle

Ischial spine

Gluteal maximus muscle

Sartorius muscle

Iliopsoas muscle

Tensor muscle

Rectus femoris muscle

Head of femur

Greater trochanter

Superior gemellus muscle

Figure 9-15 On Figure 9-15, the superior ramus of the pubic bone is now apparent. The size of the obturator internus muscle has increased significantly, an indication that the obturator foramen will soon appear.

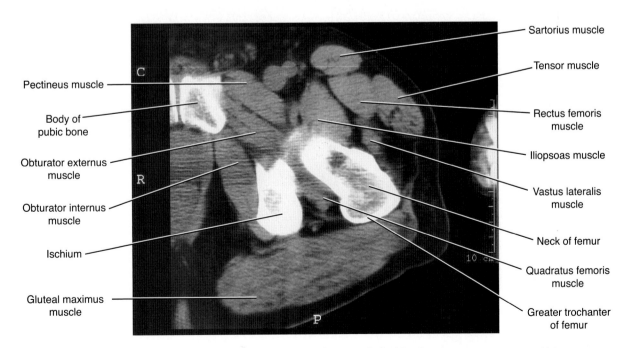

Pectineus muscle

Body of pubic bone

Obturator externus muscle

Obturator internus muscle

Ischium

Gluteal maximus muscle

Sartorius muscle

Tensor muscle

Rectus femoris muscle

Iliopsoas muscle

Vastus lateralis muscle

Neck of femur

Quadratus femoris muscle

Greater trochanter of femur

Figure 9-16 Evident on Figure 9-16 is the obturator foramen, flanked by the obturator externus and internus muscles. The ischium is seen posteriorly and the pubic bone anteriorly. Labeled again are the anterior group of muscles that move the femur, flexing the thigh at the hip joint: the iliopsoas, sartorius, and rectus femoris.

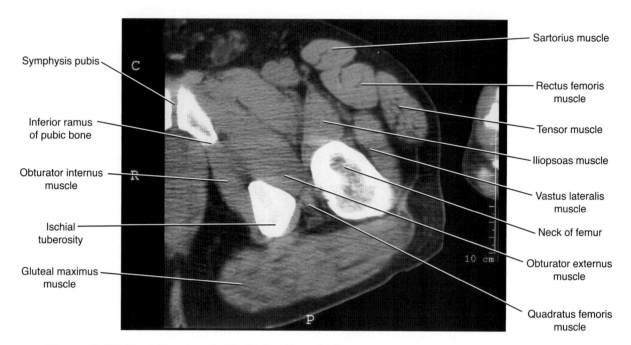

Symphysis pubis

Inferior ramus
of pubic bone

Obturator internus
muscle

Ischial
tuberosity

Gluteal maximus
muscle

Sartorius muscle

Rectus femoris
muscle

Tensor muscle

Iliopsoas muscle

Vastus lateralis
muscle

Neck of femur

Obturator externus
muscle

Quadratus femoris
muscle

Figure 9-17 The ischial tuberosity, identified on Figure 9-17, bears the weight of the body in the sitting position. The vastus lateralis, which appeared on Figure 9-16, is also identified on this figure. It originates on the anterior inferior root of the greater trochanter and superior linea aspera and is one of the four heads of the quadriceps femoris. The quadriceps femoris is involved in moving the lower leg.

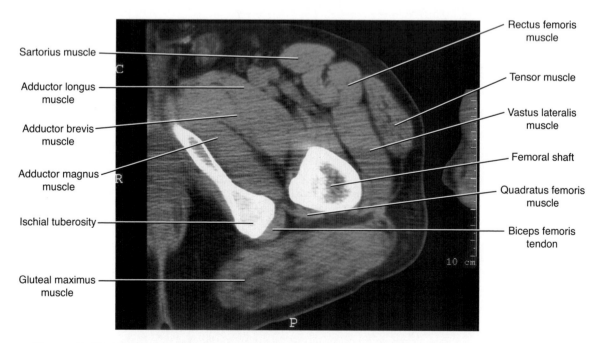

Sartorius muscle

Adductor longus
muscle

Adductor brevis
muscle

Adductor magnus
muscle

Ischial tuberosity

Gluteal maximus
muscle

Rectus femoris
muscle

Tensor muscle

Vastus lateralis
muscle

Femoral shaft

Quadratus femoris
muscle

Biceps femoris
tendon

Figure 9-18 Figure 9-18 is the last image in this series of axial CT images of the hip. Labeled are the adductor brevis and longus muscles. Grouped with the medial muscles that move the femur, along with the pectineus, they adduct the thigh at the hip joint. Also seen is the tendon of the biceps femoris muscle, which originates on the inferior ischial tuberosity. This muscle, along with the other muscles in the posterior group of muscles that move the femur, is responsible for lateral rotation.

MR Images of the Hip

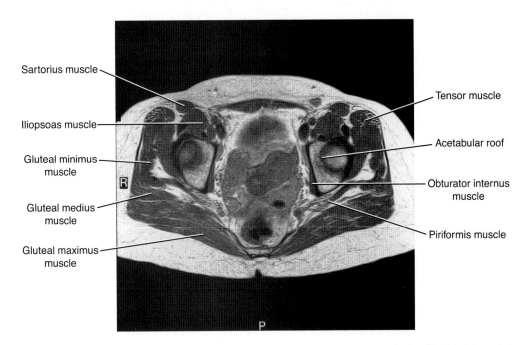

Sartorius muscle

Iliopsoas muscle

Gluteal minimus
muscle

Gluteal medius
muscle

Gluteal maximus
muscle

Tensor muscle

Acetabular roof

Obturator internus
muscle

Piriformis muscle

Figure 9-19 Figure 9-19 is an axial MR image at the level of the roof of the acetabulum. The hip joint, a ball and socket joint, is a type of synovial or diarthrodial joint. All the muscles labeled are involved in moving the femur. The iliopsoas and sartorius muscles flex the thigh at the hip joint. The obturator internus and pyriformis muscles laterally rotate the femur, and the gluteal and tensor muscles act as abductors.

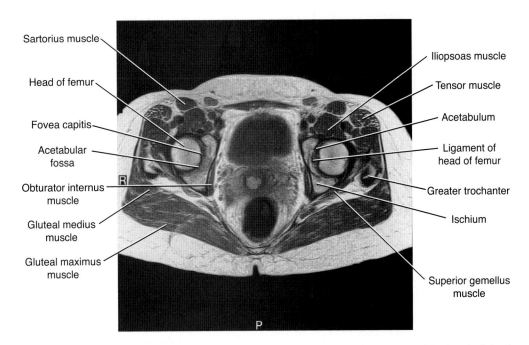

Sartorius muscle

Head of femur

Fovea capitis

Acetabular
fossa

Obturator internus
muscle

Gluteal medius
muscle

Gluteal maximus
muscle

Iliopsoas muscle

Tensor muscle

Acetabulum

Ligament of
head of femur

Greater trochanter

Ischium

Superior gemellus
muscle

Figure 9-20 Figure 9-20 demonstrates structures within the hip joint. The ligament of the head of the femur extends from the fovea capitis. It inserts onto the acetabular notch, located inferiorly on the acetabulum. Also identified is the acetabular fossa, the fossa within the acetabulum containing a fat pad covered with a synovial membrane. There is no articular cartilage in this region of the acetabulum, nor is there articulation with the head of the femur.

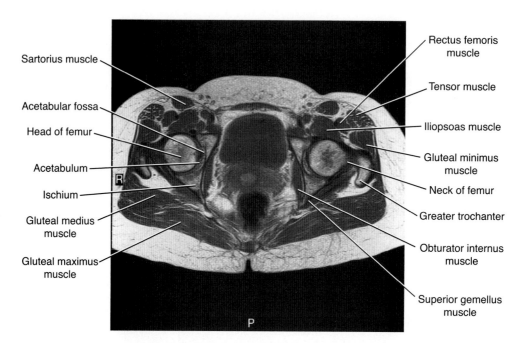

Sartorius muscle

Acetabular fossa

Head of femur

Acetabulum

Ischium

Gluteal medius muscle

Gluteal maximus muscle

Rectus femoris muscle

Tensor muscle

Iliopsoas muscle

Gluteal minimus muscle

Neck of femur

Greater trochanter

Obturator internus muscle

Superior gemellus muscle

Figure 9-21   On Figure 9-21, the greater trochanter of the femur is evident. Between the head of the femur and the greater trochanter is the neck of the femur. By studying the previous images of the hip, the location of the numerous muscles should now present a pattern with respect to their position relative to the hip joint.

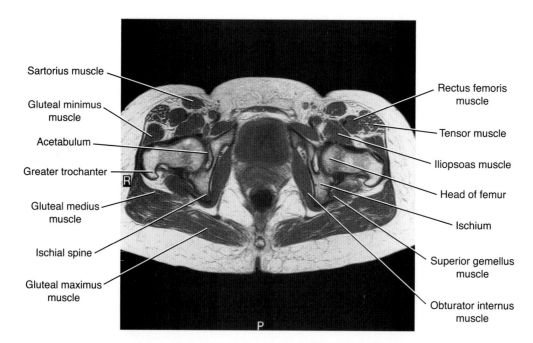

Sartorius muscle

Gluteal minimus muscle

Acetabulum

Greater trochanter

Gluteal medius muscle

Ischial spine

Gluteal maximus muscle

Rectus femoris muscle

Tensor muscle

Iliopsoas muscle

Head of femur

Ischium

Superior gemellus muscle

Obturator internus muscle

Figure 9-22   The last axial MR image of the hip joint (Figure 9-22) is at the lower level of the hip joint. Little of the acetabulum remains to be seen. Identified is the ischial spine, the point of origin for the superior gemellus muscle. The gluteal medius and minimus muscles are still evident but would not be visible at a lower cut as they insert onto the greater trochanter.

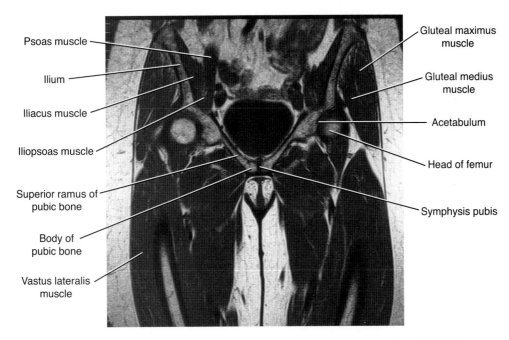

Psoas muscle

Ilium

Iliacus muscle

Iliopsoas muscle

Superior ramus of pubic bone

Body of pubic bone

Vastus lateralis muscle

Gluteal maximus muscle

Gluteal medius muscle

Acetabulum

Head of femur

Symphysis pubis

Figure 9-23 The next three MR images of the hip are from a coronal perspective. Figure 9-23 is the most anterior, demonstrating the body of the pubic bone, involved in forming the symphysis pubis, and the superior ramus of the pubic bone, forming the anterior inferior one-fifth of the acetabulum. The head of the femur is seen within the acetabulum. Superior to the lateral hip joints are the gluteal muscles; medial to the ilia are the iliopsoas muscles.

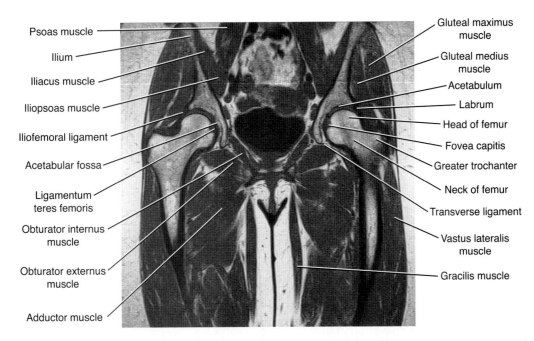

Psoas muscle

Ilium

Iliacus muscle

Iliopsoas muscle

Iliofemoral ligament

Acetabular fossa

Ligamentum teres femoris

Obturator internus muscle

Obturator externus muscle

Adductor muscle

Gluteal maximus muscle

Gluteal medius muscle

Acetabulum

Labrum

Head of femur

Fovea capitis

Greater trochanter

Neck of femur

Transverse ligament

Vastus lateralis muscle

Gracilis muscle

Figure 9-24 Figure 9-24 is on the same plane as the hip joint. On this image, the formation of the iliopsoas muscles by the bilateral psoas and iliacus muscles is visible. The head of the femur is seen within the acetabulum. Identified is the fovea capitis in which the ligamentum teres femoris is anchored. Muscles medial to the proximal femur include the obturator, adductor, and gracilis; the vastus lateralis is seen laterally. The vastus lateralis is one of the four heads of the quadriceps femoris muscle.

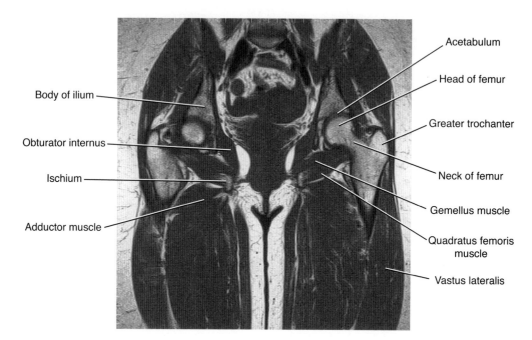

Body of ilium

Obturator internus

Ischium

Adductor muscle

Acetabulum

Head of femur

Greater trochanter

Neck of femur

Gemellus muscle

Quadratus femoris muscle

Vastus lateralis

Figure 9-25 Figure 9-25 is the most posterior cut in this series of coronal MR images. The head, neck, and greater trochanter of the femur are seen, along with the acetabulum and the ilium. The body of the ilium forms the superior two-fifths of the acetabulum, while the body of the ischium forms the remaining two-fifths, posteriorly and inferiorly.

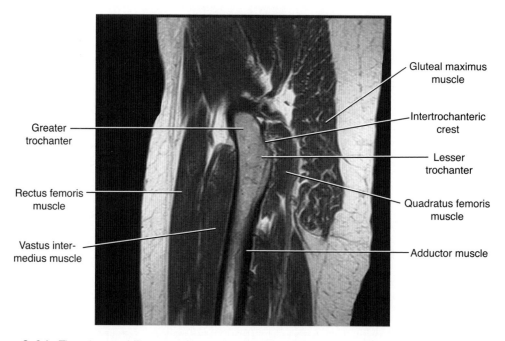

Greater trochanter

Rectus femoris muscle

Vastus inter-medius muscle

Gluteal maximus muscle

Intertrochanteric crest

Lesser trochanter

Quadratus femoris muscle

Adductor muscle

Figure 9-26 These last two MR images of the hip are from a sagittal perspective. Figure 9-26 is more lateral. Iden-tified are the greater and lesser trochanters on the proximal femur, connected by the intertrochanteric crest. The rec-tus femoris and vastus intermedius muscles are located anteriorly, while the quadratus femoris and gluteal muscles are posterior.

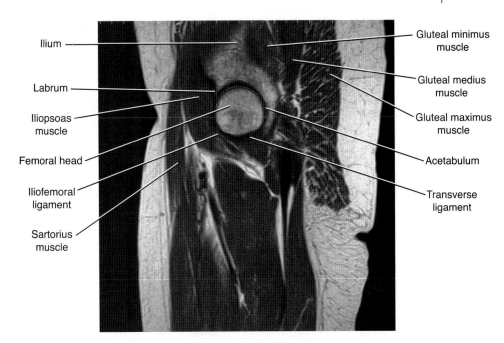

Ilium

Labrum

Iliopsoas
muscle

Femoral head

Iliofemoral
ligament

Sartorius
muscle

Gluteal minimus
muscle

Gluteal medius
muscle

Gluteal maximus
muscle

Acetabulum

Transverse
ligament

Figure 9-27 Figure 9-27 is on the same plane as the hip joint, with the head of the femur within the acetabulum. Anterior to the ilium and hip is the iliopsoas muscle. The iliofemoral ligament, extending from the anterior inferior iliac spine of the ilium to the intertrochanteric line of the femur, is seen. The iliofemoral ligament is one of the strongest ligaments of the hip.

KNEE JOINT

The **knee** or **tibiofemoral joint** is a diarthrodial joint because a synovial membrane encloses it, although its complexity is atypical. It is the largest synovial joint in the body. Within the synovial cavity, three separate joints exist: the articulation between the patella and femoral patellar surface located distally and anteriorly on the femur; the articulation between the lateral femoral and tibial condyles; and the articulation between the medial femoral and tibial condyles. The three articulations can best be classified as condyloid joints, although the movement between the femur and tibia is a modified hinge joint. The articulating surfaces of the bones involved are covered with articulating cartilage.

Although a traditional articular capsule does not encase the joint, it is enclosed by a number of ligaments and extended expansions of tendons. The capsular ligament serves to fill in gaps.

Ligaments

The ligaments involved in the knee joint can be categorized as either external or intracapsular. The external liga-

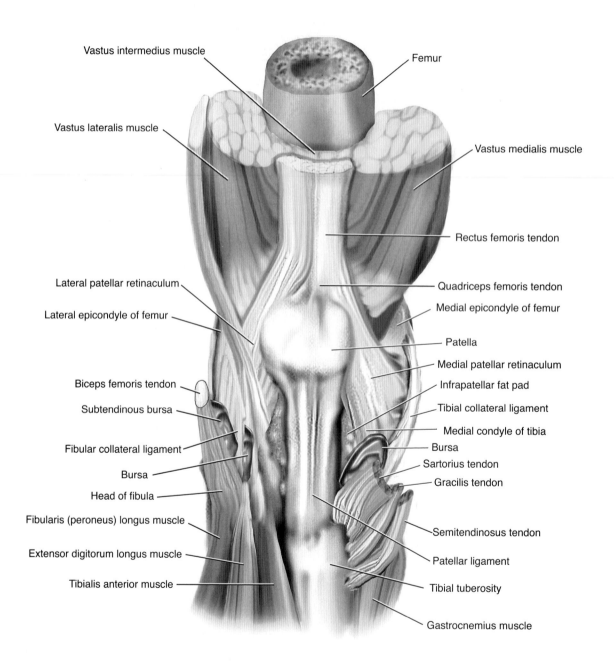

A.

Figure 9-28 Ligaments of the knee (A) anterior view *(continues)*

ments, most of which are identified on Figure 9-28 A and B, are the patellar, tibial or medial collateral, fibular or lateral collateral, capsular, medial and lateral patellar retinacula, arcuate popliteal, and oblique popliteal or posterior. The patellar ligament begins as the quadriceps femoris muscular tendon insertion and extends from the patella to the tibial tuberosity. The tibial or medial collateral ligament passes from the medial femoral condyle to the tibial condyle and proximal medial tibial shaft. The fibular collateral ligament connects the lateral condyle of the femur to the lateral aspect of the head of the fibula. A thin membrane, the capsular ligament, fills the spaces between the patellar

ligament and the collateral ligaments. In the same area are the medial and lateral patellar retinacula ligaments, the fusion of the tendons of the quadriceps femoris muscle with the deep fascia of the thigh, medial and lateral to the patella. The arcuate popliteal ligament is an extension of the capsule in the intercondylar and lateral femoral condylar region, arching over the popliteal muscle in a postero-lateral direction and attaching to the styloid process of the fibula. The oblique popliteal (posterior) ligament extends from the intercondylar fossa to the head of the tibia.

The intracapsular ligaments are the anterior and posterior cruciate and the transverse, all shown on Figure 9-29.

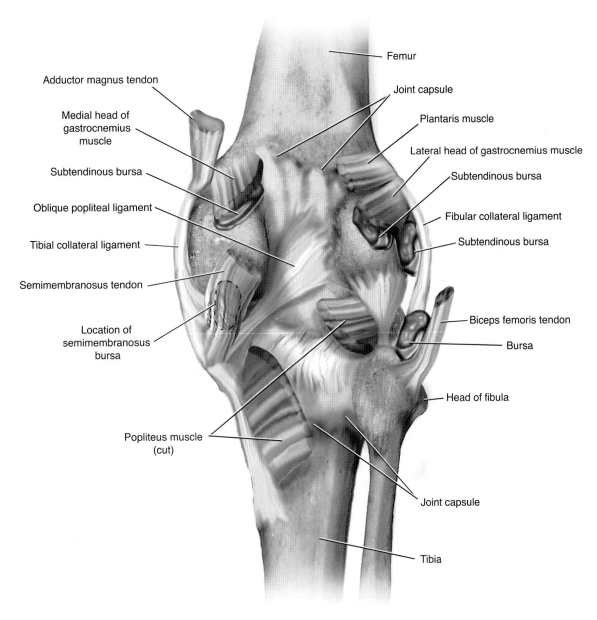

B.

Figure 9-28 (continued) (B) posterior view

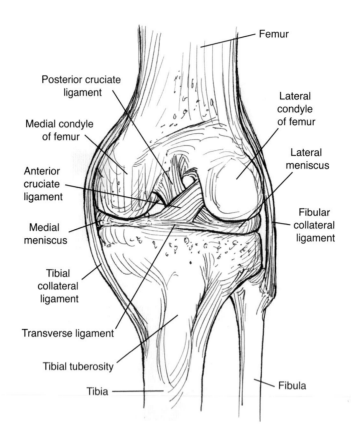

Figure 9-29 Ligaments of the knee, intracapsular, anterior view

The anterior cruciate ligament (ACL) extends from the medial aspect of the femoral lateral condyle to a point anterior to the tibial intercondylar eminence, while the posterior cruciate ligament (PCL) extends from the lateral aspect of the medial femoral condyle to the intercondylar area of the posterior proximal tibia. The transverse ligament connects the lateral and medial menisci anteriorly.

Bursae

There are as many as ten bursae in the knee preventing friction between the numerous ligaments, tendons, bone, and skin. Anteriorly, as labeled on Figure 9-30, they include the suprapatellar, subcutaneous prepatellar, and subcutaneous and deep (subtendinous) infrapatellar. The suprapatellar is an extension of the knee joint found between the anterior distal femur and the undersurface of the quadriceps femoris tendon. The subcutaneous prepatellar separates the patella and skin. Situated between the patellar ligament and skin is the subcutaneous infrapatellar bursa; the deep or subtendinous infrapatellar bursa lies under the undersurface of the patellar ligament and anterior to the proximal tibia.

Fat Pad

Underneath the patellar ligament but external to the synovial membrane is the infrapatellar fat pad, also identified on Figure 9-30.

Menisci

The medial and lateral **menisci** are crescent-shaped pads of fibrocartilage between the femoral condyles and tibial plateaus. The bilateral menisci are connected anteriorly by the transverse ligament (see Figure 9-29).

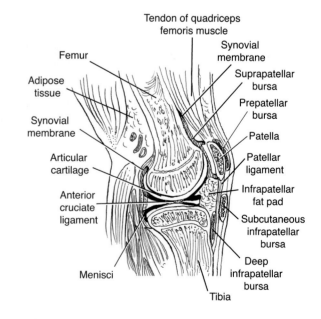

Figure 9-30 Knee joint, sagittal perspective

CT Images of the Knee

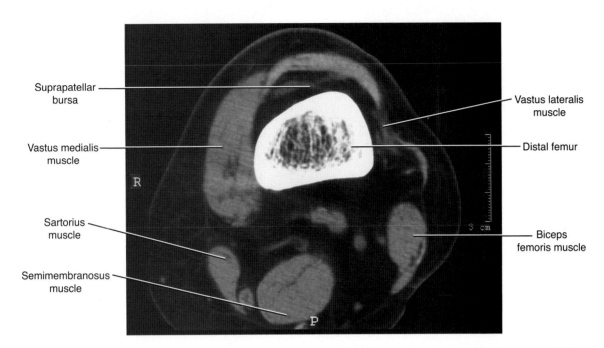

Suprapatellar bursa

Vastus medialis muscle

Sartorius muscle

Semimembranosus muscle

Vastus lateralis muscle

Distal femur

Biceps femoris muscle

R

P

Figure 9-31 The first image (Figure 9-31) is proximal to the knee joint, at the level of the distal femoral shaft. The suprapatellar bursa lies beneath the quadriceps femoris tendon. Labeled are two of the heads of the quadriceps femoris muscle, the vastus lateralis and vastus medialis. The muscles flexing the leg at the knee joint are seen posteriorly: the sartorius, semimembranosus, and biceps femoris. The semimembranosus and biceps femoris are two of the three muscles categorized as hamstring muscles.

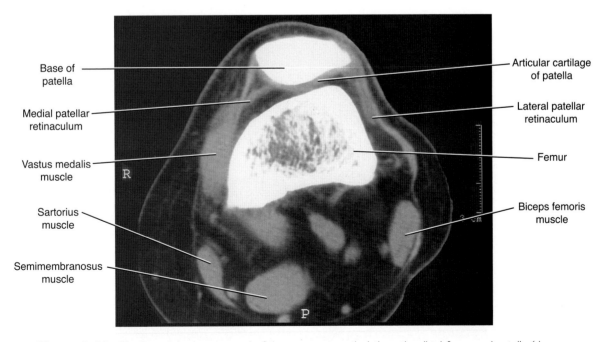

Base of patella

Medial patellar retinaculum

Vastus medalis muscle

Sartorius muscle

Semimembranosus muscle

Articular cartilage of patella

Lateral patellar retinaculum

Femur

Biceps femoris muscle

R

P

Figure 9-32 The knee joint is composed of three separate articulations: the distal femur and patella (demonstrated on Figure 9-32), and the articulations between the distal femur and lateral and medial tibial condyles. Articular cartilage covers the articulating surfaces of the bones. On either side of the patella are the lateral and medial patellar retinacula ligaments, fusions of the quadriceps femoris tendons with the deep fascia of the thigh, bilaterally.

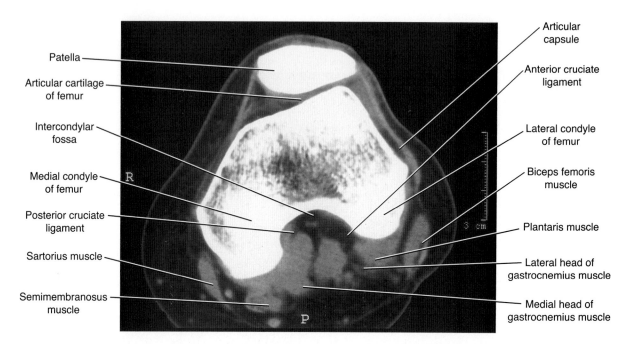

Patella

Articular cartilage of femur

Intercondylar fossa

Medial condyle of femur

Posterior cruciate ligament

Sartorius muscle

Semimembranosus muscle

Articular capsule

Anterior cruciate ligament

Lateral condyle of femur

Biceps femoris muscle

Plantaris muscle

Lateral head of gastrocnemius muscle

Medial head of gastrocnemius muscle

Figure 9-33 Evident on Figure 9-33 are the lateral and medial femoral condyles along with the intercondylar fossa, located posteriorly on the distal femur. New on this image are the lateral and medial heads of the gastrocnemius muscle, a muscle found in the posterior compartment and involved in moving the foot. Also noted are the anterior and posterior cruciate ligaments, intracapsular ligaments.

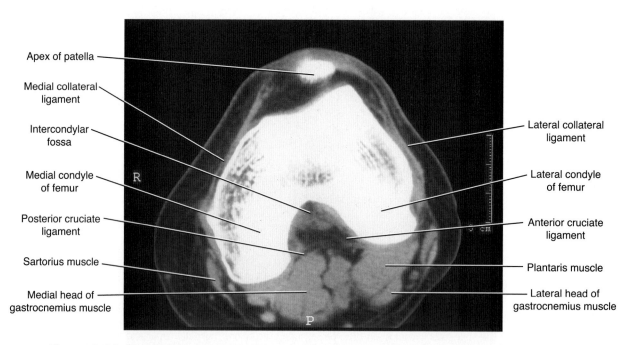

Apex of patella

Medial collateral ligament

Intercondylar fossa

Medial condyle of femur

Posterior cruciate ligament

Sartorius muscle

Medial head of gastrocnemius muscle

Lateral collateral ligament

Lateral condyle of femur

Anterior cruciate ligament

Plantaris muscle

Lateral head of gastrocnemius muscle

Figure 9-34 Figure 9-34 is at the level of the apex of the patella, the lateral and medial femoral condyles, and the intercondylar fossa. The intracapsular anterior and posterior cruciate ligaments are identified. Note the lateral and medial collateral ligaments, joining the lateral and medial femoral condyles with the proximal fibula and tibia, respectively.

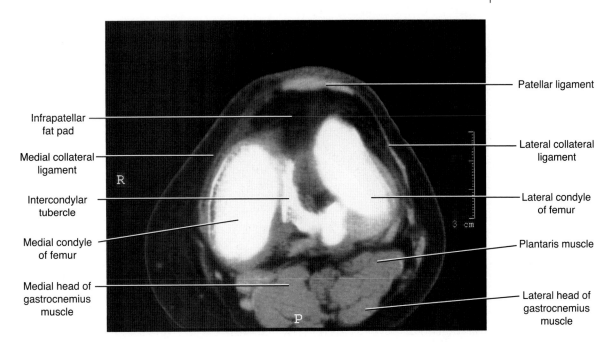

Patellar ligament

Infrapatellar
fat pad

Medial collateral
ligament

Lateral collateral
ligament

Intercondylar
tubercle

Lateral condyle
of femur

Medial condyle
of femur

Plantaris muscle

Medial head of
gastrocnemius
muscle

Lateral head of
gastrocnemius
muscle

Figure 9-35   Figure 9-35 is at the level of the joint between the distal femur and proximal tibia. The intercondylar tubercles of the tibia are identified. The patellar ligament, a continuation of the quadriceps femoris tendon, extending from the patella to the tibial tuberosity, is visible.

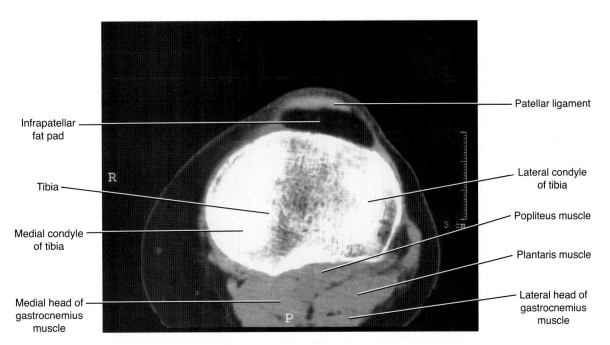

Patellar ligament

Infrapatellar
fat pad

Tibia

Lateral condyle
of tibia

Popliteus muscle

Medial condyle
of tibia

Plantaris muscle

Medial head of
gastrocnemius
muscle

Lateral head of
gastrocnemius
muscle

Figure 9-36   Figure 9-36 is an axial image of the lateral and medial condyles of the proximal tibia. The popliteus muscle is found posteriorly, a muscle originating on the lateral femoral condyle and inserting on the proximal posteromedial tibia. The lateral and medial heads of the gastrocnemius muscle are again labeled. The gastrocnemius and soleus muscles form a single tendon, the Achilles, which inserts onto the calcaneus.

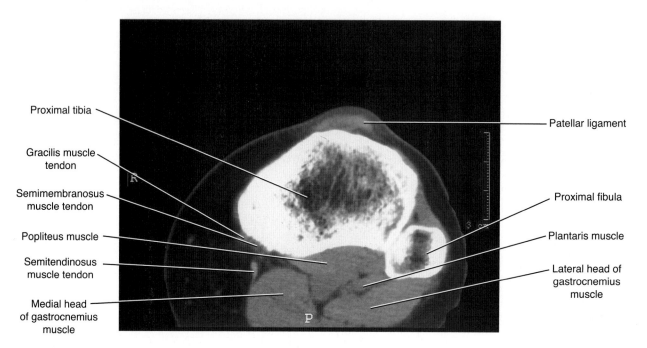

Proximal tibia

Gracilis muscle tendon

Semimembranosus muscle tendon

Popliteus muscle

Semitendinosus muscle tendon

Medial head of gastrocnemius muscle

Patellar ligament

Proximal fibula

Plantaris muscle

Lateral head of gastrocnemius muscle

Figure 9-37   The last image in this series (Figure 9-37) is distal to the knee joint, demonstrating the articulation between the proximal tibia and fibula. Along the medial border are the tendons of three muscles flexing the leg at the knee joint: the gracilis, semimembranosus, and semitendinosus.

MR Images of the Knee

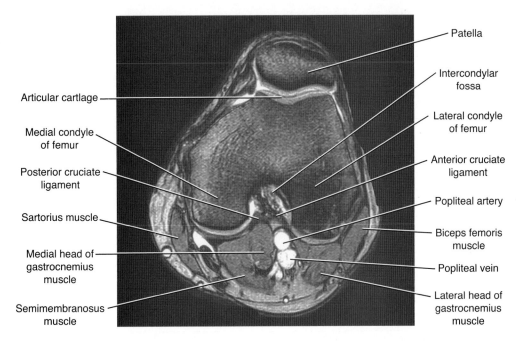

Patella

Intercondylar fossa

Articular cartilage

Lateral condyle of femur

Medial condyle of femur

Anterior cruciate ligament

Posterior cruciate ligament

Popliteal artery

Sartorius muscle

Biceps femoris muscle

Medial head of gastrocnemius muscle

Popliteal vein

Semimembranosus muscle

Lateral head of gastrocnemius muscle

Figure 9-38 Figure 9-38 is an axial image of the knee demonstrating the articulation of the distal femur and patella. Notice the articular cartilage on the surfaces of the posterior patella and anterior femur. The intracapsular ligaments are posterior to the intercondylar fossa. Muscles involved in flexing the leg at the knee joint are identified: the biceps femoris, sartorius, and semimembranosus. The biceps femoris and semimembranosus are muscles categorized as hamstring muscles. The gastrocnemius muscle moves the foot.

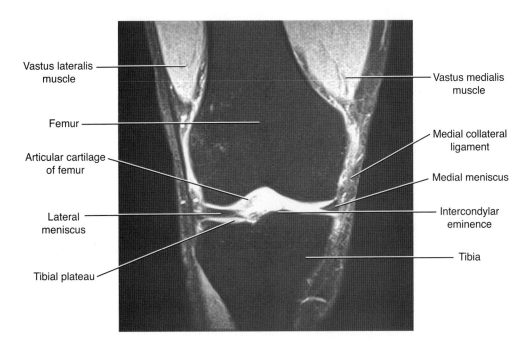

Vastus lateralis muscle

Vastus medialis muscle

Femur

Medial collateral ligament

Articular cartilage of femur

Medial meniscus

Lateral meniscus

Intercondylar eminence

Tibia

Tibial plateau

Figure 9-39 The next image (Figure 9-39) is one of two coronal MR images of the knee. It is a cut of the anterior knee joint that demonstrates the articulation of the distal femur and proximal tibia. The articular cartilage on the articulating surface is labeled. Note the lateral and medial menisci, pads of fibrocartilage between the femoral condyles and tibial plateaus. The medial or tibial collateral ligament can be identified.

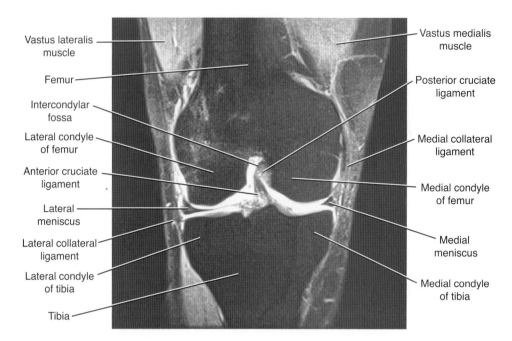

Vastus lateralis muscle
Femur
Intercondylar fossa
Lateral condyle of femur
Anterior cruciate ligament
Lateral meniscus
Lateral collateral ligament
Lateral condyle of tibia
Tibia

Vastus medialis muscle
Posterior cruciate ligament
Medial collateral ligament
Medial condyle of femur
Medial meniscus
Medial condyle of tibia

Figure 9-40 Figure 9-40 allows visualization of the intracapsular ligaments, the anterior and posterior cruciate ligaments. The vastus lateralis and medialis muscles are on either side of the distal femur. Along with the vastus intermedius and rectus femoris they form the quadriceps femoris muscle, having a single tendinous point of insertion on the patella. That tendon continues as the patellar ligament, inserting on the tibial tuberosity.

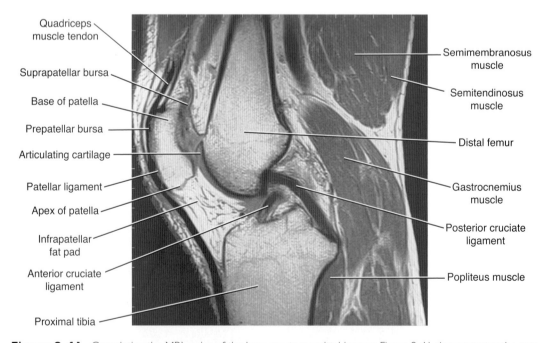

Quadriceps muscle tendon
Suprapatellar bursa
Base of patella
Prepatellar bursa
Articulating cartilage
Patellar ligament
Apex of patella
Infrapatellar fat pad
Anterior cruciate ligament
Proximal tibia

Semimembranosus muscle
Semitendinosus muscle
Distal femur
Gastrocnemius muscle
Posterior cruciate ligament
Popliteus muscle

Figure 9-41 Completing the MRI series of the knee are two sagittal images. Figure 9-41 demonstrates the anterior and posterior cruciate ligaments, intracapsular ligaments. Visible is the articular cartilage on the posterior surface of the patella and anterior surface of the distal femur. The suprapatellar bursa is superior to the patella, the subcutaneous prepatellar bursa is anterior to the patella, and the infrapatellar fat pad is inferior to the apex of the patella.

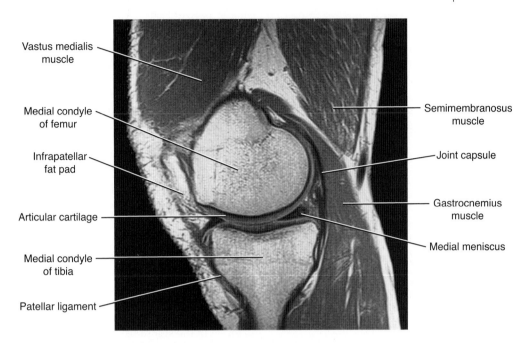

Vastus medialis
muscle

Medial condyle
of femur

Infrapatellar
fat pad

Articular cartilage

Medial condyle
of tibia

Patellar ligament

Semimembranosus
muscle

Joint capsule

Gastrocnemius
muscle

Medial meniscus

Figure 9-42 Figure 9-42 is a more medial sagittal cut of the knee joint demonstrating the medial femoral and tibial condyles and the medial meniscus. The patellar ligament is anterior to the tibia; the joint capsule is apparent posteriorly. Note the medial head of the gastrocnemius muscle. The gastrocnemius muscle and soleus muscle form a single tendinous point of insertion on the calcaneus.

ANKLE JOINT

The ankle joint is formed by the lateral and medial malleoli of the distal fibula and tibia, respectively, and the talus. It is a synovial or diarthrodial joint, specifically a hinge joint. Surfaces of the bones involved are covered with articulating cartilage. A separate fibrous capsule encloses the subtalar joint, also a synovial joint, but a gliding or planar joint.

The muscles that move the foot and ankle, drawn on Figures 9-7 and 9-8 A and B, have as points of attachment tendons that can be classified according to location in the ankle region: anterior, posterior, medial, and lateral groups. Anteriorly the tendons are the extensor digitorum longus, extensor hallucis longus, and tibialis anterior.

Posteriorly, the attaching tendons are the Achilles, the thickest and strongest in the human body, and the plantaris, which attaches to the calcaneus alongside the medial aspect of the Achilles.

The lateral group has in it the fibularis or peroneus brevis and longus.

The medial group includes most of the tendons of the deep posterior muscles: the flexor digitorum longus, flexor hallucis longus, and tibialis posterior.

Ligaments

Numerous ligaments bind the ankle. Their groupings consist of a medial, lateral, and interosseous. Figure 9-43 shows the lateral ligaments, which include the anterior talofibular and tibiofibular, calcaneofibular, and posterior talofibular and tibiofibular. The point of origination for each is the lateral malleolus of the fibula; the point of attachment is identified in the first part of each term.

The medial group includes the strongest ligament in the ankle, the deltoid, and the spring ligament, both identified on Figure 9-44. The deltoid originates from the medial malleolus of the tibia and forms three separate branches of fibers: the tibiocalcaneal, tibionavicular, and tibiotalar ligaments. The tibiotalar ligament subsequently splits into an anterior and posterior branch. The latter part of each term identifies the point of attachment. The spring (plantar) ligament passes from the sustentaculum tali to the posterior navicular bone.

The remaining interosseous or talocalcaneal ligament is found in the sinus tarsi and connects the talus and calcaneus (see Figures 9-43 and 9-44).

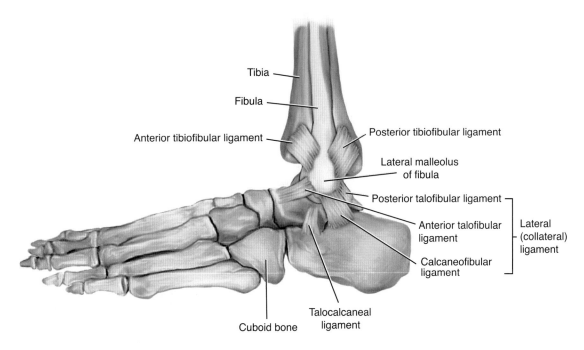

Figure 9-43 Ligaments of the ankle, lateral view

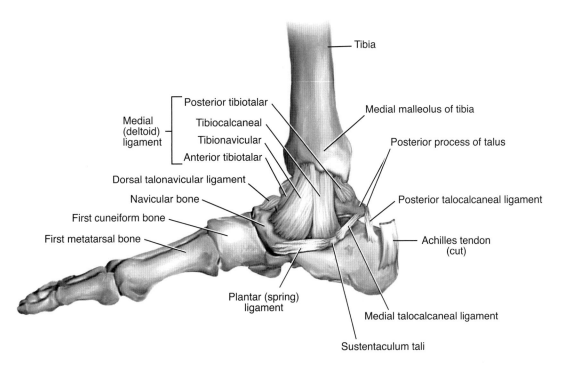

Figure 9-44 Ligaments of the ankle, medial view

Retinacula

Also involved in stabilizing the ankle joint are several retinacula (bands holding an organ in place) external to all the tendons except the Achilles. They are the superior and inferior extensor retinacula, both located anteriorly, the superior and inferior peroneal retinacula, located laterally, and the flexor, located medially (refer to Figure 9-45 A and B).

Bursae

Associated with the ankle joint are four bursae: the subcutaneous over the medial and lateral malleoli of the tibia and fibula, and the subcutaneous and subtendinous, external and internal to the Achilles tendon. They are seen on Figure 9-45 A and B.

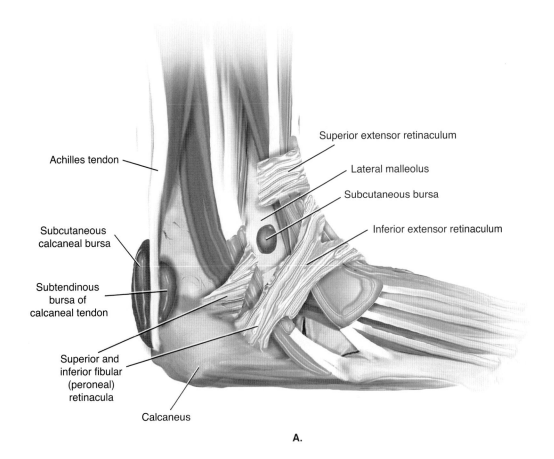

Achilles tendon

Superior extensor retinaculum

Lateral malleolus

Subcutaneous bursa

Inferior extensor retinaculum

Subcutaneous
calcaneal bursa

Subtendinous
bursa of
calcaneal tendon

Superior and
inferior fibular
(peroneal)
retinacula

Calcaneus

A.

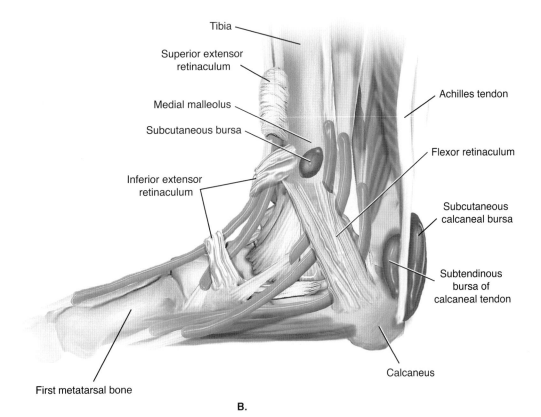

Tibia

Superior extensor
retinaculum

Medial malleolus

Subcutaneous bursa

Inferior extensor
retinaculum

Achilles tendon

Flexor retinaculum

Subcutaneous
calcaneal bursa

Subtendinous
bursa of
calcaneal tendon

First metatarsal bone

Calcaneus

B.

Figure 9-45 Ankle joint retinacula, (A) lateral view (B) medial view

CT Images of the Ankle

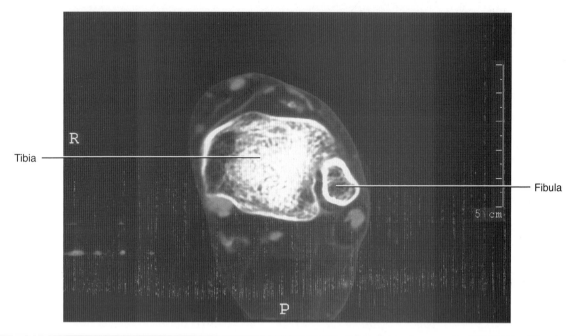

Tibia

Fibula

Figure 9-46   This first CT axial image of the ankle (Figure 9-46) is just above the ankle or mortise joint, and demonstrates the distal tibia and fibula. Visible are muscles that move the foot from each of the three compartments: anterior, posterior, and lateral or peroneal.

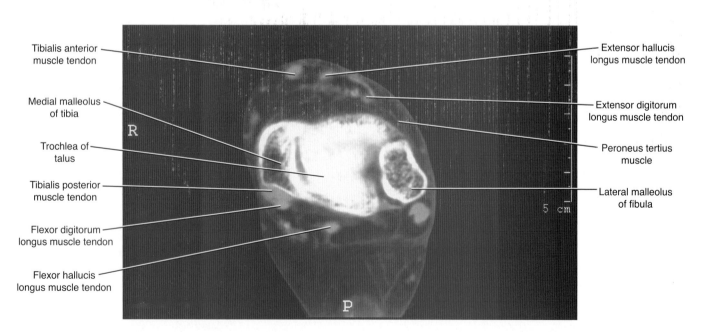

Tibialis anterior muscle tendon

Medial malleolus of tibia

Trochlea of talus

Tibialis posterior muscle tendon

Flexor digitorum longus muscle tendon

Flexor hallucis longus muscle tendon

Extensor hallucis longus muscle tendon

Extensor digitorum longus muscle tendon

Peroneus tertius muscle

Lateral malleolus of fibula

Figure 9-47   Figure 9-47 is an image of the ankle or mortise joint, involving the articulation of the lateral malleolus of the fibula, the trochlea of the talus, and the medial malleolus of the tibia. Muscles identified from the anterior compartment are the extensor hallucis longus and tibialis anterior, while the deeper muscles of the posterior compartment visible include the flexor digitorum longus and tibialis posterior.

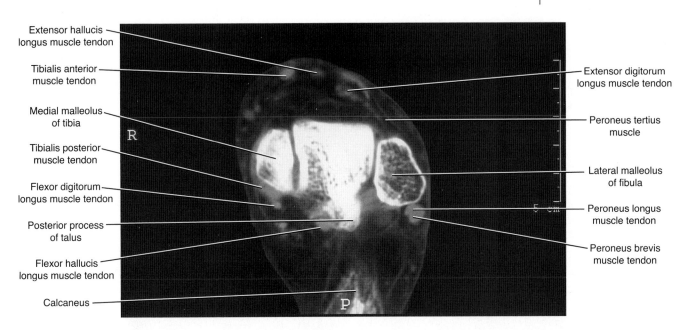

Extensor hallucis longus muscle tendon

Tibialis anterior muscle tendon

Medial malleolus of tibia

Tibialis posterior muscle tendon

Flexor digitorum longus muscle tendon

Posterior process of talus

Flexor hallucis longus muscle tendon

Calcaneus

Extensor digitorum longus muscle tendon

Peroneus tertius muscle

Lateral malleolus of fibula

Peroneus longus muscle tendon

Peroneus brevis muscle tendon

Figure 9-48 Starting to appear on Figure 9-48 is the calcaneus, found posteriorly. Notice the peroneus brevis and longus muscles. They are listed with the muscles in the lateral or peroneal compartment

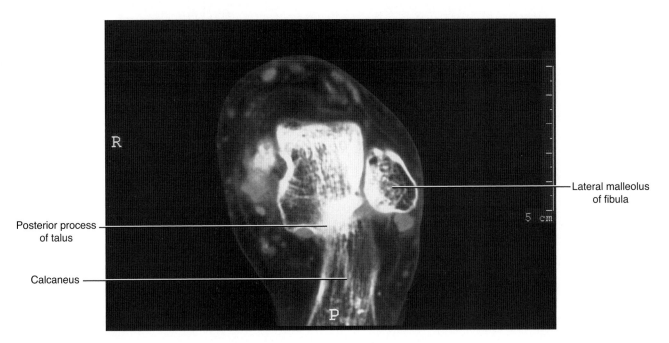

Posterior process of talus

Calcaneus

Lateral malleolus of fibula

Figure 9-49 As more of the calcaneus becomes visible the posterior process of the talus can be identified. Between the previous figure and Figure 9-49, the medial malleolus of the tibia has almost disappeared. The lateral malleolus extends more inferiorly than the medial malleolus.

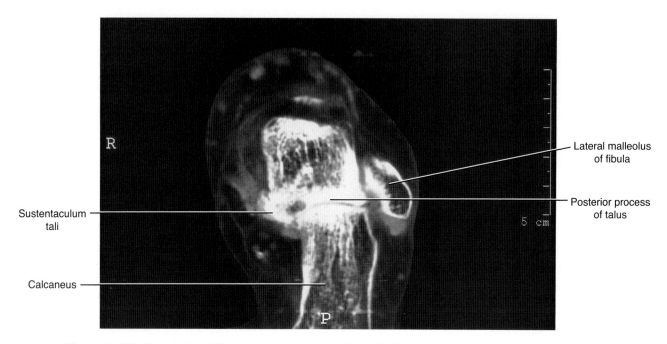

Lateral malleolus
of fibula

Posterior process
of talus

Sustentaculum
tali

Calcaneus

Figure 9-50   There is little difference between this image (Figure 9-50) and the previous but a glimpse of the sustentaculum tali is now visible on the medial calcaneus. The sustentaculum tali is the shelf of bone extending medially from the calcaneus and supporting the middle talar articulating surface.

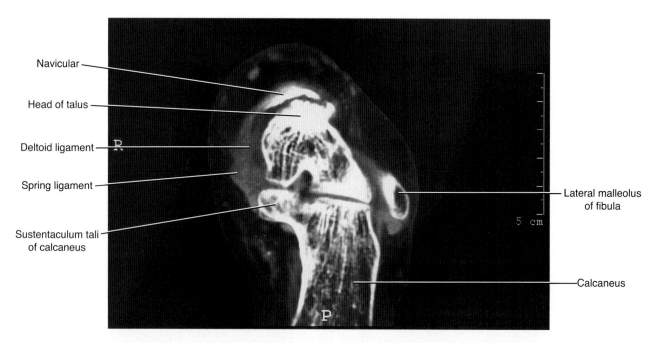

Navicular

Head of talus

Deltoid ligament

Spring ligament

Sustentaculum tali
of calcaneus

Lateral malleolus
of fibula

Calcaneus

Figure 9-51   Numerous structures have appeared as this series of CT images of the ankle continues. On Figure 9-51, along the medial border the sustentaculum tali of the calcaneus is labeled. Anterior to the head of the talus the navicular bone, one of the 7 tarsal bones, is starting to emerge. The deltoid ligament, the strongest ligament in the ankle joint, can be easily identified. Also labeled is the spring ligament, which extends from the sustentaculum tali to the posterior navicular bone.

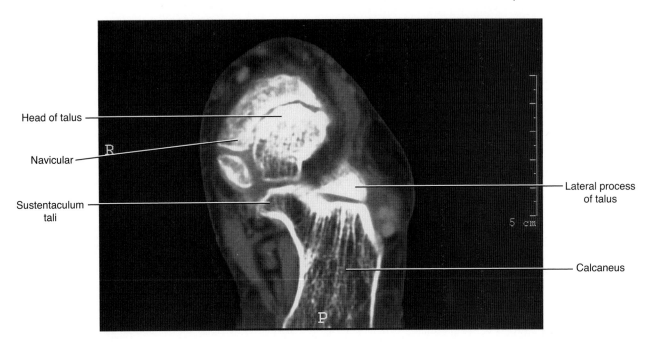

Head of talus

Navicular

Sustentaculum tali

Lateral process of talus

Calcaneus

Figure 9-52 Having moved distal to the lateral malleolus of the fibula, the lateral process of the talus is seen on Figure 9-52. The head of the talus is posterior to the navicular bone.

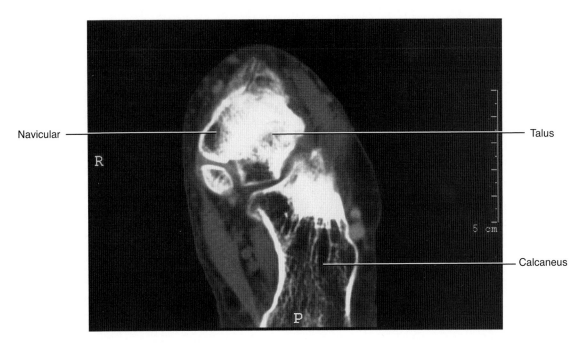

Navicular

Talus

Calcaneus

Figure 9-53 Notice the order of the tarsal bones on Figure 9-53. The navicular is anterior to the talus. The calcaneus is the most posterior tarsal bone.

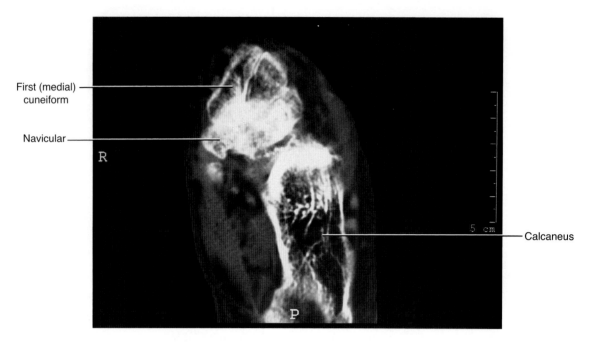

Figure 9-54 As the cuts descend, the talus disappears. On Figure 9-54, still evident are the navicular and calcaneus. New to this image is the first cuneiform.

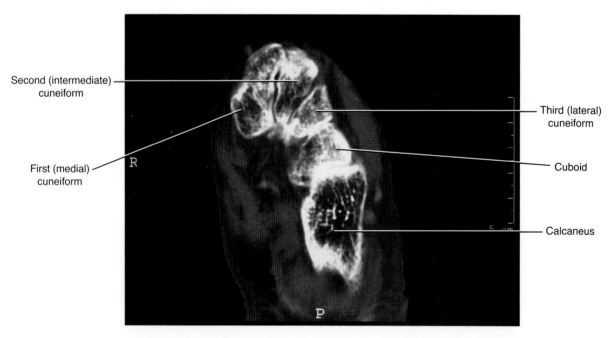

Figure 9-55 Figure 9-55 allows visualization of the first, second, and third cuneiforms, cuboid, and calcaneus. The cuneiforms are numbered starting on the medial aspect of the foot.

MR Images of the Ankle

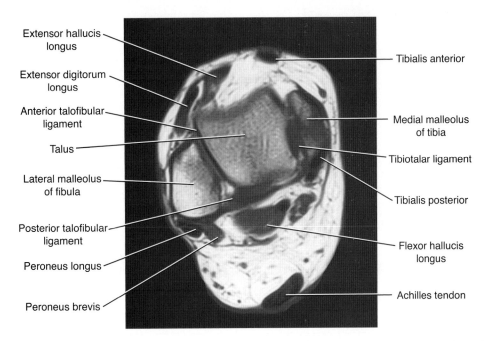

Extensor hallucis longus
Extensor digitorum longus
Anterior talofibular ligament
Talus
Lateral malleolus of fibula
Posterior talofibular ligament
Peroneus longus
Peroneus brevis

Tibialis anterior
Medial malleolus of tibia
Tibiotalar ligament
Tibialis posterior
Flexor hallucis longus
Achilles tendon

Figure 9-56 This axial MR image (Figure 9-56) is at the level of the ankle joint, and demonstrates the articulation of the lateral and medial malleoli of the fibula and tibia with the talus. The flexor muscles of the foot and ankle are found posteriorly and the extensor tendons are anterior. The Achilles tendon is identified, a shared tendon for the gastrocnemius and soleus muscle, inserting on the calcaneus.

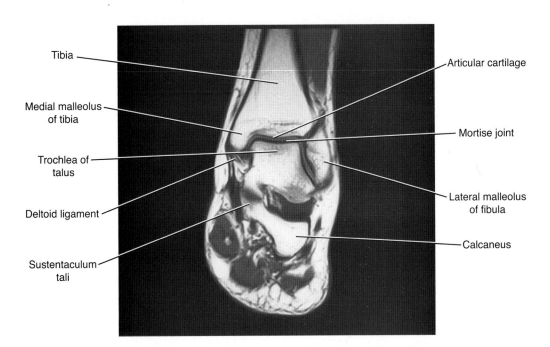

Tibia
Medial malleolus of tibia
Trochlea of talus
Deltoid ligament
Sustentaculum tali

Articular cartilage
Mortise joint
Lateral malleolus of fibula
Calcaneus

Figure 9-57 Figure 9-57 is a coronal MR image of the ankle or mortise joint that demonstrates the articulating cartilage on the surface of the bones involved. Along the medial aspect, notice the deltoid ligament, the strongest ligament of the ankle. It has three branches: the tibiocalcaneal, tibionavicular, and tibiotalar.

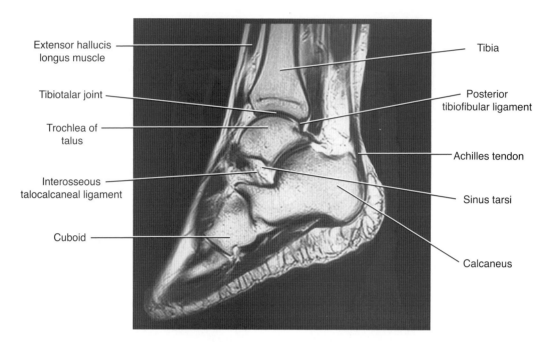

Extensor hallucis longus muscle
Tibiotalar joint
Trochlea of talus
Interosseous talocalcaneal ligament
Cuboid

Tibia
Posterior tibiofibular ligament
Achilles tendon
Sinus tarsi
Calcaneus

Figure 9-58   The remaining two MR images of the ankle are from a sagittal perspective. Figure 9-58 is more lateral, evident by the appearance of the cuboid bone, anterior to the calcaneus. Ligaments identified are the interosseous talocalcaneal, found within the sinus tarsi, and the posterior tibiofibular. Again the Achilles tendon is visible. It is the thickest and strongest tendon in the human body.

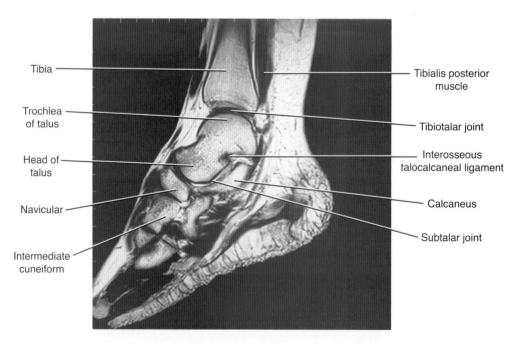

Tibia
Trochlea of talus
Head of talus
Navicular
Intermediate cuneiform

Tibialis posterior muscle
Tibiotalar joint
Interosseous talocalcaneal ligament
Calcaneus
Subtalar joint

Figure 9-59   Figure 9-59 is a sagittal MR image of the medial ankle. The inferior surface of the tibia is articulating with the trochlea of the talus, while the head of the talus is articulating with the navicular. Also visible is the subtalar joint, the joint involving the calcaneus and talus. Both the ankle joint and subtalar joint are synovial joints, but the ankle joint is a hinge joint and the subtalar joint is a gliding joint.

REVIEW QUESTIONS

1. Identify the four heads of the quadriceps femoris muscle.

    _____

    _____

    _____

    _____

2. Which of the following is *not* considered a hamstring muscle?
    a. Semimembranosus
    b. Biceps femoris
    c. Semitendinosus
    d. Rectus femoris
    e. a, b, c, and d are all considered hamstring muscles.

Match the following ligaments or muscle tendons with the correct associated sectional image.

____ 3. Patellar ligament

____ 4. Quadriceps femoris muscle tendon

____ 5. Anterior/posterior cruciate ligaments

____ 6. Ligamentum teres femoris

____ 7. Achilles tendon

    a. Hip joint
    b. Knee joint
    c. Ankle joint

8. With which joint is the zona orbicularis associated?
    a. Hip
    b. Knee
    c. Ankle
    d. a, b, and c
    e. None of the above.

9. The anterior inferior one-fifth of the acetabulum is formed by the
    a. ilium.
    b. ischium.
    c. pubic bone.
    d. None of the above.

10. On sectional images, which ligament is seen connecting the lateral and medial menisci of the knee?
    a. Anterior cruciate
    b. Transverse
    c. Arcuate popliteal
    d. Patellar

11. Which muscle tendons merge to form the Achilles tendon?
    a. Gastrocnemius and plantaris
    b. Soleus and plantaris
    c. Gastrocnemius and soleus
    d. Gastrocnemius, soleus, and plantaris

12. Which ligament of the ankle is seen medially on sectional images?
    a. Deltoid
    b. Callaneofibular
    c. Talofibular
    d. They are all seen medially.
    e. None of the above is seen medially.

13. Involved in forming the ankle or mortise joint are the medial surface of the lateral malleolus of the fibula, lateral surface of the medial malleolus of the tibia, inferior surface of the tibia, and the head of the talus.
    a. True
    b. False

14. Which articulating surface of the calcaneus rests on the sustentaculum tali?
    a. Anterior
    b. Middle
    c. Posterior
    d. a, b, and c
    e. None of the above.

15. On sectional images the sinus tarsi is between the
    a. talus and navicular.
    b. navicular and cuboid.
    c. first cuneiform and navicular.
    d. talus and calcaneus.
    e. third cuneiform and cuboid.

Key to Review Questions

CHAPTER 1

1. 8
2. b
3. b
4. c
5. b
6. b
7. e
8. a
9. c
10. c
11. b
12. d
13. c
14. a
15. a
16. b
17. b
18. d
19. respiratory, cardiac, and vasomotor centers; decussation of pyramids of medulla with crossing of nerve pathways
20. a
21. a
22. e
23. d
24. a
25. b
26. d
27. c
28. a
29. c
30. c
31. a
32. d
33. a
34. equalize blood pressure in brain; provide alternative source of blood if vessel involved in formation of circle of Willis is compromised
35. d

CHAPTER 2

1. b
2. b
3. a
4. divide nasal fossae into compartments so incoming air can be warmed, filtered, and moistened
5. d
6. a
7. b
8. c
9. d
10. a
11. b
12. c
13. d
14. c
15. lighten head; give resonance to voice

CHAPTER 3

1. d
2. cricoid
3. d
4. c
5. a

6. d
7. b
8. b
9. a
10. naturally contains iodine
11. a
12. localization purposes
13. b
14. a
15. c

CHAPTER 4

1. d
2. c
3. b
4. a
5. e
6. a
7. d
8. c
9. b
10. b
11. d
12. b
13. c
14. a
15. d
16. b
17. c
18. to the left and posterior
19. b
20. a
21. d
22. e
23. c
24. b
25. a
26. b
27. b
28. e
29. a
30. a

CHAPTER 5

1. d
2. a, c, d, b
3. splenic artery, left gastric artery, common hepatic artery
4. c
5. a
6. b
7. c
8. b
9. SMV, splenic vein
10. a
11. a
12. a
13. a
14. c
15. duodenum
16. c
17. b
18. d
19. b
20. a
21. c
22. c
23. b
24. b
25. d

CHAPTER 6

1. a
2. d
3. e
4. b
5. d
6. b
7. b
8. a
9. produce 60% of seminal fluid—energy for sperm
10. produces 25% of seminal fluid; prevents urine from mixing with semen during ejaculation
11. produce seminal fluid; lubricate end of penis during intercourse
12. c

13. d
14. accessory parts of an adjacent, related structure
15. a
16. c
17. b
18. a
19. c
20. b

CHAPTER 7

1. a
2. c
3. a
4. C1
5. b
6. e
7. d
8. b
9. d
10. a

CHAPTER 8

1. a
2. c
3. d
4. a
5. b
6. a

7. c
8. b
9. subscapularis, infraspinatus, supraspinatus, teres minor
10. a
11. c
12. b
13. b
14. d
15. c

CHAPTER 9

1. vastus intermedius, vastus lateralis, vastus medialis, rectus femoris
2. d
3. b
4. b
5. b
6. a
7. c
8. a
9. c
10. b
11. c
12. a
13. b
14. b
15. d

Suggested Readings

PRINCIPLES AND PHYSICS OF CT

Blanck, C. (1998). *Understanding helical scanning.* Baltimore: Williams & Wilkins.

Fishman, E. K., & Jeffrey, Jr., R. B. (1998). *Spiral CT: Principles, techniques and clinical applications.* Philadelphia: Lippincott-Raven.

Kalender, W. A. (2000). *Computed tomography.* Somerset, NJ: John Wiley & Sons.

Lee, J. K. T., Sagel, S. S., Stanley, R. J., & Heiken, J. P. (1998). *Computed tomography with MRI correlation* (3rd ed.). Philadelphia: J.B. Lippincott.

Seeram, E. (2001). *Computed tomography: Physical principles, clinical applications, and quality control* (2nd ed.). Philadelphia: W. B. Saunders Co.

Silverman, P. M. (1998). *Helical (spiral) computed tomography: A practical approach to clinical protocols.* Philadelphia: Lippincott-Raven.

Webb, W. R., Brant, W. E., & Helms, C. A. (1998). *Fundamentals of body CT* (2nd ed.). Philadelphia: W. B. Saunders.

PRINCIPLES AND PHYSICS OF MRI

Bushong, S. C. (2003). *Magnetic resonance imaging physical & biological principles.* St. Louis, MO: Elsevier Science.

Faulkner, W., & Seeram, E. (2002). *Rad tech's guide to MRI: Basic physics, instrumentation, and quality control.* Malden, MA: Blackwell Science.

Hannel, J. W., Dryst-Widzgowska, T., & Klinowski, J. W. (1998). *A primer of magnetic resonance imaging.* River Edge, NJ: World Scientific Publishing.

McRobbie, D. W., Moore, E. A., Graves, M. J., & Prince, M. R. (2002). *MRI from picture to proton.* West Nyack, NJ: Cambridge University Press.

Mitchell, D. G. (1999). *MRI principles.* Philadelphia: W. B. Saunders.

Westbrook, C. (1999). *Handbook of MRI technique* (2nd ed.). Malden, MA: Blackwell Science.

Westbrook, C. (2002). *MRI at a glance.* Malden, MA: Blackwell Science.

Woodward, P. (2000). *MRI for technologists* (2nd ed.). New York: McGraw-Hill/Appleton & Lange.

Glossary

(synonym [syn.]; abbreviation [abbr.]; adjective [adj.]; plural [pl.])

abdominal descending aorta — that portion of the descending aorta that is a continuation of the thoracic descending aorta from the level of the diaphragm until its bifurcation into the right and left common iliac arteries at approximately L4.

accessory nasal sinus — see paranasal sinus.

acetabulum — the cup-shaped lateral portion of the innominate bone articulating with the head of the femur; it is formed by the three bones making up the hip bone: the ilium, ischium, and pubis.

adnexa — accessory parts of another nearby related structure such as ovaries and fallopian tubes of uterus.

adrenal gland — endocrine gland found on top of each kidney; syn. — suprarenal gland.

afferent neuron — a nerve cell carrying impulses from a receptor to the central nervous system; syn. — sensory neuron.

ala — wing-shaped structure.

ALL — see anterior longitudinal ligament.

alveolar process — ridge in which the upper and lower teeth are attached on the maxillae and the mandible, respectively; syn. — alveolar ridge.

alveolar ridge — see alveolar process.

alveolus (pl. — alveoli) — air-filled sacs found in the lungs.

amphiarthrosis — a cartilaginous or slightly movable joint such as the articulation between two vertebrae.

ampulla of Vater — dilatation at end of common bile duct where it enters the duodenum.

amygdaloid nucleus — found at the tail end of the caudate nucleus, it is one of four basal ganglia located in the cerebrum; the others are the caudate and lentiform nuclei and the claustrum.

ankle joint — the hinge joint formed by the tibia, fibula, and talus; syn. — mortise joint.

annulus fibrosus — the ring-shaped outer edge of an intervertebral disk.

anterior cerebellar notch — anterior notch of cerebellum accommodating fourth ventricle.

anterior cerebral artery — branch off internal carotid artery supplying blood to anterior and medial aspect of cerebral hemispheres, bilaterally.

anterior communicating artery — a vessel joining the anterior cerebral arteries; involved in forming circle of Willis.

anterior horn of lateral ventricle — see frontal horn.

anterior jugular vein — one of two veins found in the neck that eventually drain into the bilateral external jugular veins.

anterior longitudinal ligament (abbr. — ALL) — a ligament running along the anterior aspect of the bodies of the vertebrae.

anus — the external opening of the gastrointestinal tract distal to the rectum.

aorta — the largest vessel in the body; carries oxygenated blood from the left ventricle of the heart with branches to all parts of the body.

aortic hiatus — the most posterior opening in the diaphragm through which passes the aorta.

aortic semilunar valve — valve controlling the flow of blood between the left ventricle of the heart and the aorta.

apex (pl. — apices) — the pointed end of a cone-shaped structure.

apophyseal joint — see zygoapophyseal joint.

appendicular skeleton — the appendages of the axial skeleton including the upper and lower extremities and the shoulder and pelvic girdles.

appendix — an appendage; a wormlike process extending off the first part of the large intestines, the cecum; syn. — vermiform appendix.

arachnoid — the middle or intermediate meninx covering the brain and spinal cord.

arch of aorta — curved part of aorta from which brachiocephalic, left common carotid, and left subclavian arteries arise.

arch of the azygos — the arch whereby the azygos vein empties into the superior vena cava in the thoracic cavity.

arm — anatomically, that part of the skeleton between the shoulder and elbow joint, composed of the humerus; more commonly used to refer to the upper extremity.

articular capsule — the two-layered enclosure of a diarthrodial or synovial joint with an outer fibrous capsule lined by a synovial membrane.

articular cartilage — hyaline cartilage found on the articulating surfaces of bones.

arytenoid — shape of a ladle or pitcher mouth; paired pieces of cartilage that are part of the larynx.

ascending aorta — the first segment of the aorta arising from the left ventricle of the heart and heading in a superior direction.

ascending colon — the segment of the colon or large intestines located on the right side rising in a superior direction from the cecum and ending at the hepatic flexure.

ascending lumbar vein — one of bilateral branches of the common iliac veins; the right continues as the azygos vein and the left as the hemiazygos vein.

atlas — the first cervical vertebra.

atrioventricular valve — valve between the atria and ventricles of the heart with the tricuspid on the right and bicuspid or mitral on the left.

atrium (pl. — atria) — bilateral superior chamber of the heart acting as a receiving chamber of blood.

axial skeleton — the axis of the skeleton constructed by the skull, three auditory ossicles, hyoid bone, sternum, ribs, and bones of the vertebral column.

axis — the second cervical vertebra.

axon — the process of a neuron that conducts impulses away from the cell body.

azygos vein — continuation of right ascending lumbar vein eventually draining into the SVC.

ball and socket joint — a type of synovial joint in which a rounded head of one bone fits into a cup-shaped cavity of another, permitting virtually unlimited movement.

basal ganglion (pl. — basal ganglia) — one of four masses of gray matter located deep in cerebral hemispheres including the caudate, lentiform, amygdaloid nuclei, and the claustrum; syn. — cerebral nucleus.

base — the flattened part of a structure.

basilar artery — a vessel formed by the merger of the two vertebral arteries; it eventually supplies the posterior portion of brain with blood.

belly — the main part of a muscle.

bicuspid valve — a valve having two cusps or flaps found on the left side of the heart between the left atrium and left ventricle; syn. — mitral valve.

bladder — hollow sac into which urine drains from the kidneys.

blood-brain barrier — barrier between blood, brain, and ventricles selectively prohibiting certain substances from entering brain and cerebrospinal fluid.

body — principal mass of any structure.

brachiocephalic artery — first of three major vessels arising off arch of aorta; provides the right side of the head, neck, and right arm with blood; syn. — innominate artery.

brachiocephalic vein — bilateral vessel draining deoxygenated blood from the head, neck, and arms.

brain stem — composed of the medulla, pons, and midbrain, it connects the spinal cord with the cerebrum.

bronchus (primary) (pl. — bronchi) — one of two divisions of the trachea entering right and left lungs; acts as an airway.

bulbourethral gland — bilateral accessory reproductive gland in the male located on either side of the prostate gland; produces a small amount of seminal fluid; syn. — Cowper's gland.

bursa — a sac of fluid lined by a synovial membrane serving as a cushion in the vicinity of joints between tendons and bones or other points of friction.

calyx (pl. — calyces) — cup-shaped structure.

capillary — the tiniest blood vessel in the body with walls only one cell thick, which acts as an intermediary between an arteriole and venule.

carbon dioxide — a gas composed of carbon and oxygen that is a byproduct of cellular activity and is toxic to the body at high levels; it is eliminated from the body primarily through the lungs.

cardiac notch — a large indentation along the medial left lung accommodating the heart.

cardiac orifice — opening where the esophagus empties into the stomach.

carina — the ridge separating the right and left primary bronchi at the distal end of the trachea.

carpal bone — one of eight bones in the wrist including the scaphoid, lunate, triquetrum, and pisiform in the proximal row and the trapezium, trapezoid, capitate, and hamate in the distal row.

cauda equina — the hairlike nerve roots extending from the tapered end of the spinal cord.

caudate lobe — one of four lobes of the liver; located anterior to the IVC in the upper liver.

caudate nucleus — one of two bilateral basal ganglia that are part of the corpus striatum; conforms to shape of lateral ventricle.

caval hiatus — the most anterior opening in the diaphragm through which passes the inferior vena cava.

cecum — a blind pouch making up the first part of the large intestines into which the ileum empties.

celiac artery — see celiac axis.

celiac axis — first artery branching off abdominal descending aorta; trifurcates into left gastric, splenic, and common hepatic arteries; syn. — celiac artery or trunk.

celiac trunk — see celiac axis.

cell body — the main part of a cell.

central fissure — deep groove or furrow in brain separating the frontal lobe of the cerebrum from the parietal lobe.

central lobe — see insula.

centrum semiovale — mass of white matter at center of each cerebral hemisphere.

cerebellum — largest part of the hindbrain; composed of right and left hemispheres connected by the vermis; it communicates with the other parts of the brain via the superior, middle, and inferior peduncles.

cerebral aqueduct — passageway connecting the third and fourth ventricles of brain; syn. — sylvian aqueduct.

cerebral nucleus — see basal ganglion.

cerebrospinal fluid — a watery solution secreted by the choroid plexus, it is found in the ventricles, cisterns, subarachnoid spaces of the brain, and central canal of the spinal cord.

cerebrum — the most superior and largest part of the brain; it is divided into two hemispheres separated by the longitudinal fissure and connected by the corpus callosum.

cervix — narrowed inferior portion of the uterus that leads to the vagina.

cholelith — gallstone.

choroid plexus — capillary network in four ventricles of brain producing cerebrospinal fluid by filtration and secretion.

circle of Willis — arterial anastomosis formed by internal carotid arteries, posterior cerebral arteries, anterior cerebral arteries, posterior communicating arteries, and anterior communicating artery.

cistern — a reservoir for storing fluid.

cistern pontine — cistern in the brain found anterior and inferior to pons.

cisterna magna — largest cistern in brain, it is located between the medulla oblongata, inferior aspect of cerebellar hemispheres, and occipital bone.

claustrum — one of four basal ganglia located in the cerebrum; the others include the caudate, lentiform, and amygdaloid nuclei; the claustrum is separated from the lentiform nucleus by the external capsule.

clavicle — the bilateral slender bone running transversely along the upper anterior thorax, articulating medially with the manubrium of the sternum and laterally with the acromion process of the scapula; along with the scapula forms the shoulder girdle.

clinoid (anterior and posterior) — processes of sphenoid bone found at base of skull; they form the anterior and posterior borders of the sella turcica.

coccyx — most inferior portion of the vertebral column, usually composed of four fused bones.

collateral trigone — angle where posterior and inferior horns of ventricles meet; site of heavy concentration of choroid plexus.

colliculus (pl. — colliculi) — a little eminence.

common bile duct — duct formed by the merger of the cystic duct and common hepatic duct through which bile passes into the duodenum.

common hepatic artery — one of three branches off the celiac axis; supplies liver with oxygenated blood.

common hepatic duct — the bile duct formed by the merger of the hepatic ducts; the common hepatic duct then merges with the cystic duct to form the common bile duct.

common iliac artery — bilateral artery created by the bifurcation of the descending aorta at L4.

common iliac vein — bilateral vessel draining deoxygenated blood from legs; the right and left common iliac veins merge to form the IVC.

concha (pl. — conchae) — shell-shaped; bilateral superior, middle, and inferior structures that divide the two nasal cavities into compartments; the superior and middle conchae are part of the ethmoid bone and the inferior conchae are separate facial bones; syn. — turbinates.

condyloid joint — a type of synovial joint where a condyle of one bone fitting into an elliptical cavity of another permits movement in two axes (e.g., up and down and side to side but not axial rotation).

condyloid process of mandible — posterior superior portion of mandible involved in temporomandibular joint.

cone — one of two types of receptors for vision; sensitive to color.

conus medullaris — cone-shaped or tapered end of the spinal cord.

convolution — fold; fold on surface of cerebrum.

corniculate — horn-shaped projection; paired pieces of cartilage that are part of the larynx.

coronary artery — one of two immediate branches off the ascending aorta providing the heart with oxygenated blood.

coronary sinus — the venous channel draining the deoxygenated blood from the heart into the right atrium of the heart.

corpora quadrigemina — see quadrigeminal plate.

corpus callosum — portion of brain composed of white matter connecting the two cerebral hemispheres.

corpus striatum — basal ganglia composed of caudate and lentiform nuclei, which are separated by the internal capsule.

cortex — an outer layer of a body organ or structure.

Cowper's gland — see bulbourethral gland.

cranial bone — one of eight bones of the skull encasing the brain, consisting of one frontal, two parietal, one occipital, two temporal, one ethmoid, and one sphenoid bone.

crest of the ilium — the superior ridge of the ilium bounded by the anterior and posterior superior iliac spines.

cribiform plate — horizontal superior part of ethmoid bone fitting into the ethmoidal notch of the horizontal portion of the frontal bone.

cricoid cartilage — ring-shaped; the most inferior of the nine pieces of cartilage making up the larynx and the only one to completely surround the pharynx.

crista galli — superior projection of the cribiform plate of the ethmoid bone.

crus (pl. — crura) — structure resembling a leg; crus of diaphragm — point of attachment of diaphragm to vertebra.

cuneiform — wedge-shaped; paired pieces of cartilage that are part of the larynx.

cystic duct — duct draining bile from the gallbladder that merges with the common hepatic duct to form the common bile duct.

decussation of pyramids of medulla — a crossing of fibers in the anterior inferior aspect of medulla resulting in the right half of the brain controlling the left half of the body and vice versa.

dendrite — the process of a neuron conducting impulses toward the cell body.

dens — see odontoid process.

descending aorta — segment of aorta that is a continuation of the arch of the aorta to approximately L4 where it bifurcates into the right and left common iliac arteries; it can be divided into the thoracic or abdominal descending aorta.

descending colon — the segment of the colon or large intestines extending down on the left from the splenic flexure and ending at the sigmoid colon.

diaphragm — a dome-shaped muscle separating the thoracic cavity from the abdominal cavity.

diarthrodial joint — a freely movable joint having an enclosed joint cavity lined by a synovial membrane; syn. — synovial joint.

diencephalon — part of the forebrain; composed primarily of the thalamus and hypothalamus; it forms the lateral and ventral walls of the third ventricle.

diploe — spongy bone found between two layers of compact bone in skull.

dorsum sellae — posterior surface of sella turcica.

ductus vas deferens — a continuation of the epididymis carrying sperm from the testis to the ejaculatory duct.

ductus venosus — a branch of the umbilical vein in the fetus diverting blood directly into the inferior vena cava; transformed into the ligamentum venosum in the adult.

duodenum — first part of the small intestines distal to the stomach into which the common bile and pancreatic ducts empty.

dura mater — the tough outermost meninx of the brain and spinal cord.

dural sinus — channel located between two layers of dura mater that drain blood and cerebrospinal fluid.

efferent neuron — nerve cell conveying impulses away from the central nervous system.

ejaculatory duct — a continuation of the bilateral ductus vas deferens that is joined by the duct leading from the seminal vesicle, eventually draining into the urethra.

elbow joint — the hinge joint formed by the articulation of the distal humerus and proximal radius and ulna.

endocardium — the inner lining of the chambers of the heart in direct contact with the myocardium.

ensiform process — see xiphoid process.

epicardium — the innermost layer of the serous pericardium.

epididymis — the posterior portion of the testis where sperm maturation occurs; continues as ductus vas deferens.

epidural space — the space outside the dura mater of the brain and spinal cord.

epiglottis — the most superior of the nine pieces of cartilage making up the larynx; its function is to cover the airway when eating or drinking to prevent aspiration into the lungs.

epimysium — the outermost covering of a muscle.

erector spinae muscle — bilateral muscle found posterior to the vertebral column on either side of the spinous process.

esophageal hiatus — centrally located opening in the diaphragm through which passes the esophagus.

esophagogastric junction — the union of the esophagus and stomach.

esophagus — the tubular structure originating at the distal larynx through which food and liquids pass to reach the stomach.

estrogen — one of two female hormones produced by ovaries in females and adrenal cortex in males and females; responsible for female sexual characteristics and maintenance of pregnancy.

ethmoid bone — one of eight cranial bones; containing the ethmoidal sinuses, it is located between the eyes; the perpendicular plate of the ethmoid bone forms the superior part of the bony nasal septum.

ethmoid sinus — paranasal sinus contained in the ethmoid bone.

external carotid artery — branch off common carotid artery that supplies blood to face, scalp, and most of neck and throat, bilaterally.

external iliac artery — one of two terminal branches of common iliac artery; it eventually becomes the femoral artery in the thigh, bilaterally.

external iliac vein — a continuation of the femoral vein; it merges with the internal iliac vein to form the common iliac vein, bilaterally.

external jugular vein — bilateral vein found in the neck draining the blood from the area of the head supplied by the external carotid arteries.

external oblique muscle — bilateral muscle that is the most lateral of the three lateral abdominal muscles.

facial bone — one of the 14 bones making up the face: 2 maxillary, 2 zygomatic, 2 lacrimal, 2 nasal, 2 inferior nasal conchae, 2 palatine, 1 vomer, and 1 mandible.

falciform ligament — a ligament separating the right and left lobes of the liver anteriorly and attaching the liver to the diaphragm.

fallopian tube — bilateral tube extending laterally from uterus that serves as a site for fertilization of a female ovum or egg by the male sperm; syn. — uterine tube, oviduct.

false pelvis — cavity found above and anterior to the pelvic inlet.

falx cerebelli — fold of dura mater that forms a vertical partition between hemispheres of the cerebellum.

falx cerebri — dip of dura mater into longitudinal fissure separating two hemispheres of cerebrum.

femoral — pertinent to the femur.

femur — the long bone between the hip and knee; the longest and strongest bone in the human body; syn. — thigh.

fibrous pericardium — the outermost layer of the pericardium.

fibula — the slender long bone in the lateral lower leg, articulating proximally with the tibia and distally with the tibia and talus.

filium terminale — an extension of the pia mater beyond the conus medullaris anchoring the spinal cord to the coccyx.

fimbria (pl. — fimbriae) — one of many fingerlike processes extending from the infundibulum of the uterine tube; resembles a fringe.

foot — the part of the lower extremity distal to the tibia and fibula; composed of 7 tarsal bones, 5 metatarsals, and 14 phalanges.

foramen magnum — literally "large opening"; located on inferior portion of occipital bone.

foramen of Luschka (pl. — foramina of Luschka) — bilateral opening from fourth ventricle connecting it with subarachnoid space; syn. — lateral aperture.

foramen of Magendie — median opening of fourth ventricle draining cerebrospinal fluid into central canal of spinal cord and subarachnoid space; syn. — median aperture.

foramen of Monro — see interventricular foramen.

foramen ovale — an opening between the right and left atria of the heart in the fetus.

forearm — that portion of the upper extremity between the elbow and wrist composed of the ulna medially and radius laterally.

forebrain — anterior portion of the brain in embryo evolving into cerebrum and diencephalon.

fornix — archlike structure; white matter lying below splenium of corpus callosum of cerebrum and constructing inferior margin of septum pellucidum; recess where cervix meets vagina.

frontal bone — one of the eight cranial bones; forms the forehead and contains the frontal sinuses.

frontal horn — hornlike projection of lateral ventricle found in frontal lobe of cerebrum; syn. — anterior horn.

frontal lobe — anterior portion of each cerebral hemisphere lying beneath frontal bone.

frontal process of maxillary bone — superior, medial extension of maxillary bone articulating with frontal bone.

frontal sinus — paranasal sinus contained in the frontal bone.

fundus — the larger part of a hollow organ farthest from the opening.

gallbladder (abbr. — GB) — organ found on the undersurface of the liver storing bile manufactured by the liver.

genitalia — reproductive or sex organs; syn. — genitals.

genitals — see genitalia.

genu — the knee or any angular structure resembling the flexed knee; anterior portion of corpus callosum.

gladiolus — the body of the sternum.

glenohumeral joint — the shoulder joint, formed by the head of the humerus and the glenoid fossa of the scapula.

globus pallidus — one part of lentiform nucleus, the other being the putamen; they are both found lateral to the thalamus, with the globus pallidus being most medial.

gluteal muscle — bilateral muscle in buttocks; includes gluteal minimus, medius, and maximus.

gonadal — referring to the gonads or sex glands: testes in males; ovaries in females.

gray matter — nervous tissue composed mainly of cell bodies rather than neurons with myelinated processes.

great vessel — one of the major vessels entering and exiting the heart including the SVC, IVC, pulmonary trunk, and aorta.

greater curvature of the stomach — convex curvature located along lateral border of stomach.

greater sciatic notch — a large indentation located posteriorly and inferiorly on the ilium.

gyrus (pl. — gyri) — see convolution.

hand — that portion of the upper extremity distal to the forearm composed of eight carpal and five metacarpal bones and the fourteen phalanges.

hard palate — bony roof of the mouth formed anteriorly by the palatine process of the maxillary bones and posteriorly by the palatine bones.

head — proximal end; alternative term for one of multiple origins of muscle.

heart — the organ in the mediastinum responsible for pulmonary and systemic circulation.

hemiazygos vein — continuation of the left ascending lumbar vein draining into the azygos vein.

hemisphere — either half of cerebrum or cerebellum.

hepatic duct — one of two ducts emptying bile from the right and left lobes of the liver that merge to form the common hepatic duct.

hepatic flexure — bend at superior aspect of ascending colon where it meets transverse colon inferior to the liver.

hepatic vein — one of three vessels leaving the liver carrying deoxygenated blood to the IVC.

hilum (pl. — hila) — a concave indentation in a structure through which vessels, nerves, or other structures enter or exit.

hindbrain — division of the brain composed of the pons, medulla oblongata, and the cerebellum.

hinge joint — a type of synovial joint in which the articulating bones can move in only one plane, anteriorly and posteriorly, with each bone moving in opposite direction.

hip bone — see innominate bone.

hip joint — the ball and socket joint formed by the articulation of the head of the femur with the acetabulum of the hip bone.

humerus — that part of the skeleton between the shoulder and elbow joint; syn. — arm.

hydrocephalus — abnormal increased accumulation of cerebrospinal fluid in ventricles of brain.

hyoid bone — U-shaped bone in the anterior neck.

hypothalamus — one of two primary sections of the diencephalon, the other being the thalamus; the hypothalamus, found inferior to the thalamus, is connected to the posterior lobe of the pituitary gland by way of the infundibulum and comprises the ventral wall of the third ventricle.

ileocecal valve — the valve connecting the distal portion of the small intestines, the ileum, with the first part of the large intestines, the cecum.

ileum — the third and last segment of the small intestines preceded by the jejunum and emptying into the cecum, the first part of the large intestines.

iliac spine — one of four sharp processes found on the ilium: anterior superior, posterior superior, anterior inferior, and posterior inferior.

iliacus muscle — bilateral muscle medial to ilium that eventually merges with psoas muscle to form the iliopsoas muscle.

iliopsoas muscle — bilateral muscle formed by the merger of the psoas and iliacus muscles within the pelvic region.

ilium — the most superior of the three bones making up the innominate bone, the other two being the ischium and pubis.

IMA — see inferior mesenteric artery.

IMV — see inferior mesenteric vein.

inferior articulating process — the name for two of the seven processes attached to the vertebral arch; articulates with the superior articulating process of the vertebra below to form a zygoapophyseal joint.

inferior horn of lateral ventricle — see temporal horn.

inferior mesenteric artery (abbr. — IMA) — most inferior branch off the abdominal descending aorta; supplies left half of transverse colon, descending colon, sigmoid, and most of the rectum with oxygenated blood.

inferior mesenteric vein (abbr. — IMV) — vessel draining deoxygenated blood from those organs supplied by the IMA; it empties into the splenic vein, contributing blood to what eventually becomes the portal vein.

inferior vena cava (abbr. — IVC) — one of the two largest veins in the body draining almost all the deoxygenated blood from below the level of the heart into the right atrium.

infundibulum — funnel-shaped structure or passageway; a stalk connecting the hypothalamus with the posterior lobe of the pituitary gland; the lateral end of the uterine or fallopian tube.

innominate artery — nameless; alternative term for brachiocephalic artery.

innominate bone — one of two bones making up the pelvic girdle; each innominate bone originates as three separate bones, which eventually fuse: the ilium, ischium, and pubis; syn. — hip bone, os coxae.

insertion — the movable point of attachment of a muscle.

insula — division of each cerebral hemisphere found medial to lateral sulcus or central fissure; syn. — central lobe.

interatrial septum — the wall of the heart separating the two atria.

intermediate mass — a bridge of gray matter passing through the third ventricle connecting the thalamus.

internal carotid artery — branch of common carotid artery that primarily supplies blood to anterior, medial, and lateral aspects of brain.

internal iliac artery — one of two terminal branches of the common iliac artery; it remains within the pelvic area.

internal iliac vein — a vessel that drains deoxygenated blood from the pelvic area and merges with the external iliac vein to form the common iliac vein.

internal jugular vein — bilateral vein found in the neck draining the dural sinuses of the brain.

internal oblique muscle — bilateral muscle on the lateral abdominal region medial to the external oblique muscle.

interventricular foramen — point of communication between lateral ventricles and third ventricle; syn. — foramen of Monro.

interventricular septum — a wall of the heart separating the two ventricles.

intervertebral disk — a fibrocartilaginous structure located between the bodies of two adjacent vertebrae, composed of the outermost annulus fibrosus and innermost nucleus pulposus.

intervertebral foramen (pl. — foramina) — bilateral foramen formed by the vertebral notches of two adjacent articulating vertebrae through which pass spinal nerves.

ischial spine — bilateral medial extension of the ischium.

ischial tuberosity — the large protuberance forming the inferior ischium upon which the body rests when seated.

ischium — the inferior posterior bone involved in forming the innominate bone, the other two being the ilium ad pubis.

IVC — see inferior vena cava.

jejunum — the second segment of the small intestines bounded proximally by the duodenum and distally by the ileum.

jugular notch — the indentation along the superior aspect of the manubrium of the sternum; syn. — suprasternal notch.

kidney — one of two bilateral organs found in the posterior abdomen that are largely responsible for controlling the volume of body fluid by urine production.

knee joint — the modified hinge joint formed by the articulation of the distal femur, proximal tibia, and patella; syn. — tibiofemoral joint.

kyphosis — an exaggerated posterior convex curvature of the spinal column in the thoracic region.

labrum — a liplike structure; a rim of fibrocartilage extending beyond the edge of the glenoid fossae and acetabula.

lacrimal bone — one of a pair of bones included in the fourteen facial bones; involved in forming the anterior medial wall of the orbit.

lamina — posteromedial extension of the bilateral pedicles of a vertebra involved in forming the vertebral arch.

large intestine — the wider distal portion of the gastrointestinal system beginning with the cecum, into which the ileum empties, and ending at the anus; composed of the cecum, vermiform appendix, ascending, transverse, descending, and sigmoid colon, and rectum.

laryngopharynx — distal portion of pharynx surrounded by larynx.

larynx — "voicebox"; surrounds distal portion of pharynx.

lateral aperture — see foramen of Luschka.

lateral fissure — fissure or sulcus separating frontal and parietal lobes from temporal lobe of cerebrum; syn. — Sylvian fissure.

lateral mass — bilateral inferior extension of cribiform plate that contains ethmoid sinuses; bilateral section of the sacrum lateral to the foramina; bilateral projection off neural arch of C1.

left common carotid artery — second of three major vessels arising off arch of aorta; provides left side of neck and head with blood.

left gastric artery — one of three branches off the celiac axis; supplies stomach with oxygenated blood.

left gastric vein — vessel draining deoxygenated blood from the stomach into the splenic vein, contributing blood to what eventually becomes the portal vein.

left subclavian artery — third and last vessel to arise off arch of aorta; supplies blood to left arm and posterior aspect of head.

lens — the transparent, convex structure in the eye through which light passes and is refracted before reaching the retina.

lentiform nucleus — one of two bilateral basal ganglia making up corpus striatum; found lateral to thalamus and consisting of the globus pallidus (the medial aspect) and the putamen (the lateral aspect).

lesser curvature of stomach — concave curvature located along medial border of stomach.

levator ani muscle — paired muscle originating at symphysis pubis and inserting onto coccyx; forms the pelvic floor.

ligament — band of fibrous tissue binding bones together.

ligamentum flava — a ligament running along the medial aspect of the laminae of the vertebrae.

ligamentum nuchae — a ligament running along the tips of the spinous processes of the vertebrae from C7 to the occipital bone.

ligamentum teres — a remnant of the umbilical vein arising from the umbilicus and joining the free edge of the falciform ligament on the inferior liver, eventually separating the quadrate and left lobes of the liver; syn. — round ligament.

ligamentum venosum — remnant of fetal ductus venosus in an adult separating the caudate and left lobes of the liver.

linea alba — a tendinous membrane that separates the bilateral rectus abdominis muscles; created by the convergence of the three lateral abdominal muscles.

liver — the largest organ in the body; located in the right upper quadrant it extends into the left upper quadrant and manufactures bile.

longitudinal fissure — deep groove or furrow in brain separating the cerebral hemispheres; fissure seen along the posterior liver separating the right and left lobes.

longus capitis — a muscle found in the neck in front of the bodies of the cervical vertebrae.

longus colli — a muscle found in the neck in front of the bodies of the cervical vertebrae.

lordosis — a normal or exaggerated anterior concave curvature of the spinal column, usually in the lumbar region.

lung — bilateral organ located on either side of the thorax involved in intake of oxygen and elimination of carbon dioxide.

malar bone — see zygomatic bone.

mammary gland — bilateral accessory reproductive gland in females responsible for lactation or milk production.

mandible — one of the fourteen facial bones; it forms the lower jaw and is the only movable bone in the skull; its anterior superior alveolar ridge accommodates the lower teeth.

manubrium — a handle-shaped structure; the upper segment of the sternum that articulates with the two clavicles and 1½ pairs of ribs; the jugular notch is the superior aspect.

maxillary bone — one of a pair of the bones included in the fourteen facial bones; involved in forming the oral and nasal cavities as well as the orbits; its inferior alveolar ridge accommodates the upper teeth.

maxillary sinus — paranasal sinus contained in the maxillary bone.

median aperture — see foramen of Magendie.

mediastinum — cavity found between the right and left lungs containing heart, its great vessels, trachea, esophagus, thymus, lymph nodes, and connective tissue.

medulla — inner or central portion of an organ; abbreviated term for medulla oblongata.

medulla oblongata — most inferior part of the brain stem and hindbrain, which continues as the spinal cord below the level of the foramen magnum and contains many vital reflex centers.

meninx (pl. — meninges) — one of three membranes covering the brain and spinal cord including the dura mater, arachnoid, and pia mater.

meniscus (pl. — menisci) — a crescent-shaped pad of fibrocartilage found in the knee joint.

menstruation — periodic external discharge of blood from vagina as a result of the sloughing off of the uterine lining if pregnancy does not occur.

mentum — chin.

metacarpal — one of five bones found in the palm of the hand articulating proximally with the distal row of carpal bones and the proximal phalanges distally.

metatarsal — one of five bones between the tarsal bones and phalanges of the foot, numbered I through V, starting on the medial foot.

midbrain — middle portion of the embryonic brain that evolves into the cerebral peduncles and the corpora quadrigemina.; the cerebral aqueduct passes through the midbrain.

middle cerebral artery — branch off internal carotid artery supplying blood to lateral portion of brain.

mitral valve — see bicuspid valve.

mixed nerve — a nerve having both sensory and motor fibers.

mortise joint — see ankle joint.

motor neuron — a nerve cell conveying impulses from the central nervous system to initiate muscular contraction; a type of efferent neuron.

muscle — a structure composed of muscle cells that cause movement of a bone, organ, or other part of the body through contraction and relaxation.

myocardium — cardiac muscle forming the walls of the heart.

myofilament — filament making up a muscle; may be thick or thin.

nasal bone — one of a pair of bones included in the fourteen facial bones; involved in forming the bridge or arch of the nose.

nasal fossa (pl. — nasal fossae) — bilateral cavity of the nose.

nasal septum — wall dividing the right and left nasal cavities, composed of cartilage anteriorly and bone posteriorly; the bony nasal septum is formed superiorly by the perpendicular plate of the ethmoid bone and inferiorly by the vomer.

neck — constricted part of a structure often adjacent to the head.

neural arch — see vertebral arch.

neuron — a nerve cell; the basic structural and functional unit of the nervous system.

nucleus pulposus — the center of an intervertebral disk.

obturator foramen — one of two apertures of the hip formed by the pubic and ischial bones.

obturator muscle — bilateral paired muscle in vicinity of obturator foramen; includes obturator internus and externus.

occipital bone — one of eight cranial bones; forms the posteroinferior portion of skull.

occipital horn — hornlike projection of lateral ventricle found in occipital lobe of cerebrum; syn. — posterior horn.

occipital lobe — posterior region of right and left cerebral hemisphere lying beneath occipital bone.

odontoid process — a toothlike process projecting superiorly from C2 articulating with C1 allowing for rotation of the head; syn. — dens.

optic chiasma — an X-shaped crossing of some optic nerve fibers in the brain.

optic nerve — nerve exiting the back of the orbit carrying the sensory information received by the retina to the brain.

orbit — conical cavity containing the eyeball.

origin — beginning; the fixed point of attachment of a muscle.

os coxae — see innominate bone.

ovary — paired sex gland in female producing ovum, the female egg, and the female hormones, estrogen and progesterone.

oviduct — see fallopian tube.

ovum — a mature female egg or germ cell produced by the ovaries.

oxygen — a gas essential to human life received into the lungs through respiration (breathing).

palatine bone — one of a pair of bones included in the fourteen facial bones; involved in forming the posterior part of the hard palate.

palatine process — inferior horizontal portion of maxillary bone forming anterior part of roof of mouth.

pancreas — a mixed gland found behind the stomach; the exocrine portion produces pancreatic juice, which exits through the pancreatic duct into the duodenum to aid in digestion; the endocrine portion produces hormones including insulin and glucagon.

pancreatic duct — duct passing through the pancreas transporting pancreatic enzymes.

paranasal sinus — one of many air-filled cavities that communicate with each other and the nasal cavity; includes the maxillary, frontal, ethmoidal, and sphenoidal sinuses, named for the bones containing them; syn. — accessory nasal sinus.

pararenal space — the space near the kidneys.

parietal — the wall of a cavity.

parietal bone — one of a pair of bones included in the eight cranial bones; forms roof and sides of skull.

parietal lobe — division of right and left cerebral hemisphere lying beneath each parietal bone.

parotid gland — one of three pairs of salivary glands; found near the ear.

patella — a sesamoid bone anterior to the distal femur; the largest sesamoid bone in the human body.

pectineus muscle — muscle originating at pubic bone and inserting onto lesser trochanter.

pedicle — bilateral posterior extension of the body of a vertebra involved in forming the vertebral arch.

peduncle — a band of fibers connecting parts of the brain.

pelvic girdle — one of the bilateral innominate or hip bones to which the lower extremity is attached.

pelvic inlet — the superior opening to the true pelvis with an anterior border of the superior symphysis pubis and a posterior border of the superior anterior sacrum.

pelvis (adj. — pelvic) — structure composed of the sacrum, coccyx, and the two innominate or hip bones joined at the symphysis pubis.

pericardium — the sac enclosing the heart and great vessels constructed of two layers, the fibrous and serous pericardium.

perirenal space — the space around the kidneys.

peritoneum — a membrane lining the abdominal cavity encasing and enfolding many abdominal organs.

perpendicular plate of the ethmoid bone — portion of the ethmoid bone forming the superior bony nasal septum.

phalanx (pl. — phalanges) — one of 14 bones forming the fingers of the hand and toes of the foot.

pharynx — common passageway for food, liquid, and air, which originates behind the nose and terminates at the distal larynx; its three divisions include the nasopharynx, oropharynx, and laryngeal pharynx.

pia mater — the innermost meninx of the brain and spinal cord.

pineal gland — endocrine gland located in brain superior to cerebellum and beneath the splenium of the corpus callosum; frequently calcifies.

piriformis muscle — see pyriformis muscle.

pituitary gland — an endocrine gland secreting a number of hormones, some of which are tropic, stimulating the other endocrine glands to secrete their hormones; it is considered the "master gland of the body" because of the importance and number of hormones it secretes; it is divided into two lobes, anterior and posterior, with the posterior lobe connected to the hypothalamus via the infundibulum.

pivot joint — a type of synovial joint allowing for rotation only where an extension of one bone fits in a bony/ligamentous ring of another.

platysma — a thin muscle found in the anterior neck.

pleura — the double-layered lining encasing the lungs; the outermost layer is the parietal pleura and the innermost layer is the visceral pleura.

PLL — see posterior longitudinal ligament.

pons — the rounded superior anterior part of the hindbrain.

porta hepatis — a fissure in the liver where the portal vein and common hepatic artery enter and the hepatic ducts exit.

portal vein — vessel going to the liver carrying deoxygenated blood formed by the union of the splenic vein and the SMV; prior to its formation the IMV and gastric vein empty into the splenic vein.

posterior cerebellar notch — posterior notch of cerebellum accommodating the falx cerebelli.

posterior cerebral artery — bilateral branch off basilar artery supplying right and left posterior portion of brain with blood.

posterior communicating artery — bilateral vessel that joins the posterior cerebral arteries with the internal carotid arteries; involved in forming circle of Willis.

posterior horn of lateral ventricle — see occipital horn.

posterior longitudinal ligament (abbr. — PLL) — a ligament running along the posterior aspect of the bodies of the vertebrae.

progesterone — one of two female hormones produced by ovaries in females that are responsible for maintenance of pregnancy.

prostate gland — an accessory reproductive gland in the male surrounding the urethra whose functions include producing some of the seminal fluid and preventing urine from entering the urethra during ejaculation.

psoas muscle — bilateral muscle on either side of vertebral body in abdominal region, which eventually merges with iliacus muscle in pelvic region to form the iliopsoas muscle.

pterygoid process — bilateral medial and lateral process extending inferiorly from the sphenoid bone.

pubis (adj. — pubic) — the inferior anterior bone involved in forming the innominate bone, the other two being the ilium and ischium.

pudendum — see vulva.

pulmonary artery — bilateral vessel arising from the pulmonary trunk carrying deoxygenated blood from the heart to the lungs.

pulmonary circulation — the blood flow from the heart to the lungs and back whereby carbon dioxide is removed from the blood and replaced with oxygen.

pulmonary semilunar valve — valve controlling the flow of blood between the right ventricle of the heart and the pulmonary trunk.

pulmonary trunk — a major vessel leaving the right ventricle of the heart carrying deoxygenated blood to the lungs.

pulmonary vein — vein carrying oxygenated blood to the left atrium of the heart from the right or left lung.

putamen — one part of the lentiform nucleus, the other being the globus pallidus; they are both found lateral to the thalamus with the putamen being most lateral.

pyloric antrum — a bulge found in the distal portion of the stomach.

pyloric sphincter — a circular muscle found at the distal pylorus of the stomach controlling the movement of the stomach contents into the duodenum.

pyriformis muscle — bilateral pear-shaped muscle originating on anterior surface of sacrum and inserting on greater trochanter; syn. — piriformis.

quadrate lobe — one of four lobes of the liver; located anterior to the gallbladder in the lower liver.

quadratus lumborum muscle — bilateral muscle lateral to the transverse process of the vertebrae in the abdominal region.

quadrigeminal cistern — enlarged area posterior to quadrigeminal plate storing cerebrospinal fluid.

quadrigeminal plate — the dorsal portion of the midbrain consisting of two superior and two inferior colliculi; syn. — tectum or corpora quadrigemina.

radius — the long bone found laterally in the forearm involved in forming the elbow joint proximally and wrist joint distally.

ramus (pl. — rami) — a branch.

rectum — distal end of gastrointestinal tract preceded by the sigmoid colon and terminating in the anal canal.

rectus abdominis muscle — bilateral muscle found on the anterior abdominopelvic wall separated by the linea alba.

rectus femoris muscle — muscle extending from the anterior inferior iliac spine to the patella.

rectus muscle — one of four muscles involved in moving the eye including the superior, inferior, medial or internal, and lateral or external rectus muscles.

renal artery — bilateral artery branching off abdominal descending aorta inferior to SMA, which supplies right and left kidneys with oxygenated blood.

renal pelvis — the collecting area for the urine draining from the large calyces in the kidney.

renal vein — vessel draining deoxygenated blood from each kidney into inferior vena cava.

retina — the innermost covering of the posterior portion of the eye, which contains rods and cones, the nerve cells involved with vision.

retinaculum (pl. — retinacula) — a band or structure holding an organ in place.

retromandibular vein — vein found behind lower jaw that continues as external jugular vein.

retroperitoneal space — the space behind the peritoneum.

rib — one of 12 pairs of curved flat bones involved in forming the bony thorax; articulate with the thoracic vertebrae posteriorly; the first seven ribs are considered true ribs as they articulate indirectly with the lateral margin of the sternum via cartilage; ribs eight through twelve are false ribs as they do not articulate with the sternum; ribs eleven and twelve are floating ribs, having no articulation anteriorly.

right common carotid artery — branch off brachiocephalic artery providing blood to right side of neck and head.

right subclavian artery — branch off brachiocephalic artery supplying blood to left arm; syn. — innominate artery.

rod — one of two types of receptor cells for vision; sensitive to dim light.

root of the lung — the collection of blood vessels, bronchi, lymphatic vessels, and nerves entering and exiting the lungs.

round ligament — see ligamentum teres.

sacral foramina — bilateral openings found on the sacrum, eight on each side, four anterior and four posterior.

sacral promontory — the midline superior aspect of the sacrum, which articulates with the body of L5.

sacroiliac joint — the bilateral articulation of the lateral portion of the sacrum with the ilia of the innominate bones.

sacrum — lower triangulated portion of vertebral column composed of five fused vertebrae articulating superiorly with L5, inferiorly with the coccyx, and laterally with the two innominate bones.

sartorius muscle — longest muscle in the human body; originates at the ASIS and inserts onto the proximal medial tibia.

SC joint — see sternoclavicular joint.

scalene muscle — muscle found in the neck on either side of the body of the cervical vertebrae; includes the anterior, middle, and posterior.

scapula (pl. — scapulae) — one of two flat triangular bones found in the upper posterior thoracic region providing points of attachment for the humerus to form the shoulder joint and the clavicle to form the acromioclavicular joint; along with the clavicle forms the shoulder girdle.

scrotum — external sac that contains two testes in males.

sella turcica — a bony saddle found on the floor of the cranium in the sphenoid bone, which accommodates the pituitary gland.

semen — see seminal fluid.

semilunar — crescent or half-moon shape.

seminal fluid — the fluid containing sperm excreted during ejaculation; syn. — semen.

seminal vesicle — bilateral gland in males found behind the bladder producing a large percentage of seminal fluid.

sensory neuron — see afferent neuron.

septum — wall that divides two cavities.

septum pellucidum — sheet of nervous tissue separating the two lateral ventricles.

serous membrane — a membrane or layer of tissue lining a cavity that produces serous fluid.

serous pericardium — the innermost layer of the pericardium having two layers: the parietal and visceral; the visceral layer of the serous pericardium (epicardium) is the innermost layer and is in direct contact with the myocardium or heart muscle.

shoulder girdle — a protective structure for the upper thorax that also provides a point of attachment for the humerus and sternum, bilaterally.

shoulder joint — the ball and socket joint formed by the articulation of the head of the humerus with the glenoid fossa of the scapula.

sigmoid colon — the S-shaped segment of the colon or large intestines beginning at the distal end of the descending colon and ending at the rectum.

skeletal — referring to the skeleton.

SMA — see superior mesenteric artery.

small intestine — the first part of the intestines emptying into the large intestines; composed of three segments: the duodenum, jejunum, and ileum.

SMV — see superior mesenteric vein.

sperm — male germ cell.

sphenoid bone — one of the eight cranial bones; serves as anchor for the remaining cranial bones and is found on the floor of the skull; contains the sphenoid sinuses.

sphenoid sinus — paranasal sinus contained in the sphenoid bone.

spinal canal — see vertebral canal.

spinal cord — continuation of medulla oblongata below level of foramen magnum; all ascending and descending nerve tracts travel through the spinal cord to enter and exit the brain.

spinal nerve — one of the 31 pairs of nerves attached to the spinal cord.

spinous process — one of the seven processes attached to the vertebral arch of a vertebra; extends posteriorly from the midline union of the bilateral laminae.

spleen — organ in left upper posterior quadrant of the abdomen that filters and stores blood and produces lymphocytes and monocytes after birth.

splenic artery — one of three branches off the celiac axis; supplies spleen with oxygenated blood.

splenic flexure — bend near spleen where transverse colon meets start of descending colon.

splenic vein — vessel leaving the spleen carrying deoxygenated blood; it merges with the SMV to form the portal vein.

splenium — thickened posterior portion of corpus callosum.

squamous — platelike.

sternal angle — the palpable joint between the manubrium and body or gladiolus of the sternum.

sternoclavicular joint (abbr. — SC joint) — the union of the manubrium of the sternum and the medial aspect of the clavicle.

sternocleidomastoid — a muscle found in the neck attaching to the mastoid superiorly and sternum and medial aspect of clavicle inferiorly.

sternohyoid/sternothyroid — muscles found in neck attaching to thyroid cartilage and hyoid bone at one end and sternum at other end.

sternum — the flat bone located midline on the anterior aspect of the thoracic cage constructed of three segments: the manubrium, body or gladiolus, and xiphoid process or ensiform process.

stomach — a hollow gastrointestinal organ in the left upper quadrant situated between the esophagus and duodenum; involved in the digestion of food.

striated — "striped"; a particular type of muscle cell that has a striped appearance.

subarachnoid space — the space between the arachnoid and the pia mater.

subclavian vein — vein draining the arm; unites with internal jugular to form brachiocephalic or innominate vein.

subdural space — the space between the dura mater and arachnoid.

sublingual gland — one of three pairs of salivary glands; found beneath the tongue.

submandibular gland — one of three pairs of salivary glands; found beneath the rami of the mandible.

sulcus (pl. — sulci) — a furrow or groove; especially on brain surface.

superior articulating process — the name for two of the seven processes attached to the vertebral arch of a vertebra; articulates with the inferior articulating process of the vertebra above to form a zygoapophyseal joint.

superior mesenteric artery (abbr. — SMA) — second artery to arise from abdominal descending aorta; supplies most of small intestines, ascending and right half of transverse colon with oxygenated blood.

superior mesenteric vein (abbr. — SMV) — vessel draining deoxygenated blood from those organs supplied by the SMA; it merges with the splenic vein to form the portal vein.

superior vena cava (abbr. — SVC) — one of the two largest veins in the body draining all deoxygenated blood from above the level of the heart into the right atrium.

suprarenal gland — see adrenal gland.

supraspinous ligament — a ligament running along the tips of the spinous processes of the vertebrae from C7 to the sacrum.

suprasternal notch — see jugular notch.

SVC — see superior vena cava.

sylvian aqueduct — narrow canal between third and fourth ventricle of brain; syn. — cerebral aqueduct.

sylvian fissure — see lateral fissure.

symphysis pubis — the slightly movable fibrocartilaginous midline joint between the two pubic bones.

synovia — see synovial fluid.

synovial fluid — clear viscous lubricating fluid secreted by synovial membranes lining synovial joints, bursae, and tendon sheaths; syn. — synovia.

synovial joint — a freely movable joint having an enclosed joint cavity lined by a synovial membrane; syn. — diarthrodial joint.

synovial membrane — a membrane secreting synovial fluid found lining synovial joints, bursae, and tendons.

systemic circulation — the blood flow to all parts of the body (other than the lungs) and back whereby oxygen is delivered and carbon dioxide is removed.

tarsal bone — one of seven ankle bones including the talus, calcaneus or oscalcis, cuboid, navicular, first, second, and third cuneiforms.

tectum — see quadrigeminal plate.

temporal bone — one of a pair of bones included in the eight cranial bones; forms inferior lateral skull.

temporal horn — hornlike projection of lateral ventricle found in temporal lobe of cerebrum; syn. — inferior horn.

temporal lobe — division of each cerebral hemisphere lying beneath each temporal bone.

temporomandibular fossa — a depression found along the inferior edge of the temporal bone articulating with the condyloid process of the mandible to form the temporomandibular joint.

temporomandibular joint — articulation of condyloid process of mandible with temporomandibular fossa of temporal bone.

tendon — the tapered cordlike extension of a muscle allowing for attachment to a bone or other part.

tensor muscle — muscle originating at ASIS and inserting onto lateral thigh.

tentorium cerebelli — extension of dura mater between the cerebrum and cerebellum.

testicle — see testis.

testis (pl. — testes) — one of two sex glands located in the scrotal sac responsible for the production of sperm and the male hormone testosterone; syn. — testicle.

testosterone — male hormone produced in the testes in males and the adrenal cortex in males and females; responsible for male sexual characteristics.

thalamus — one of two primary sections of the diencephalon, the other being the hypothalamus; the thalamus forms the wall of the third ventricle.

thebesian valve — the valve controlling blood flow from the coronary sinus into the right atrium of the heart.

thigh — see femur.

thoracic descending aorta — that portion of the descending aorta originating at the distal portion of the arch of the aorta and extending to the diaphragm.

thymus — organ of endocrine system located behind manubrium of the sternum; involved in maturation of T cells.

thyroid cartilage — largest of the nine pieces of cartilage making up the larynx; forms the "Adam's apple."

thyroid gland — an endocrine gland found anterior to the lower larynx.

tibia — the long weight-bearing bone in the medial lower leg, articulating proximally with the femur to form the knee joint and distally with the talus to form the ankle joint.

tibiofemoral joint — see knee joint.

trachea — the airway originating at the distal larynx and bifurcating at the carina to form the two primary bronchi.

tracheal cartilage — U-shaped pieces of cartilage found in front of the trachea.

transverse colon — the segment of the colon or large intestines extending crosswise between the hepatic flexure on the right and the splenic flexure on the left.

transverse fissure — deep groove or furrow in brain separating cerebellum and cerebrum.

transverse process — the name for two of the seven processes attached to the vertebral arch of each vertebra.

transversus abdominis muscle — bilateral muscle that is the most medial of the three lateral abdominal muscles.

tricuspid valve — a valve having three cusps or flaps found on the right side of the heart between the right atrium and right ventricle.

tropic — having an influence on.

true pelvis — cavity found beneath the pelvic inlet.

trunk — body.

turbinate — see concha.

ulna — the long bone found medially in the forearm involved in forming the elbow joint proximally and the wrist joint distally.

umbilical notch — indentation on the anterior inferior liver.

ureter — tube draining urine from kidney to bladder.

urethra — passageway for external drainage of urine from bladder in males and females; in males also passageway for semen during ejaculation.

urethral orifice — external opening of urethra.

uterine tube — see fallopian tube.

uterus — female reproductive organ in which fetal development occurs; the sloughing off of its lining in the absence of pregnancy is responsible for menstruation.

vagina — passageway in females for penile insertion during coitus, delivery of infant at end of pregnancy, and flow of blood during menstruation.

vaginal orifice — external opening of vagina.

valve — a mechanism or structure controlling the direction of flow.

ventricle — a cavity; a cavity in the brain filled with cerebrospinal fluid: either one of the two lateral ventricles, the third ventricle or fourth ventricle; a chamber on either side of the lower heart acting as a pumping chamber of blood.

vermiform appendix — see appendix.

vermis — bridge connecting right and left hemispheres of cerebellum.

vertebra (pl. — vertebrae) — one of 33 bones involved in forming the backbone; there are 7 cervical, 12 thoracic, 5 lumbar, 5 sacral, and 4 coccygeal.

vertebra prominens — the seventh cervical vertebra, which has a prominent spinous process.

vertebral arch — the posterior portion of a vertebra formed by the two pedicles and two laminae; syn. — neural arch.

vertebral artery — bilateral branch off right and left subclavian artery; the right and left vertebral arteries merge to form the basilar artery, and eventually supply the posterior portion of brain with blood.

vertebral canal — the passageway for the spinal cord created by the collective vertebral foramina; syn. — spinal canal.

vertebral foramen — the foramen formed by the vertebral arch and body of a vertebra.

vertebral notch — a concavity above and below each pedicle of the vertebrae.

visceral — referring to a viscus or organ within a cavity.

vocal cord — bilateral ligament in the larynx; movement results in the production of sound.

vomer — one of 14 facial bones; forms the inferior part of the bony nasal septum.

vulva — external female genitalia; syn. — pudendum.

white matter — nervous tissue composed principally of nerve fibers with myelinated axons.

wrist — the region between the forearm and metacarpals that includes eight carpal bones: the scaphoid, lunate, triquetrum, and pisiform in the proximal row and the trapezium, trapezoid, capitate, and hamate in the distal row.

xiphoid process — the inferior segment of the sternum; syn. — ensiform process.

zygoapophyseal joint — an intervertebral joint between the inferior articulating process of one vertebra and the superior articulating process of the vertebra below; syn. — apophyseal joint.

zygomatic bone — one of a pair of bones included in the 14 facial bones; involved in forming the cheekbone; syn. — malar bone.

Index

Note: Page numbers in bold text indicate figures. Where multiple CT or MR images in a chapter show the same structure, only the first image is listed in the index.